SIGMUND FREUD AND OSKAR PFISTER ON RELIGION

Sigmund Freud and Oskar Pfister on Religion examines the dialogue between psychoanalysis and religion through the encounters of two men: the "unfaithful Jew" who founded psychoanalysis, and a pastor of profound religious faith and proven psychoanalytic conviction.

Carlos Domínguez-Morano analyses the original encounters between Freud and Pfister and their respective positions, noting the incidences, impasses and progress of their discussions. The complex interactions between psychoanalysis and religion over time are considered, and Domínguez-Morano assesses the fundamental parameters of each perspective, with reference to Catholicism. The book explores the relationship between psychoanalysis and religion as a rich, on-going, and unending dialogue and sheds new light on the origins of psychoanalysis.

Sigmund Freud and Oskar Pfister on Religion will be of great interest to academics and scholars of psychoanalytic studies, religion, the history of psychology, and the history of ideas.

Carlos Domínguez-Morano, PhD, is a psychotherapist, emeritus professor at the Faculty of Theology of Granada, and vice-director of the master's degree in Transcultural Spirituality at the Loyola Andalusia University, Spain.

SIGMUND FREUD AND OSKAR PFISTER ON RELIGION

The Beginning of an Endless Dialogue

Carlos Domínguez-Morano
Translated by Francisco Javier Montero

Routledge
Taylor & Francis Group
LONDON AND NEW YORK

Designed cover image: Getty

First published in English 2024
by Routledge
4 Park Square, Milton Park, Abingdon, Oxon OX14 4RN

and by Routledge
605 Third Avenue, New York, NY 10158

Routledge is an imprint of the Taylor & Francis Group, an informa business

Translated by Francisco Javier Montero

Published in Spanish as *Psicoanálisis y religión: diálogo interminable* by Trotta, Madrid 2000

British Library Cataloguing-in-Publication Data
A catalogue record for this book is available from the British Library

ISBN: 9781032482637 (hbk)
ISBN: 9781032482620 (pbk)
ISBN: 9781003389804 (ebk)

DOI: 10.4324/9781003389804

Typeset in Bembo
by KnowledgeWorks Global Ltd.

To my friends María José Úbeda and Juan Piñero,
companions in thought, work, and heart.

CONTENTS

PREFACE

My work on Oskar Pfister, *Psicoanálisis y religión: diálogo interminable,* published by Trotta in Spain (2000) and presented here in English, became possible only after the fall of solid inner resistances. My psychoanalytical training in Paris with Louis Beirnaert, Jacques Pohier, Philippe Julien, and Jacques Sedat marked me with a distinct position when approaching the dialogue between Freud's work and the Christian faith. Staying clear of any concordist temptation, the aim was to examine critically what the unconscious could mean for religious belief. From this position, Oskar Pfister looked to me particularly suspicious of a defensive concordism to be avoided at all costs.

However, having later found myself under suspicion from my own ecclesial institution because of my Freudian allegiance (for example, I was denied by Rome access to the chair at the Faculty of Theology for "problematic assertions" in the Spanish original of my *Belief after Freud,* Routledge, 2017), and, with the feeling that I was also under suspicion from certain psychoanalytical circles as a priest and a believer, I became interested in Oskar Pfister, who, we know, was also the subject of similar mistrust as much from the ecclesial part as from the emerging psychoanalytic movement. Little by little, an unexpected identification with the pastor from Zurich made its way once the suspicions of concordism melted away along with my resistances. From there, the question was in what terms the dialogue between psychoanalysis and any religious belonging should be established.

The critical study of the first confrontation between psychoanalysis and faith, as shown in Pfister's relationship with Freud, underlines the excessive dependency both parties kept on the rationalist principles of the Enlightenment. They seemed to fail to find a more psychoanalytic sense when approaching religious matters. At least the way these are shown in Freud's *The future of an Illusion* and Pfister's reply, *The Illusion of a Future.* The atheist position of the first and the second's conciliatory efforts swept away the more decisive matters to tackle. Among them, still felt today, is the need that psychoanalysts cease to be *particularly blind to the theme of religion,* as Bion said. And the need for the believers to shred their unconscious resistances and allow that dialogue to proceed satisfactorily.

The present work, in two parts, tries to give an account of that initial exchange between Freud and Pfister, then, in the second part, takes a panoramic look at what the debate between psychoanalysis and faith has brought until today. The conclusion tries to formulate the most favourable conditions for that dialogue, overcoming sterile attack and defence positions, to leave space for courageous questioning of what the unconscious poses to any subject holding religious beliefs. It does not correspond to psychoanalysis to take a stand on the content of any belief, but only, not least, to ask what each subject means when saying "I believe" or "I do not believe". In this light, the dialogue between psychoanalysis and religion will never have an end. It will always be endless, not by chance, but by its essence, as long as a subject says "I believe". And, as Jean Baptiste Pontalis noted, only the dead do not believe ("*il n'y a que les morts pour ne croire à rien*").

The interminable character of the psychoanalysis and faith dialogue is duly shown in the immense literature on the theme, which still flows today. Therefore, when reviewing the work for the present English edition, the need to account for the most significant of the published contributions, in English and in Spanish, French, Italian, Portuguese, German… Finally, a Bibliography Subject Index is offered to guide the reader in such a vast bibliographic wood.

The extension of this work's reach to such a comprehensive and significant public as the English-speaking one gives me particular satisfaction, opening new possibilities of exchange and reflection. I vividly thank Routledge, their Publishers and Editors for that. I also wish to especially thank my good friend, Francisco Javier Montero, for the translation he has completed with rigour and commitment, without which the present edition would not have happened.

Granada, 4 November 2022.

ACKNOWLEDGEMENTS

As already said in the Preface, my deep thanks go to Francisco Javier Montero, my translator and friend, for his work of translation, advice and friendly backing all along the way. I cannot forget my appreciation and gratitude to the Library of the Granada Faculty of Theology for the wealth of their bibliographic material and their willingness to provide me with any text I could be interested in throughout the development and revision of the present work.

PART I

The History of a Friendship

1

THE ENCOUNTER OF TWO WORLD VIEWS

On Sunday, 25 April 1909, Freud's family home saw the arrival of a visitor who seemed to come from another planet in that setting. It was not usual to find a figure like Oskar Pfister, with the clothing of a Protestant Pastor, the courteous manners of a good cleric and, particularly, close and affectionate attention to every family member, especially the younger ones. As described by W. Hoffer (Hoffer, 1958, pp. 216–226), he was a tall and vigorous man with a full and thick moustache and eyes that were kind and enquiring at the same time.

The memory of that visit remained impressed on whom would later be an eminent figure in psychoanalysis, Anna Freud, then the youngest family member ("The little girl who took care of the lizards, who now writes very serious papers for the International Psycho-Analytical Association, was still on short skirts ..." (Meng & Freud, 1963, p. 91), as recalled years later by Oskar Pfister himself). And these are Anna's words in 1962, fifty-three years later: "In the totally non-religious Freud household, Pfister, in his clerical garb, and with the manners and behaviour of a pastor, was like a visitor from another planet. In him, nothing of the almost passionately impatient enthusiasm for science caused other pioneers to regard time spent at the family table only as an unwelcome interruption of their theoretical and clinical discussions. On the contrary, his human warmth and enthusiasm, his capacity for taking a lively part in the minor events of the day, enchanted the household's children and made him at all times a most welcome guest, a uniquely human figure in his way. To them, as Freud remarked, he was not a holy man, but a kind of Pied Piper of Hamelin, who had only to play on his pipe to gather a whole host of willing young followers behind him" (Meng & Freud, 1963, p. 11).

For Oskar Pfister, who was also going through difficult times, it was also a day to remember. The warm emotions sparked by the visit to that house and that

DOI: 10.4324/9781003389804-2

family still resonated fifteen years later: "I felt as if I were in a divine, Olympian abode, and if I had been asked what the most agreeable place in the world was, I could only have replied: 'Find out at Professor Freud's …'" (Meng & Freud, 1963, p. 91). As a gift, the pastor presented the family with a silver replica of the Matterhorn peak in Switzerland, which Freud fondly kept on his desk, "as homage" – he will comment a few days later – "from the only country in which I feel a man of property, knowing that the hearts and minds of good men there are well disposed towards me" (Meng & Freud, 1963, p. 23).

Freud already had good references for Oskar Pfister through Carl G. Jung, who a few months earlier had written to Freud about "the big propaganda campaign for your ideas", the pastor was doing in Zurich (McGuire, 1974, p. 195). Shortly after that, Jung wrote to Freud again: "Pfister is a splendid fellow …. Nothing scares him, a redoubtable champion of our cause with a powerful intelligence. He will make something of it. What? I don't know yet. Oddly enough, I find this mixture of medicine and theology to my liking (…). You will shortly receive another longish paper from him. He is feverishly busy …." (McGuire, 1974, p. 197). In effect, shortly afterwards, Pfister's paper was received by Freud, who considered it highly interesting. However, the personal encounter that April Sunday added an undoubtedly warm and close human quality. A few days later, in a letter to his Hungarian friend, psychoanalyst Sandor Ferenczi, Freud comments on his impressions of the pastor: he found in him, he reports, "a charming fellow who has won all our hearts, a warmhearted enthusiast, (…). We parted as good friends" (Gay, 1988, p. 191). As O. Pfister remembers (Pfister, 1993 [1927], p. 563), after the family lunch, the meeting of the two men went on, with a long walk on the sunny Belvedere Park, exchanging views on their broad intellectual and professional interests, so different and until then so foreign to one another. There were, in effect, two worlds that met for the first time on that spring Sunday. Two cultures, sensibilities, different fields of professional activity, two nationalities and, very importantly, two ethnic and religious origins.

Pastor Oskar Pfister came from Zurich, where he did an intense pastoral activity. Up to that moment, his biography would contain references and a socio-cultural background quite different from those we would have considered describing Professor Sigmund Freud's history.

Oskar Pfister's family background

He was born in Wiedikon, a district in the Swiss city of Zurich, on 23 February 1873, the youngest of four children of the harmonious couple formed by his father, a liberal-tempered and genuinely altruistic pastor, and his mother, an unassuming woman, somewhat strict and puritanical in her view of life and, above all, her children's religious training. In his generous devotion to pastoral work, Oskar's father was outstandingly sensible to the pains of his sick and poor parishioners, especially to the high number of children suffering from diphtheria at that time. Hence, he wished to complete his education with the study of medicine, a desire he could not fulfil because of his premature death, worn out by the daunting mission as both doctor for the body and pastor for the soul. Oskar was then three years old, and the family moved to Baden, Black Forest, to take refuge in a communitary institution in Königsfeld. Four years later, they moved back to Zürich (Zulliger, 1966, p. 173).

When Oskar Pfister was born, Sigmund Freud, already sixteen years old, had graduated *summa cum laude* from the Sperl Gymnasium and had started studying chemistry and anatomy at the University of Vienna Medical School. He, too, had to change residence when he was three years old, from the small town of Freiberg, in Moravia, to the capital of the Austro-Hungarian Empire. However, the structure and background of little Sigmund's family were quite different from those of Oskar's. His father had two sons from his first marriage, and their age was close to that of Amalie, his third wife (after a childless second marriage) and Sigmund's mother. As her first son, Sigmund was also her admired favourite. However, throughout his life, he maintains a deep ambivalence towards the head of the family, made easier by the father's empty, though pompous and vain, character, an unsuccessful wool merchant. Little Sigmund's education, typical of a Jewish home of that time, was nevertheless devoid of any attention or instruction of a religious type. His father considered himself an enlightened Jew and did not seem to follow the orthodox practices of Judaism. Of the mother, we only know in this respect that she kept "some belief in the Deity" (Jones, 1953, p. 19). As Freud himself expressed years later: "I have always been an unbeliever and was brought up without any religion" (Freud, 1941e, p. 273). In the determination of Freud's atheism by his first family relationships, particularly by the ambivalent link to his father, we should underline the work by Ana-Maria Rizzuto (Rizzuto, 1998a).

These early family relationships, and the identifications coming from these familiar, cultural, and religious frames of reference, will condition, far more than they imagined and disclosed, the future debates between the two men who met on that Sunday in 1909. Moreover, the academic and intellectual environment in which they will move afterwards will undoubtedly increase their differences in their respective world views.

Academic training

At the University of Vienna, Sigmund Freud was immersed in the medical materialism of the times under positivist physiologist Ernst Brücke's teachings and direction from 1877 to 1883. Mentor of Freud, Brücke was an authentic crusader of scientism, an enthusiastic follower of Helmholtz and his materialistic and mechanicist principles applied to physiology. Freud worked as a resident under Theodor Meynert, who wanted neuro-psychiatry to follow the physics model. All these influences turned young Freud, as expressed by E. Jones, into a "radical materialist" (Jones, 1953, p. 43). As for Oskar Pfister, he studied Theology in Zürich under the influence of Hegel, Strauss, Schleiermacher, and other critical theologians such as Hermann Kutter or Leonhard Ragaz, who were introducing socialist ideas in the theological and pastoral areas.

Oskar Pfister's pursuance of theological studies was not easy, and certainly not for lack of interest or vocation. Schooled as a child in orthodox dogmatism, he had difficulty accepting it; he felt a strong antagonism towards traditional beliefs. His critical spirit in front of the established teachings was present from adolescence. Still in school, he worked to formulate a profound and sharp critical view of biblical stories, trying, for instance, to find a scientifically sound historical explanation for episodes such as the Exodus and the crossing of the Red Sea. Oskar Pfister could not forget how "he was annoyed when a conservative professor tried to ridicule his studies" (Zulliger, 1966, p. 174). In his *The illusion of a future,* he writes how at the age of twelve, after reading the biblical story of the Great Flood, he ran to the Zoological Museum "in order to compare the measurements of the ark with those of the glass cases and to base a childlike theory of evolution on this, but, at the same time, assuming a sceptical attitude toward the Bible, which later changed into frank criticism" (Pfister, 1993 [1927], p. 569). This early and deep attitude of young Pfister helps to understand the difficulties he suffered during his studies of traditional theology. His discomfort was so intense that, at a particular time, he considered abandoning his theological studies for good. However, after eight semesters, he passed his final examination and, with additional studies in Berlin, also won his title as a Doctor in Philosophy. The thesis of his choice was a problem on religious psychology and philosophy around the work of the Swiss theologian, A.E. Biedermann. This Protestant theologian was first an associate and then a full Professor of Theology at the University of Zürich. His theological work was deeply marked by the attempt to conciliate the truth of religion with the truth of reason.

Oskar Pfister felt particularly disappointed throughout his studies by the atmosphere of disquisitions and disputes between the diverse theological systems, which he described as pure quackery. He looked to philosophy to help understand the main theological problems, only to find the same atmosphere of division and dispute as in theology and a world entirely alien to what he considered the fundamental cause of human suffering. He then looked back to theology, trying to apply the religious philosophy of Rudolf Hermann Lotze (1819–1881). Thus, renewed in a certain way, he returned to theology with conviction and always remained a personal, intellectual, and apostolic requirement (Kienast, 1974).

Encounter with psychoanalysis

However, the impact of psychoanalysis on Oskar Pfister will be so strong that all his theological thought and pastoral praxis will be determined forever by the new perspective opened by his encounter with Freud. "... what a great and magnificent thing analysis is (....) It brought an unparalleled illumination into my life, and

I cannot thank you enough for all you have done for me by your discoveries and your personal kindness to me" (Meng & Freud, 1963, p. 90).

Oskar Pfister's interest in psychology was not new. He attended psychology classes while studying philosophy and theology at the University of Basel. His doctoral thesis on Theology centred on the psychological construction of Biedermann's work (Pfister, 1910a [1898]). Also, in 1903, when psychology ceased to belong to the theological studies *curriculum*, as had been the case for a long time, Pfister wrote a pointed article criticising that withdrawal, which he considered a grave "sin of omission" (*Unterlassungssünden*). The marginalization of psychology in theological training is going to contribute, he asserted with conviction, to the broader isolation of theology from the other human sciences (Pfister, 1903).

In any case, the treatises he had seen in his search for good psychology of religion appeared as blunt as most of the theology he had studied until then. So, in 1908, shortly before meeting Freud, he vehemently attacked the ineptitude and poverty of theology and psychology to offer help to relieve human suffering (Pfister, 1905). In the same year, he turned down the chair as Professor of Systematic Theology at the University of Zürich; in the same way, he declined shortly after the chair in Philosophy at the University of Riga. The reason will always be the same: to continue the pastoral work in Wald, close to Zürich, that he had started in 1897 and that he maintained after 1902 as Pastor in Predigerkirche. He will sustain pastoral action for thirty-seven years as his life's fundamental task. At the beginning of his work in Wald, in 1897, he married Erika Wunderli. They had a son who, in time, became a psychiatrist.

Hans Zulliger, who would later be one of his closest and best-known friends, encounters psychoanalysis when reading Oskar Pfister's book *The Psychoanalytic Method.* At Pfister's suggestion, he goes on to make use of psychoanalysis with children and education (Pfister, 1913). Hans Zulliger transmits Pfister's words on what pastoral action meant for him at the time: "I loved to preach from the pulpit. I loved the pastoral care of the sick and the suffering, of the lost and of the poor. Most of all I loved teaching religion. I never had the slightest difficulty keeping order among the 400 children between the ages of 12 and 16 years who came from seven different school districts. They came from many mountains to my school. The most effective method of discipline was a lively way of reaching, which described religion as salvation, as a source of joy and support in times of danger" (Zulliger, 1966, pp. 174–175).

A few weeks after having turned down the chair of Theology in order to keep his engagement with pastoral action, Pfister came across some texts by Freud. They reach him through Carl G. Jung, already well known internationally, the son of a Protestant pastor like Pfister himself, when he visits him to get advice on the case of a mother tortured by paranoid delirium. As he read through these Freudian texts, he felt "as if an old premonition had become true (...) there were no endless speculations on the metaphysics of the soul, no experimentation with minimal trivialities while the great problems of life remained untouched ... with

Freud the highest functions in life were placed under the microscope and gave evidence of their origins and connections, of their development laws and their deepest sense in the totality of psychical life" (Hahn, 1927, pp. 168–170) [translated for this edition].

Years later, in 1931, during a round table with other Swiss Reformed pastors, Pfister resumes his account of what psychoanalysis meant in his personal and professional itinerary: "How did I come to psychoanalysis? Because I simply could not do anything with the age-old methods. With psychoanalysis one can achieve success that previously would just not have been possible. One can re-activate such a lot of human destinies that previously had no way out but to go to the insane asylum, or the poorhouse or otherwise into misery. The unconscious is a powerful force and is able to cause serious aberrations. Psychoanalysis can only plough, naturally, and not plant. It is a matter of course that a positive pastoral care must augment it. That is the point that most people overlook. It is true that Freud views religion as an illusion. Therefore, it is up to us pastors to do analysis. We must enter upon these new tasks with all reverence, and we shall become *Seelsorger* (pastoral 'carers', spiritual shepherds) only when we bring people out into the sunlight – a concept given us by Jesus" (Kienast, 1974).

After his encounter with psychoanalysis, Oskar Pfister became the *Analysenpfarrer*, the *pastor of analysis* and a good friend of Freud. He used to sign his contributions to psychoanalysis as *Oskar Pfister, pastor in Zürich*. Even if inspired with hope, the task was not easy at all. On the one side, being a cleric, to obtain recognition and respect in the psychoanalytic environment. On the other side, being an optimist, passionate Christian, to conquer the sincere and even affectionate friendship of the pessimist, the destructor of illusions, who bragged as well that he was an *unfaithful Jew*. They came from two very different cultures, two very different ethnic and religious groups, so often confronted with violence to each other in the past and, in all likelihood, also in the future. They had familiar, educational, and relational stories that were very far for each of them in behaviour and style. The two schools of thought they belonged to, one in the school of science and the other in religion, confronted each other since the Age of Enlightenment. Everything was giving shape to two personal dispositions of markedly different profiles. Perhaps for this very reason – we should think – they were able to find in each other the interlocutor that, more or less inhibited, pulsed inside each of them.

Personal profile

It should not be too risky, far from any wild psychoanalysis, to draw up a kind of psychodynamic profile of Oskar Pfister from the available documents. From his letters and publications, and the comments by Freud and other pioneers of psychoanalysis on our man, we can describe the predominant traits that marked his personality. From that basis, the significant differences in character that set him apart from Freud, his mentor, appear evident.

Pfister's history drove him naturally to become what we usually call a "good man". As Freud says: "It reminds me of a remarkable man who came to see me one day, a true servant of God, a man in the very idea of whom I should have had difficulty in believing, in that he feels the need to do spiritual good to everyone he meets. You did good in this way even to me" (Meng & Freud, 1963, p. 24). There is no doubt that this distinctive trait in his personality was the basis for the unique relationship he succeeded in creating, not only with Freud but, quite unlike others among psychoanalysis pioneers, also with all the other members of the founder's family and, in a unique way, with the younger ones. At a given point, Freud wonders what pastor Pfister sets in motion with the former's children to get them so enthusiastic about the latter's person. He writes: "I do not know what promises you left behind with my children, because I keep hearing things like next year I am going with Dr Pfister, I am going climbing with him, and so on and so forth" (Meng & Freud, 1963, p. 28).

As shown by Freud's correspondence with him and other psychoanalysts, Pfister was seen on many occasions as a vehement, exalted, and even rapturous person. However, he was able to appear with perfect dominion over himself when circumstances required. In this respect, Freud's words about how Pfister can undertake criticism in his publications are significant. The difference with himself is manifest, as he writes in his letter dated 24 January 1910: "Well, I admire your ability to write like that, in such moderate, affable, considerate manner so factually and so much more for the reader than against your opponent .... I could not write like that ... I could only write to free my soul, to release my affect and, as the letter would not emerge in an edifying manner, and as our opponents would be only too delighted to see me roused, I prefer not answering at all (...) as I am incapable of artistically modifying my indignation, of giving it an aura pleasurable to others, I hold my peace. I could not lower the temperature in dealing with him" (Meng & Freud, 1963, p. 33).

In sum, Pfister was what we could call, with all the ambiguity the term may hold, a "virtuous man"; in a way which, otherwise, could even turn into difficult to undertake his work as a psychoanalyst. From his essentially superego-based disposition, he seemed to face particular difficulty in interpreting and bringing the patient's defensive systems to consciousness, with the risk of becoming the ally of those defences. That is what Freud reproaches him for, with a provocative tone, when reviewing a work that Pfister had just published (Pfister, 1910b): "I think your analysis suffers from the hereditary vice of – virtue; it is the work of too decent a man who feels himself bound to discretion (...) Thus, discretion is incompatible with a satisfactory description of an analysis". Somehow, Freud went on, the analyst "would have to be unscrupulous, give away, betray, behave like an artist who buys paints with his wives housekeeping money or uses the furniture as firewood to warm the studio for his model. Without a trace of that kind of unscrupulousness the job cannot be done" (Meng & Freud, 1963, p. 38).

Freud saw himself as very different from that highly virtuous Pfister. This seemed to cause in him a hidden but relevant ambivalence. Even though sometimes, as we have seen, he took pleasure in the provocation, on other occasions he seemed to manifest his admiration and even a kind of envy of the virtuous frame of mind of his good friend, the pastor. "This Pfister, I said to myself, is a man to whom any kind of unfairness is totally alien, you cannot compare yourself to him ..." (Meng & Freud, 1963, p. 77). The difference, which very well could have been the cause of the impossibility of maintaining the friendship, seemed not to have been strong enough for that, either because, in a latent way, there was admiration and the wish to keep the link or because, along with the difference, other conditions existed to keep the relationship strength. In any case, Freud appeared happy with the outcome: "... all I can do is belatedly express the satisfaction that a holy man like you has not allowed himself to be scared of such a heretical relationship", he says on one occasion (Meng & Freud, 1963, p. 83).

However, in all probability, it is not on the grounds of "holiness" or "heresy" (there are some play and mutual complicity in the underlining that both of them mark in this respect) where we find the basic differences between the personal tempers of Freud and Pfister, or where we could fit the eventual complementarity in their relationship. It is, essentially, in the optimistic attitude of the pastor and in the pessimistic one of the physician where we notice the main difference between the two personal profiles. In depth, there are two world views, undoubtedly determined by the individual positions of each one of them in front of religious belief, that face each other at the time of perceiving any aspect of reality.

There is no doubt it is there where they are farther from each other. "Your tendency to resignation distresses me", Oskar Pfister confesses one day. Like Freud sometimes seems to do, he cannot believe that the power of unconscious forces comes to stand as the fundamental engine of the whole existence. "If I took you literally, I should object that you had handed over to your id full power over life and death, good fortune and ill fortune, and, in the name of your charming daughter, your delightful wife, your whole family, science, and the whole pantheon of supreme powers, I should protest" .... (Meng & Freud, 1963, p. 99).

The view of the future and the possibilities it may hold is also conditioned by the acceptance or denial of the power given to *ananké*. That is why Pfister is pleased when he reads *The Ego and the Id* (Freud, 1923b), in the belief that the work, especially in its reflections on the *super-ego,* offers possibilities to elaborate as well a psychology of the highest values concerning the person and culture. But even at that point, when it is a matter of interpretation of the world of values and ideals, Pfister diverges from Freud, finding him too conservative. In his more optimistic and hopeful vision, Pfister considers we are not only in debt with what has been introjected from the parental identifications. There is also a tendency to the future, to achieve, to go further ahead of what we received from our parents. The *ego-ideal* cannot then be understood as a crude imitation of the parents. Moreover, it is precisely in that longing for improvement that we could find the essential difference between the animal world and the human world: "... in the fact that we aspire to climb higher, over the dead and the images of our parents, while the ape, in so far as he is not urged forward by the not completely conservative nature of his phylogenesis, is content to go on hanging to his father's tail?" (Meng & Freud, 1963, p. 136).

This aspect of Oskar Pfister's personality does not respond (as some profiles of hagiographic tones would pretend, including H. Zullinger's) to what we could call a desirable achievement of extraordinary maturity. It is a psychodynamic structure that allows us to see problematic elements from what we could consider a psychodiagnosis point of view. At certain times, Pfister gives us the impression of being marked by hypomanic traits. His excessive optimism on some occasions, his almost endless enthusiasm, his many times near messianic attitude, his predominant exaltation, his both spoken and written verbosity (the number of his publications was near three hundred), and his hyperactivity that gives ever-working Freud a complex: "Your productivity is beginning to put mine to shame, and I have not been in the least lazy in my time" (Meng & Freud, 1963, p. 96), lead the thoughts on that direction and at the same time force us to think that, along with many other intellectual or religious conditions, we find here an essential element of his difference with Freud, whom we manifestly should place on the opposite depressive pole.

Certainly, Pfister's life was not free from psychical conflicts, even though they did not seem to be serious ones. "Pfister is a splendid fellow" – Jung tells Freud on one of the first occasions he mentions him "a neurotic himself of course, although not a severe one" (Meng & Freud, 1963, p. 197). Indeed, we do not find in the analysis of the correspondence between the first analysts (where it is not unusual to find a malicious exchange of clinical diagnosis) any other reference to neurosis or conflict of the pastor. Admittedly it does not seem any more significant than the rest of the psychoanalysis pioneers. However, it is also true that, at least at a particular time in Pfister's life, the conflicts reached enough importance for him to undertake his own analysis finally. "Pfister" – Jung tells Freud in a confidential tone – "is presently on analysis with Riklin. He has obviously had enough of being roasted over a slow fire by his complexes" (Meng & Freud, 1963, p. 421).

In sum, Pfister comes up as a good man, a natural enthusiast, with a good intellectual capacity and personal conflicts at the average level of most human beings. In any case, his relationship with Freud certainly meant the encounter of two quite opposed world views, two different ethical temperaments and two somewhat antagonistic psychodynamic structures. "Of all Freud's friendships ...." – Peter Gay comments – "it was distinctly the least expectable ...." (Gay, 1987, p. 75). But if the Christian cleric and the unfaithful Jew, the good and virtuous man and the inveterate and heterodox provoker, or the natural optimist and the on-going pessimist, were able to establish a profound and sincere link of friendship, it was due, without any doubt, besides their complementary mutual oppositions, to the fact that they coincided at being, and seeing each other, as passionate and courageous men in search of truth. Truth searched even at the cost of personal sacrifices, not at all negligible. It is said that Oskar Pfister noted once that he preferred to go to hell rather than to heaven at the price of lying. A truly shared passion in both men enabled them to surpass the relevant differences they met in other fundamental aspects of their lives.

From this joint search for truth, they could live a friendly relationship that benefited and enriched both. As can be seen in their correspondence, their mutual trust and personal engagement grew progressively as the years went by. So did their loyalty at difficult times, either due to external circumstances in the life of one or the other or from the difficulties born of their relationship from the deep divergence in their respective world views.

References

Freud, S. (1923b), *The Ego and the Id*, S.E., 19: 3, London: Hogarth.

Freud, S. (1941e). *Address to the Members of the B'nai B'rith*, S.E., 20: 273, London: Hogarth.

Gay, P. (1987). *A Godless Jew. Freud, Atheism and the Making of Psychoanalysis*, New Haven, CT: Yale University Press.

Gay, P. (1988). *Freud: A Life for Our Time*, New York, NY: Norton.

Hahn, E. (1927). *Die Pädagogik der Gegenwart in Selbstdarstellungen II*, Leipzig: Meiner.

Hoffer, W. (1958, Nov.–Dec.). Oskar Pfister; 1873–1956. *The International Journal of Psycho-Analysis, 39(6)*: 616–617.

Jones, E. (1953–1955–1957). *Sigmund Freud: Life and Work, Volume 1–3*, New York, NY: Basic Books.

Kienast, H. W. (1974). The significance of Oskar Pfister's in-depth pastoral care. *Journal of Religion and Health, 13 (2)*: 83–95.

McGuire, W. (Ed.) (1974). *The Correspondence Between Sigmund Freud and C. G. Jung*, Princeton, NJ: Princeton University Press.

Meng, H. & Freud, E. L. (Eds.) (1963). *Psychoanalysis and Faith: The Letters of Sigmund Freud and Oskar Pfister*, New York, NY: Basic Books.

Pfister, O. (1903). Die Unterlassungssünden der Theologie gegenüber der mondernen Psychologie. *Protentantische Monatshefte*, 7: 125–140.

Pfister, O. (1905). Das Elend unserer wissenschaftlichen Glaubenslehre. *Schweizerische Theologische Zeitschrift*, *22*: 209–212.

Pfister, O. (1910a) [1898]. *Die Genesis der Religionsphilosophie A.E. Bierdermann, untersucht nach Seiten ihres psychologischen Ausbaus*, Whitefish, MT: Kessinger Publishing, LLC.

Pfister, O. (1910b). Analytische Untersuchung über die Psychologie des Hasses und der Versöhnung. *Jahrbuch für Psychoanalytische und Psychopathologische Forschungen*, *2*: 134–178.

Pfister, O. (1913). *Die Psychoanalytische Methode*. Leipzig-Berlin: Julius Klinkhardt.

Pfister, O. (1993) [1927]. The Illusion of a Future: A Friendly Disagreement with Prof. Sigmund Freud. *The International Journal of Psychoanalysis*, *74* (2): 557–599.

Rizzuto, A. M. (1998a). *Why Did Freud Reject God? A Psychodynamic Interpretation*, New Haven, CT: Yale University Press.

Zulliger, H. (1966). Oskar Pfister, Psychoanalysis and Faith. In: F. Alexandre, S. Eisenstein & M. Gotjahn (Eds.) *Psychoanalytic Pioneers* (pp. 169–179), New York, NY: Basic Books.

2

THE INS AND OUTS OF A FRIENDSHIP

To go deep into the links that made up the relationship between our two men, we rely on the basic information contained in the correspondence they maintained for thirty years, published in 1961. We find there new, direct, and ample information, even if it reaches us mutilated for several reasons (Heinrich Meng was in charge of editing the correspondence, which appeared with a preface by Ernst L. Freud and the cooperation of Anna Freud). For one thing, it was Oskar Pfister himself who asked Freud to shred part of it, probably the one where he gave an account of a close affective story which we will refer to later on. "I have just finished the hangman's job you asked me to do via Frau H", Freud writes, "The letters of 1912 have been destroyed; a few of impersonal content still remain. I have done what you asked me to do but did not do so gladly" (Meng & Freud, 1963, p. 108).

Another part of the correspondence was lost because of the incidents of Freud's exile. We find a long gap from March 1913 to October 1918. Five years for which we have to look elsewhere for the information. All this has an unfortunate effect since the information about Pfister we can get from his own letters is considerably less than what we could obtain about Freud. The direct information we get on the Swiss pastor is just the one that could be reconstructed from his shorthand notes. After having first lost and recovered Freud's letters, Pfister kept them as a treasure and approved their publication on the condition of doing so without the paragraphs that could hurt living persons.

My dear Man of God...

> ... there is a special value in personal relations which shared work and interests cannot completely make good; and we two, at this moment when we have become aware of the ultimate, fundamental differences between us, have

DOI: 10.4324/9781003389804-3

> particular occasion- and, I hope, inclination- to foster such relations". These words from Freud to Pfister are significant to what the Swiss pastor meant to him. Neither professional interests nor any convergence in their views on life was the support of that friendship. A personal, affective bond marked the relationship and gave it that singular character compared to other friendly links maintained by Freud. This friendship, as E. Jones asserts, "it lasted without a cloud to the end of his life"
>
> (Jones, 1955, p. 46).

One element that stands out when reviewing the correspondence is the beneficial impact that Pfister's figure seems to have had on the person of Freud (more than in his ideas). As the latter writes, "We have all grown very fond of Pfister. He is really an acceptable priest, and he has even helped me by exerting a modulating influence on my father complex. We were like old friends in no time; he is a little fulsome in his enthusiasm, but there is nothing false or exaggerated in his warmth" (Meng & Freud, 1963, p. 222). We will find time and again the "he has helped me" expression – not a straightforward acknowledgement for Freud about the relationship with a priest. But, as we have seen, "an acceptable priest". They are not all acceptable, in particular considering that "father complex" that Freud mentions and that Pfister successfully dealt with by "exerting a modulating influence".

Not long after having met Pfister for the first time, Freud tells him, "It reminds me of a remarkable man who came to see me one day, a true servant of God, a man in the very idea of whom I should have had difficulty in believing, in that he feels the need to do spiritual good to everyone he meets. You did good in this way even to me" (Meng & Freud, 1963, p. 24). Once again, the expression of the good that Pfister does to him. In addition, this time Freud points explicitly to the altruistic decision he took, without any doubt on his part, because of the pastor's influence. In effect, shortly after the meeting with Pfister, Freud gave up his fees in favour of some patients who were in difficult circumstances "But for you and your influence I should never have managed it; my own father complex, as Jung would call it, that is to say, the need to correct my father, would never have permitted it" (Meng & Freud, 1963, p. 24).

The letters Pfister sends him also stir positive feelings and emotions on himself and on life.: "You always make one cheerful (...) I always read your letters with pleasure, they are always so full of life, warmth and success (...) You have the gift of throwing a rosy sheen over the everyday life one takes part in so colourlessly" (Meng & Freud, 1963, pp. 27, 83, 91). Expressions like these are repeated over the years, always revealing the same beneficial influence that the idealistic and enthusiastic man projects on the one who tried to resign himself to the hard designs of *ananke*.

One day he writes to Jung: "On my arrival I found a letter from Pfister, which affected me as his letters always do. At first I believe everything, I tend to be credulous about good news – everything looks wonderful. Then after a while,

I relapse into my usual wretched state" (McGuire, 1974, p. 249). In similar terms, mentioning again the good he gets from it and calling him for the first time my dear Man of God, he comments to Pfister on that same day: "But do not believe that I believe everything or even a large part of the delightful things that you say to me and about me, i.e., I believe them of you but not of me. I do not deny that it does me good to hear that sort of thing, but after a while I recall my own self-knowledge and become a good deal more modest. What remains behind is the belief that you honestly mean what you say, and the pleasure given by your kind and enthusiastic nature" (Meng & Freud, 1963, p. 29).

An element that no doubt also played in Freud's affective link with Pfister was the positive impact the latter had on Freud's children. There are many references to this in the correspondence. The impression that Anna Freud kept of the first visit by the pastor reveals a typical attitude in Pfister's human temper, open to broader interests than those of purely intellectual or scientific character. "The reason I write to you about family matters is that no visitor since Jung has so much impressed the children and done me so much good" (Meng & Freud, 1963, p. 27). We already saw the enthusiasm that the pastor's figure stirred up among the young in the house and the phantasies of play, excursions, and fun his presence caused immediately in the family (Meng & Freud, 1963, pp. 27–28). Therefore, the prospect of a new Pfister's visit to the house was always greeted with great excitement, as expressed by Freud to the pastor one year after the first encounter: "All the young people are looking forward to seeing you again and identify you with Switzerland" (Meng & Freud, 1963, p. 32). What Freud wishes at the start of the New Year is: "My wish for myself, that in the course of it I may win the friendship of more men such as you, is probably too ambitious to have any prospect of fulfilment" (Meng & Freud, 1963, p. 31). His friend, most likely, would not have agreed.

Confidences and compromises

Pfister's confessions

Pfister, however, is always open, frank, and free from any excess of modesty when communicating with his master. His relation to Freud has an unmistakably filial tone. Moreover, even if, as we have seen, Pfister as a priest could stimulate in Freud certain "dangerous" paternal representations, the latter, as "master", assuredly activated the same kind of representations in Oskar Pfister, without causing in him, it seems, any type of resistance. Fatherless since he was three years old, as he reminds Mrs. Freud after her husband's death ("I, who grew up fatherless and suffered for a lifetime under a soft, one-sided bringing up...." (Meng & Freud, 1963, p. 145), he did not seem to have any difficulty for the bond with Freud, in whom, no doubt, he found a paternal representation made to measure. Pfister's enthusiasm, gratitude, veneration, and almost childish adoration towards Freud barely need any evidence. That becomes obvious as soon as we start to look into his person.

So Pfister does not hesitate and trusts Freud soon after the relationship is initiated. For example, after just a few months, he tells him already of the difficulties in his marriage and his intention to divorce his wife Erika Wunderli, whom he had married in 1897, having a son. In October 1911, Pfister seemed to have finally decided to take the step. So he tells Freud, who encourages him, saying that it is the right time to do it if he does not wish to waste his life. In a letter to Jung, Freud gives the news, adding *Prosit!* (McGuire, 1974, p. 448).

However, the matter will still take time. Jung meets the girl who attracts Pfister "into the ways of the ungodly. I know this charming little bird", he tells Freud, "But it seems that she only wants to lure him out of his cage, not to marry him" (McGuire, 1974, p. 450). Meanwhile, Pfister's wife, whom we gather was a difficult and probably very unbalanced woman, expresses her wish to undertake her psychoanalysis with Jung, who takes such intention as a threat. "I shall resist as long and as fiercely as I possibly can. These days I am getting practically nothing but divorce cases. To hell with them!" rounds off Jung, set against his will in this imbroglio (McGuire, 1974, p. 461). Soon after, Pfister's wife gave up her intention of entering analysis, to his relief. "This will probably start the ball rolling and, we must hope, save Pfister from the infantilism that is stultifying him. It will be a hard struggle" concludes Jung (McGuire, 1974, p. 465).

Hard, indeed, and long. Because poor Pfister gets into a situation he cannot control. His relationship with the girl is becoming known, and the enemies of psychoanalysis take advantage of it. Even his position as a pastor is in danger. Jung writes to Freud: "Pfister has no doubt told you how bad things are going with him. It may even cost him his job. I fear he is too optimistic, too trusting, despite warnings. Our opponents are wont to pick on the vulnerable spots and one of the weak points in our armour is Pfister, whom they can hurt by spreading rumours" (McGuire, 1974, p. 487).

The instability in Pfister's life at the time seems to make Freud unable to understand what is going on. "I am surprised to hear that all is not well with Pfister. In his last letter, which came shortly before yours, he was overjoyed at having finally found a woman for whose sake it would be worthwhile to put up with the drawbacks of marriage; nothing seemed amiss. I haven't heard from him since. If he is in trouble, we must do everything in our power to help him" (McGuire, 1974, p. 488).

Months later, Pfister's love story keeps going, and the purpose of divorce is maintained, to be carried out six months later. Freud writes to Ferenczi: "There is better news from Pfister; he seems to be holding his own. The photograph that he has enclosed shows the charming face of a girl, access to whom has of course been closed to him for the time being, because he has promised to postpone the divorce by half year" (Brabant et al., 1993, p. 366). However, closer to all the characters in the story, Jung sees the situation getting more and more problematic. On the one hand, Pfister's position as a pastor is progressively compromised, without his behaviour becoming more careful. On the other hand, the girl in question was too young and infantile and seemed not to realise where she was and how things were going. In a situation that was beyond his control ("his libido is in it so it might turn out well", noted Jung), Pfister seemed to behave like a child. Jung is harsh in his judgement: "First he married a mother, now it's a daughter" (McGuire, 1974, p. 493).

The situation is hazardous, and Jung prefers not to get involved unless the pastor asks for his help. Contemplating a possible change of assignment by his superiors, Pfister was thinking of working as an assistant in the psychoanalytic practice of a doctor who would accept him, although Jung questions who would do that since such a practice did not promise many opportunities. Jung also wonders how the girl would take such a change. "Now he is terribly in love and imagines he can't live without the girl. I hope it will be all right in the end. We are very worried about him", concludes Jung (McGuire, 1974, p. 493).

The ending of the story is difficult to investigate in its dénouement. The correspondence of Jung with Freud will soon be interrupted, and the letters of this period from Pfister to his master will be destroyed, as we know, at the request of Pfister himself. Also, information from other sources is scarce. However, we know the story's final chapter: Pfister kept his marriage until 1929, when his wife died, twenty years after our good pastor showed his intention to divorce. The data also tell us that Pfister got out of the amorous imbroglio (although we do not know well how he did it) and succeeded in the recovery of his personal and professional stability. A year after his wife's death, he married a widow, his cousin, Martha Zuppinger-Urner, with whom he lived happily until his death on 6 August 1956. His new wife had two children, and he raised them as his own.

The censorship of psychoanalytical circles (because strange as it might seem, it also works in such spaces) tried to hide all the episodes of the love *affaire* of the analyst pastor. They chose to draw a veil on this important chapter of his life and opt for making a genuinely hagiographic profile, such as the one written by his disciple and fellow analyst, Hans Zulliger (Zulliger, 1966).

However, Pfister's difficulties were not limited to those caused by that passionate love story. With that, without being possible for us to define where the origin was, we should point to those coming from the Lutheran institution because of his relationship and compromises with psychoanalytic circles. At the time, early in 1912, psychoanalysis was fiercely attacked in Zurich's newspapers, causing disastrous effects in psychoanalysts' offices. The press denounced the wicked theories "of Viennese origin" and expressed, at the same time, their hope that they would fail in perverting the pure souls of the Swiss. All of that contributed to troubling Pfister's relations with the Swiss theological establishment and to finding himself severely questioned by the Lutheran authorities. At one point, he tells Freud: "The well-meaning, feeling sorry for me, worried and gently reproachful, asked me why I should have acted so irresponsibly" (Gay, 1987, p. 86). As testified by Pastor

Paul Urner, friend, colleague, and brother-in-law of Oskar Pfister, the struggles that from time to time the latter suffered from the Lutheran authorities were not unusual (Stettner, 1973).

His difficulties with other psychologists and pedagogues also appear in confidence with Freud. So, for instance, at the Psychology Congress held in Breslau in 1913, he warned about the dangers of applying psychoanalysis to young people. It seems that Pfister was the victim of a smear campaign in pedagogy circles.

In the same way, Pfister takes Freud in confidence when he starts to sense that Jung and the Zurich group move progressively away from psychoanalytic theory. At one time, Freud recognises to Karl Abraham how "Bleuler has nicely developed backwards. I suspect that the last motives were the ... papers on the synaesthesias, which raised tremendous resistance in him ... A proof perhaps that Pfister and Hug are really right in this matter" (Abraham, 2002, letter 159F). The evolution of his Swiss analytical group becomes a matter of concern that appears in the exchanges with his master. He worries about the relationship between Freud and Jung falling apart and tries to find a remedy without seeing many probabilities for that on Freud's part. "Do not have too much confidence in a lasting personal agreement between me and Jung. He demands too much of me, and I am retreating from my over-estimation of him. It will be sufficient if the unity of the association is maintained" (Meng & Freud, 1963, p. 59). That unity, we know, could not be maintained. During the process to the final break, we observed how the Swiss pastor was progressively opting for Freud's side, becoming more and more ready to oppose Jung's theoretical and technical innovations. At one point, Freud tells him that he is very pleased with his opposition to Jung's innovations and affirms that Pfister will not be isolated in "this purely internal and objective battle" (Meng & Freud, 1963, p. 58).

Freud's careful confidences

To understand the personal involvement of Freud in his friendships with men, it is necessary to keep in mind the previous determinants that had taken place in this area. Freud, who had always needed a kind of Alter Ego to recognise himself since his youth, had suffered several profound disappointments in this connection. In an especially traumatic manner, his relationship with Wilhelm Fliess, revived years later in his friendship with Jung, marked his ways of communicating with men forever. As we know, Fliess was his great confidant during 1997–1900 of Freud's self-analysis. Only years later, having finished his analysis and his relationship with Fliess, was Freud able to understand the complex affective dynamics involved in such a unique and intense relationship· Very far was left that feeling one day expressed precisely to Fliess: "I do not share your contempt for friendship between men, probably because I am to a high degree party for it. In my life, as you know, woman has never replaced the comrade, the friend" (Masson, 1985, p. 447). After his break with Fliess, Freud did never allow a relationship in confidence and mutual intimacy as he had before. One incident in his relationship with S. Ferenczi is significant in this connection. In 1910, replying to the latter's complaint about the lack of reciprocity he felt in the level of personal communication, Freud writes: "Not only you noticed, but you understood that I no longer have any need to reveal my personality, and you have rightly related this fact to the traumatic reason for it. Since Fliess's case, with the overcoming of which you recently saw me occupied, that need has been extinguished. A part of homosexual cathexis has been withdrawn and made use of to enlarge my own ego. I have succeeded where the paranoiac fails" (Mannoni, 1971 [2015, p. 125]).

All of that explains how, in the relationship with Pfister, despite the closeness, warmth and deep affection that Freud always showed towards the pastor, no true reciprocity was reached regarding confidential communication. Pfister is generally the one who uncovers himself, while Freud always remains more careful and reserved and keeps appearing as "the discreet founder of the indiscreet science" [translated for this edition] (Marcuse, 1969). That did not prevent him from expressing to his friend his everyday worries and concerns, as well as his pain when life hit him. Particularly from 1918 to 1926, after the correspondence gap in the preceding years, we see a significant recovery of the yarns of a friendship that grows more and more profound and personal on the part of Freud. The relationship with Pfister was strengthened after the crisis with Jung and the Zurich group. The news and the family problems, the ups and downs of the psychoanalytical movement, and the material and moral concerns in a time of war take more space in communications. Also, as the relationship gets stronger, the differences between the two correspondents turn more frank and free.

The war brought Freud and his family a series of hardships shown in the written communications. "… the possibility of war keeps us on tenterhooks", he wrote in December 1912 (Meng & Freud, 1963, p. 58), before warfare began. Once the war is on, two of his sons (Martin and Ernst) are on the front line. In January 1919, right after the end of the war, he informed Pfister about their anxiety at home regarding his son Martin since they ignored if he had been taken prisoner. Later, they learned he had been severely ill and, finally, he was recovering in Teramo. The war hardships also appeared in his communication with Oskar: "Conditions in Vienna are undeniably very hard, and the future will perhaps be even worse" (Meng & Freud, 1963, p. 65), he comments in the same letter. However, he expresses thanks but declines the pastor's invitation to move to Zurich. Of all the difficulties involved, he points just to one of them: whoever leaves German Austria must give up between 50% and 75% of his possessions. The freedom to change residence had been practically cancelled. Years later, in 1933, when anti-Semitism was already intensifying with violence, Freud complained about his two sons and his son-in-law being forced to search for a new home out of Germany without success so far. Switzerland is not one of the most welcoming countries. "There has been little occasion for me to change my opinion of human nature, particularly the Christian Aryan variety (Meng & Freud, 1963, p. 140)".

However, in those years, the most terrible blow in Freud's life is the death of his dear daughter Sophie: "The undisguised brutality of our time weighs heavily on us", he laments with Pfister. The added difficulties so soon after the war prevented him from travelling to Berlin, where his daughter lived, to attend the burial. "Our poor Sunday child is to be cremated tomorrow! ... Sophie leaves behind two boys, one aged six and the other thirteen months, and an inconsolable husband who will have to pay dearly for the happiness of these seven years. The happiness was only between them, not in external circumstances, which were war and war service, being wounded and losing their money, but they remained brave and cheerful" (Meng & Freud, 1963, p. 75). The care with his believer friend, Pfister, prevented him from expressing himself in the terms he used with Ferenczi, to whom he writes on the same cause: "Since I am profoundly unbelieving, I have no one to blame, and I know that there is no place where one can lodge a complaint" (Brabant, 2000, p. 6). Work is the only place where he can staunch his wound: "I do as much work as I can, and am grateful for the distraction. The loss of a child seems to be a grave blow to one's narcissism; as for mourning, that will no doubt come later" (Meng & Freud, 1963, p. 74).

On another level, the correspondence with the pastor shows the problems caused by the dissent of some disciples. The Jung *affaire*, as we have seen and will have the opportunity to keep verifying, comes time and time again in the correspondence, showing concern, and disappointment ("I am retreating from my over-estimation of him") (Meng & Freud, 1963, p. 59), the sorrow and even the open aggressiveness caused by the break. Also, about another leading dissident, Alfred Adler, he says: "He forgets the saying of the apostle Paul, the exact words of which you know better than I: 'And I know that ye have not love in you'. He has created for himself a world system without love, and I am in the process of carrying out on him the revenge of the offended goddess Libido" (Meng & Freud, 1963, p. 48). Similarly, he mentions "a lot of hard nuts to crack" (Meng & Freud, 1963, p. 92) caused by the work of future dissidents Sandor Ferenczi and Otto Rank entitled *Entwicklungsziele der Psychoanalyse*. "That psychoanalysis is leading to a new outlook on life I cannot and will not admit" he says, anticipating ideas he will develop in *The Question of a Weltanschauung*. "All analysis can do is make valuable contributions to building up such an outlook" (Meng & Freud, 1963, p. 92).

Freud does neither reach any further in intimacy with Pfister, nor did he with anybody else after the break of his friendship with Fliess, which was later revived with Jung. His old need for confident friends was progressively replaced by a plural type of friendship, less affectively engaged and at a lesser risk of disappointment. The "analytic fraternity" in which his disciples, even if they were called and considered friends, never lost the condition of pupils, was the place where he was able somehow to soothe his old, frustrated desire for the confident, comrade and friend (Flem, 2003).

Tolerance in the difference

When we dealt with Oskar Pfister's personal configuration, we had the opportunity to underline the remarkable differences between his worldview and that of Freud. "Virtue" against provocation, optimist enthusiasm against resigned pessimism, idealism, and a positive vision against a sarcastic and negative spirit towards life and people. These personal differences, which probably hide a temper substrate of manic-depressive tendencies, also shape the foundations of two world views, which, in turn, determine quite diverging positions when approaching theoretical and practical problems in psychoanalysis.

Oskar Pfister welcomed the approaches that psychoanalysis could take towards the more idealist philosophy that had formed a good part of his education and provided a convenient bridge between psychoanalysis and his religious belief. To Freud, however, with his wish to keep in the more limited field of positivist science, such philosophic elucubrations caused an evident unease. That was shown, for instance, in the different reception given to the thoughts of James Putnam, the American analyst who undertook very early on a theological and moral reflection regarding psychoanalysis, starting from the Hegelian philosophy basis, which he firmly defended. In the Weimar Congress 1911, Putnam made an allegation for introducing philosophy in psychoanalysis (Putnam, 1911). Courteous and reserved, Freud wrote: "Putnam's philosophy is like a decorative centrepiece, everyone admires it but no one touches it" (Jones, 1953–1957, vol. 2, pp. 85–86). In other words, the speculative system is useless beautiful fiction. Not even dangerous. Pfister, however, was fascinated with the philosopher, although he always managed to keep a critical attitude in front of the calls to submit psychoanalysis to philosophy: "I can still vividly remember— he would write years later—the impression that was made by Putnam's paper. The audience, under the spell of a profound spiritual achievement, was glowing with the noblest sentiments; but the copious rush of thoughts left behind a certain bewilderment (….) this obscure metaphysics which advances with victorious mien and haughtily demands that empirical science shall follow in its triumphant train" (Pfister, 1923, pp. 178–179).

Pfister wisely avoided the speculative temptation to reduce psychoanalysis to a philosophy or a worldview. However, the divergences (recognised or not) between Freud and himself about their respective philosophic positions and the appreciation of the philosophical thought each one made were also evident. "The only thing I cannot pack into my rucksack is your joke about philosophy … If my philosophy amuses you …, we are quits, and you come off the better …" (Meng & Freud, 1963, p. 76), he told Freud on one occasion, expressing well the distance between them in this field. And even if Pfister recognised the Freudian idea of the unconscious determination in building up philosophic systems, he did not reduce these in the way Freud tended to do it. "The unconscious determines the direction and the general result of the thought" [translated for this edition], he recognised in one of his works (Pfister, 1934a). However, philosophic thought also had great significance for him as a rationalised credo, as a basis for logic, epistemology, and ontology, and even for comprehension of sense, values, and norms (Pfister, 1949).

The diverse views in the appreciation of philosophy resulted in diverse positions in psychoanalytic theorisation. The radical Freudian pessimism that showed in the theory of the death instincts was almost allergically rejected by a markedly idealistic vision of life and a deep and hopeful religious conviction. Pfister clearly expresses that in his critical comment on Freud's *Civilization and its Discontents* (Freud, 1930a): "I gladly make use of the opportunity freely to criticise your book (…) contains a tremendous number of deep and important ideas but, so it seems to me, is not right in everything. (…) In instinctual theory you are a conservative while I am a progressive. As in the biological theory of evolution, I see an upward trend, as in Spitteler's Olympian spring, in which the laborious ascent of the gods continues, in spite of obstacles and reverses, and occasional slippings back. I regard the 'death instinct', not as a real instinct, but only as a slackening of the 'life force' (…) I see civilisation as full of tensions. Just as in the individual with his free will there is a conflict between the present and the future to which he aspires, so is it with civilisation. Just as it would be mistaken to regard the actual, existing facts about an individual as the whole of him, ignoring his aspirations, it would be equally mistaken to identify with civilisation its existing horrors, to which its magnificent achievements stand out in contrast" (Meng & Freud, 1963, pp. 130–131).

Nevertheless, Freud defends, to his regret, he believes, the fatality of the death instincts in the conviction that it is an obligated thesis because of the data imposed by biology and psychology. To think otherwise would be to fall squarely in the illusory: "If I doubt man's destiny to climb by way of civilisation to a state of greater perfection, if I see in life a continual struggle between Eros and the death instinct, the outcome of which seems to me to be undeterminable, I do not believe that in coming to those conclusions I have been influenced by innate constitutional factors or acquired emotional attitudes. I am neither a self-tormentor nor I am cussed and, if I could, I should gladly do as others do and bestow upon mankind a rosy future, and I should find it much more beautiful and consoling if we could count on such a thing. But this seems to me to be yet another instance of illusion (wish fulfilment) in conflict with truth. The question is not what belief is more pleasing or more comfortable or more advantageous to life, but of what may approximate more closely to the puzzling reality that lies outside us. The death instinct is not a requirement of my heart; it seems to be only an inevitable assumption on biological and psychological grounds. The rest follows from that. Thus, my pessimism seems a conclusion, while the optimism of my opponents seems an *a priori* assumption. I might also say that I have concluded a marriage of reason with my gloomy theories, while others live with theirs in a love-match. I hope they will gain greater happiness from this than I" (Meng & Freud, 1963, pp. 132–133).

Such a different view on existence had to be also seen in the approach to morality. Both personalities, marked by a solid moral disposition towards life, had very different views on the foundations of morality and its final goals. Much less different, probably, in its essential content.

From his open position as a liberal Protestant, Oskar Pfister minimises the differences at certain moments, trying to make Freud realise he is not so far from his position. "The (ethical) difference between your outlook and mine is perhaps not so great as my calling might suggest", he says early in the correspondence, before they had met, and goes immediately to refer to certain aspects of sexual morality. The attitude of the Protestant Church, in particular that of de Zurich liberals, is very different from the position of the Catholic Church, closer to Freud's living environment. As Pfister explains: "Protestant ethics .... removed the odium of immorality from sexual relations. For the Reformation was fundamentally nothing but an analysis of Catholic sexual repression, unfortunately, a totally inadequate one, hence the anxiety neurosis of church orthodoxy and the concomitant phenomena— the witch trials, political absolutism, the social rigidity of the guild system, etc. We, modern Evangelical pastors, feel ourselves to be completely Protestant and we are sure (?) that we are much too little reformed. We are searching for a new land. Our Church leaves us Zürichers complete liberty. In ethical matters we are able to be free thinkers without being heroes".

From there, in the same letter, Pfister goes on to an analysis of the social conditions that determine sexuality. This analysis shows surprising parallelism with a paper published by Freud shortly before on "*'Civilised' Sexual Morality and Modern Nervous Illness*" (Freud, 1908d). The brave words tried by Pfister to show his proximity to Freud on this matter are as follows: "Sexual conditions, particularly in our towns, are full of hypocrisy and therefore of uncleanness. The dreadful combination of monogamy and lies and the plague of prostitution are completely clear and intolerable to us. The ideal of free love glows in us too. But what we do not see is how really free love can be combined with marriage. The dividing line between 'free' and 'wild' is very hard to draw ... We shall be freed from the mass misery of neurosis and vice, not by better theories about the marriage tie, but only by an improvement in social conditions, healthier education, and a healthier outlook on life. In the meantime my only recourse is to put forward the ideal of marriage and leave it to the individual and his conscience to decide how far he will depart from it. The more one abides by the doctrine of Jesus and refrain from judgement and confines oneself quietly and energetically to fighting one's own battle for the ideal, the easier one makes sublimation to the weak ..." (Meng & Freud, 1963, p. 18).

Nonetheless, the diverse disposition of each of them in the moral sphere appeared repeatedly, particularly when it was necessary to be specific on psychoanalytical theory and praxis. We have seen that before. To be an analyst, Freud says provokingly, "one would have to be unscrupulous .... Without a trace of that kind of unscrupulousness the job cannot be done" (Meng & Freud, 1963, p. 38). Also, Pfister's position regarding analytical tasks frequently shows a moralising attitude that Freud repeatedly denounces. Thus, for instance, when, upon receiving a work by Pfister on love relations and child development (Pfister, 1922b), he writes that he senses that the book will be for him one of the best, but if he must be frank, he should tell him "Complete objectivity requires a person who takes less pleasure in life than you do; you insist in finding something edifying in it. True, it is only in old age that one is converted to the grim heavenly pair *logos kai ananké*" (Meng & Freud, 1963, p. 86).

Pfister, however, does not let himself be convinced. Or rather, he cannot be convinced. His attitude towards the educative task fundamentally marks him: it is dominated by an ethical project regarding the pupils. And that, Pfister thinks, cannot be renounced. "You yourself used to insist that children have to be educated", Pfister replies. "And, when analysis is over and done with, the little beasts and angels with whom we have to deal have to be filled with honourable intentions. Not that one should blow upon them with the breath of the spirit and blow one's soul into them, but they must have a bit of mental and social hygiene and practice it with healthy love. But analysis as such should take all witch's brews seriously, adorn the devil with no fig leaves, and do full justice to the parable of the tares among the wheat ..." (Meng & Freud, 1963, p. 87). In sum, there is no point in looking for ethical motivations in the unconscious, as in Jung's proposal. However, the ethical dimension that education and psychoanalysis should carry cannot be ignored either. In his turn, Freud answers that both dimensions should be well differentiated in the practice, at all costs avoiding any moralising of the analytical work: "Of course there must be an education, and it can even be strict; it does it no harm if it is based on analytic knowledge, but analysis itself is after all something quite different and is in the first place an honest establishment of the facts" (Meng & Freud, 1963, p. 87). Pfister had great difficulty fully understanding and accepting this approach in a matter which directly affected the neutrality principle of analysis.

When Pfister publishes his *Psychoanalysis in the Service of Education*, Freud contests the nonconformity that Pfister shows with his ethics and sexual theory. On the first of these matters, Freud does not seem to feel much interest: "One thing I dislike is your objection to my 'sexual theory and my ethics'. The latter I grant you; ethics are remote from me, and you are a minister of religion. I do not break my head very much about good and evil, but I have found little that is 'good' about human beings on the whole. In my opinion, most of them are trash, whether they publicly subscribe to this or that ethical doctrine or to none. This is something that you cannot say aloud, or perhaps even think, though your experiences of life can hardly have been different from mine. If we are to talk of ethics, I subscribe to a high ideal from which most of the human beings I have come across departs most lamentably". The second matter, however, seems relevant to him since it concerns very directly psychoanalytic theory: "Why on earth do you dispute the splitting up of the sex instinct into its component parts which analysis imposes on us every day? Your arguments against this are really not very strong. Do you not see that the multiplicity of these components derives from the multiplicity of the organs, all of which are erotogenic (...)? In science one must take apart before one can put together. It looks to me as if you want a synthesis without a previous analysis. In the technique of psycho-analysis there is no need of any special synthetic work; the individual does that for himself better than we can" (Meng & Freud, 1963, pp. 61–62). It seems evident that Pfister's hurry to reach the plenitude of love led him to go too fast through the analysis of the primary components on which that love could stand up. The analysis will have to deal with features by detecting them in the adult's imaginary life streams. The basic, primary, instinctual dimensions of love were hardly recognisable in his theorisation and probably, disregarded in practice.

Freud loses patience sometimes when clashing with the same difficulty in Pfister. At a given moment, he confesses he has been late in his reply because he has needed time to dispel the annoyance caused by "the scant success of my effort to put you right in the matter of sexual theory" (Meng & Freud, 1963, pp. 132–133). He rebuked Pfister for his rather pusillanimous approach, at least verbally, in matters of sexuality. In his turn, Oskar Pfister reproached Freud for underestimating the importance of sublimation, thanks to which the psychoanalytic cure could have a high educational value. The divergence on this matter was visible. Different sensibilities caused opposite reactions in one and the other.

The same differences were also shown in a book by Georg W. Groddeck published by the psychoanalysis publishing house in 1921 with the title *Der Seelensucher* (*The Soul Searcher*) (Groddeck, 1921). The book is a quixotic story of a retired bachelor who loses his fight against the bugs that have infested his house and wanders out into the world searching for the meaning of life. The work had a spicy tone, with some openly obscene passages. Oskar Pfister was not the only one who considered the book unsuitable for a severe and scientific publication. Ernest Jones, for instance, was very critical of the book. Sandor Ferenczi, however, compared it with works by Balzac for "unmasking the devoutly hypocritical spirit of our times" [translated for this edition] (Rodrigué, 1996, p. 253). The Swiss Society for Psychoanalysis held a special meeting to deal with the matter and expressed their discomfort and protest (Jones, 1957, p. 78). Freud, however, had found the book very entertaining and, as he tells Pfister, "I energetically defend Groddeck against your respectability. What would you had said if you had been a contemporary of Rabelais?" he finishes off (Meng & Freud, 1963, pp. 80–81). Pfister, however, does not change his position at all and expresses it to Freud in total clarity: "I understand very well that it is impossible for you to think otherwise (...). But, with the best will in the world, I cannot adopt your view, as indeed you do not expect me to. But there is a great difference between Rabelais and Groddeck: The former remains within his role as a satirist and avoids the error of putting himself forward as a savant. Groddeck, however, wavers between science and *belles lettres*. You say yourself that his trend is definitely scientific, but I dislike his spicing it with jokes. I like a clean sheet of paper, and I also like fresh butter, but butter-stains on a sheet of paper satisfy neither my eye nor my belly" (Meng & Freud, 1963, p. 81). The opposite positions were thus clearly stated in this respect, and the issue showed how the divergence could be freely expressed without letting it disturb the existing deep bond. So Freud understands when he writes: "I was delighted with your remarks about Groddeck. We really must be able to tell each other home truths, i.e. incivilities, and remain firm friends, as in this case. I am not giving up my view on Groddeck either, I am usually not so easily taken in by anybody. But it does not matter" (Meng & Freud, 1963, p. 82).

Nevertheless, the most problematic issue regarding divergences between Freud and Pfister concerns the practical aspects of psychoanalytic technique. The world-views, the questions of philosophy, morality, or religion could be understood as dependent on different personal dispositions or life options far from anything specifically psychoanalytic. However, the matters relating to fundamental psychoanalytic concepts and, even more, to the ways of carrying out psychoanalytic practice were the object of higher preoccupation and care by Freud and most pioneering psychoanalysts.

There is a critical principle of neutrality in analytic technique: the psychoanalyst must remain apart from any consideration about values. Pfister questioned this principle in theory and practice because he tended to blur the boundaries of therapeutic practice and cure of souls (Freud, 1912e, pp. 117–119). Educational concerns and the wish to reconcile the patient with ethical or moral ideals got in the way of his work, preventing it from reaching an authentically psychoanalytic approach to the interpretation of symbols. He had thus a tendency to come too close to Jung's vision.

Some years before his death, Pfister expressed a meaningful thought in joint work on psychoanalyst and pedagogue A. Aichhorn (1878–1949). He wrote: "The ethical content of analytic therapy fully coincides with the original Christian message, except in two points. In the first place, Jesus has produced his morality, not in a scientific, empirical way, but in an intuitive way. He founded his *Weltanschauung* philosophically on the ultimate reasons for being, that is, on absolute values, while Freud, a positivist, has rejected all philosophy and all ontology. In the second place, Freud has negatively conceived his task: its goal is to redress the adaptations of unconscious origins and suppress neurosis. It is not concerned about how the patient will take charge of his existence. He considers it out of the analyst domain, regardless of the morality or immorality of the patient's path. On this last point, all those disciples of Freud who dealt with pedagogy (except Melanie Klein) have adopted a different point of view. Going beyond his master, they consider the individual a social being and that establishing social relationships is an essential element of the treatment" [translated for this edition] (Widlöcher, 1966, pp. 40–41). So, we see that the misunderstanding persisted at this crucial point in analytic technique despite Freud's efforts. An ideal of adaptation and normality presides over Pfister's project beyond the mere discovery goal assigned to the analytical task.

The same neutrality principle used to be also hindered by the attitude of warm, friendly, and personal closeness Pfister tried to maintain with his patients, more in tune with the type of relationship appropriate for the cure of souls.

At one point, Pfister poses to Freud the question of the type of relations which would be convenient to establish with the analysand. Specifically, it happened about the successful treatment he carried out with H. Schjelderup (a brilliant professor of philosophy and psychology who would later write one of the best treaties on the psychology of religion) (Schjelderup & Schjelderup, 1932), whom he relieved from horrific migraine attacks. During the treatment, Pfister is active, with abundant interpretations and stimulating the personal activity of the analysand. This way, he thinks, a healthy transference is established. To him, a close and friendly attitude seems more natural and convenient than the distant and cold detachment prescribed by most psychoanalysts. Pfister writes to Freud, "... I am really not concerned with making friends of my analysands, but for their good; hence this is a therapeutic question. In your paper on *The Ego and the Id* you mention in the footnote on page 64 the importance of the analyst's personality permitting him to take the place of the patient's ego-ideal (...) it is also important that the analyst should transmit values that over-compensate for the patient's gain from illness or guilt feelings" (This idea is very dear to Oskar Pfister; as a fundamental principle, moral education should always seek compensation for the immoral behaviour that should be eradicated) (Pfister, 1931). Finally, he brings up with Freud how important it would be not to break the relationship with the patient entirely and keep it once the transference has been cleansed. "You will no doubt approve of my being always ready to be of assistance in making use of every kind of human value in regard to which the patient is not always able to help himself, because that is my duty as an educator and a minister" (Meng & Freud, 1963, p. 112). Like in other important matters, Freud did not hesitate to express his view clearly in reply: "You as a minister naturally have the right to call on all the reinforcements at your command, while we as analysts must be more reserved, and must lay the chief accent on the effort to make the patient independent, which often works out to the disadvantage of the therapy. Apart from that, I am not so far from your point of view (...). It should not be concluded from this instance that analysis should be followed by a synthesis, but rather that thorough analysis of the transference situation is of special importance. What then remains of the transference may, indeed should, have the character of a cordial human relation" (Meng & Freud, 1963, p. 113). So, the effort to do a completed task would instead be placed in the area of the cure of souls.

Pfister is conscious of the difference that sets him apart from Freud on this point and does not seem ready to change his view and his particular way of practising analysis from positions that would seriously compromise the analytic principle of neutrality. It can be argued that such a principle is a utopian ideal in that pure asepsis in moral, religious, and political terms will never be possible for any analyst. However, the commitment to maintain such aspiration (as ideal as it might be) and to keep a critical attitude to follow that principle will be inexcusable for the exercise of authentically psychoanalytic therapy. Pfister, however, from a scant delimitation between cure of souls and psychotherapy, did not seem convinced of the need for that technical principle of neutrality. He wrote to Freud: "Thus there remains between us the great difference that I practice analysis within a plan of life which you indulgently regard as servitude to my calling, while I regard this philosophy of life, not only as a powerful aid to treatment (in the case of most people), but also as the logical consequence of a philosophy that goes beyond naturalism and positivism, is well based on moral and social hygiene, and is in accordance with the nature of mankind and the world. In all this it is the patient's business to what extent he will strike out on a road in harmony with his social and individual characteristics, and the amount of aid he requires to find what is the right road for him depends on himself alone" (Meng & Freud, 1963, p. 116).

The question of brief therapies (which will become ample space for debate and development) is already present in Pfister's technical procedures. The opposition of some analysts was unequivocal from the beginning. In 1927, the nonconformist practice by Pfister on this point was contested by some Swiss colleagues, rightly considering that the pastor did not observe the standard rules set by the International Psychoanalytic Association. The question was also affected by the fact that Pfister was not a physician, a matter which, as we will see, was the object of a bitter controversy in those years. Obelhozer and R. Braun left the Swiss Society for Psychoanalysis. Raymond de Saussure stopped short of leaving, clearly showing his opposition to Pfister's technique: "You practice very brief psychoanalysis that does not fit what Freud understand today as psychoanalysis. That causes difficulties in local doctors who observe the of the Viennese master´s technique" [translated for this edition] (Roudinesco & Plon, 1997). Freud, in effect, was also against shortening the analytic processes. Only the special closeness he felt towards the pastor made him tolerant of something on which he could not but leave a record of his dissent. Eventually, the conflict in the relationship of Pfister with another Swiss analyst became insurmountable, and there was a breakup. Freud feels sorry and asks Pfister to reconsider. He writes: "I have been very sorry to hear what a large part was played in his departure by critical dissatisfaction with your analytical practices and your therapeutic optimism. Sorry, because on these points I am to a large extent on his side and, with all my personal liking for you and all my appreciation of your work, I cannot approve of your enthusiastically abbreviated analyses and the ease with which you accept new members and followers. I would prefer not to choose (…), and I should like you to get on with and become more moderate towards each other" (Meng & Freud, 1963, p. 121). Tolerance is thus Freud's proposal to Pfister and is also what he displayed in their relationship. As Marthe Robert affirms, Freud's relationship with Oskar Pfister shows how untrue the alleged intellectual intolerance of Freud towards his followers is. Pfister never gave in to his scientific and religious ideas without ever seeing his friendship or his belonging to the psychoanalytic movement in question. Freud preferred a clear divergence to the adulation, often hiding authentic aggressiveness (Robert, 1964, vol. 1, p. 229).

Loyalty in the difficulties

It was a proven friendship, first, in the loyalty they knew how to keep at difficult times. In a particularly significant way, the loyalty Pfister pledged to Freud at the time of the separation of Jung and the Swiss group. Only the pastor-analyst remained on Freud's side in Switzerland. Moreover, the points of divergence between Pfister and his Viennese master seemed to foster the scales to tip in favour of Jungian psychology. The concept of sexuality and the different appreciation of religion were, in effect, the two crucial points in which Jung y Freud found the ground for their separation. Also, those were precisely the two matters in which Freud y Pfister most diverged.

Freud had found special support in the Swiss group in Zurich, facing the Vienna group closer to him. The Swiss group, enjoying a prestigious international recognition, offered a better perspective opening out into the world than the Vienna one, weaker and more provincial. Zurich represented for Freud the key to getting free from the claustrophobic atmosphere of the Viennese psychoanalytic circle. The Zürichers were not old, were not Viennese, and were not Jews, as Peter Gay remarks very well (Gay, 1987, p. 78). So, from an early date, already at the first Salzburg Congress in 1910, the Swiss group showed more specific weight than the Vienna one. "What will happen if my Zürichers desert me?" exclaimed Freud (Clark, 1980, p. 296).

The divergences, as we know, did not take long to come. In July 1912, Freud wrote to Pfister: "It is a pity that you did not meet or speak to Jung. You could have told him from me that he is at perfect liberty to develop views divergent from mine, and that I ask him to do so without a bad conscience" (Meng & Freud, 1963, pp. 56–57). That is the first hint we find in the correspondence with the Swiss of any divergence with whom had been, till then, his favourite. On the same day, Freud tells Ferenczi: "Now he (Jung) is preaching against the analytic activity of laymen, after he himself led Pfister to analysis" (Brabant et al., 1993, p. 389).

Once Jung published *Wandlungen und Symbole der Libido (1912)* (Jung, 1916), the divergence which Freud had refused to recognise turned unquestionable (Rivers of ink have run on the relationship between Freud and Jung, starting with their own views (Donn, 1988; Freud, 1914d; Freud, 1925d; Gay, 1998; Jung, 1962). In that work, the Swiss psychiatrist considered that the libido was not limited to sexuality but should be understood as unspecific energy that enlivens all the vital forces of the individual. The *Urlibido*, the proto-libido, is progressively desexualised over the development stages. An idea, no doubt, not far from the Freudian concept of sublimation. However, the difference was remarkable: Freud was not ready to admit that sublimation would be a true desexualisation. Still, the rest of the Swiss group considered that the options taken by Jung were in better concordance with Christian anthropology, and nearly all followed him. Freud then writes to Ferenczi: "... the untenable relationship with the Zürichers, I certainly won't continue the polemic" (Brabant et al., 1993, p. 562). He informs Abraham that he does not expect any Swiss representative at the coming Dresden Congress. Pfister, however, remained at his side.

Nevertheless, the obvious similarities between Pfister's theories and those of Jung caused suspicion more than once about the pastor's actual position. Especially Karl Abraham, who, as Peter Gay says, played the "watchdog" role, warns Freud that Pfister was diverting towards clearly Jungian notions. Freud refused to think so despite having learned to trust Abraham judgment of people. He had not usually misjudged as he did with Jung. Freud always believed Pfister's adhesion was sincere. But Abraham, for all that, was insistent. In his letter to Freud on 16 July 1914, he says: "On the other hand, dear Professor, I take a completely opposite view from yours about Pfister". However, this time, it was Abraham who was wrong. Pfister remained loyal, and Freud had the opportunity to confirm it through specific contacts held in 1914. In February 1915 Freud wrote to Abraham: "Pfister is drawing very close to us, and has contributed a critical paper on the 'arson' of the splendid Z. Schmid; he has also sent us a short essay by a new worker, who draws an analogy between our libido and Plato's theory of Eros" (Freud was referring to M. Nachmannshon's work (Nachmannshon, 1915).

After the communication returns after the war, Freud confesses to Pfister: "Your complete and ever more manifest defection from Jung and Adler has given me great satisfaction for a long time past". Because of that, he asks the pastor not to reject his own work, *The Psychoanalytic Method (1917),* even if impregnated in many concepts by the theory of the Swiss psychiatrist, but to revise it (Meng & Freud, 1963, p. 88).

Knowing Pfister's character traits, we would not be surprised that his estrangement from Jung on theory did not involve a break in their relationship. As reported by Elisabeth Bollag, a colleague of Oskar Pfister, he kept maintaining occasional contact with Jung. That Freud knew about this can be inferred from a postcard from him in February 1921: "I am very glad that you have had things out in such a friendly way with Rank. I hope it leaves no trace behind" (Meng & Freud, 1963, p. 80). Things were different with Adler when the latter came to propose Pfister a common cause against Freud, and "This manoeuvre has been rebuffed with indignation here" (McGuire, 1974, p. 545).

The loyalty was confirmed even after Freud's passed away. In 1952, a few years before his own death, Pfister still crossed his sword with Karl Jaspers, replying to a publication by the renowned philosopher and psychiatrist in which he likened psychoanalysis with a worldview comparable to Marxism and considering both pure ideologies. In Jasper's understanding, psychoanalysis derived from a nihilistic psychological principle that destroyed science and philosophy. Pfister argues in his reply on the influence of Freud in medicine and philosophy and proclaims his importance in both fields (Jaspers, 1998; Pfister, 1952).

In turn, Oskar Pfister could also feel the loyalty of his friend and master, not only with closeness and support at the times when he conveyed his innermost problems but also when he found difficulties inside the psychoanalytic movement, either because of his lay condition or because of the opposition his theories or technical practices met. We already saw how Freud placed himself on Pfister's side, even when he agreed more with the theoretical reasons of the opponents, like in the brief therapies case. However, above all, stands the issue of Emil Oberholzer, President of the Swiss Society for Psychoanalysis and the primary opponent of Pfister in Zurich, whom Freud confronted in defence of his friend, the pastor, advising the latter to forget that "stubborn fool whom one best leaves alone" (Gay, 1988, pp. 490, 716).

Also of importance was the conflict Pfister had with Hans Sachs, who did trust neither the psychology of the Swiss nor Jung's influence on them. Pfister had applied to join the International Psychoanalytical Association when the new Swiss Psychoanalytic Society replaced the old one chaired by Jung. In front of the difficulties he found, he wrote a seven-page letter to Sachs complaining of the latter's demand for him to withdraw his application. Freud intervened, assuring Pfister of his admission and membership in the Society, while at the same time he tried to make Pfister understand the reservations existing in his regard. The matter was finally solved, and the relationship with Hans Sachs was restored (Meng & Freud, 1963, pp. 68–71).

A friendship made of confidences and mutual commitment, extreme tolerance of important differences, and proven loyalty throughout many years. A friendship for mutual enrichment, both in the intellectual and professional areas and in the more personal approaches to life. Unlike other relationships maintained by Freud after those of Fliess and Jung, perhaps the one he enjoyed with Pfister was among the most relevant at that strictly personal level. At least, it was on that ground where it found its most solid foundation.

References

Abraham, K. (2019), The *Complete Correspondence of* Sigmund Freud and Karl Abraham: 1907–1925. London/New York, NY: Routledge.

Brabant, E., Falzeder, E. & Giampieri-Deutsch, P. (Eds.) (1993). *The Correspondence of Sigmund Freud and Sandor Ferenczi Volume 1, 1908–1914*, Cambridge, MA: Harvard University Press.

Brabant, E., Falzeder, E. & Giampieri-Deutsch, P. (Ed.) (2000). *The Correspondence of Sigmund Freud and Sandor Ferenczi Volume 3, 1920-1932*. Cambridge, MA: Harvard University Press.

Clark, R. W. (1980). *Freud, the Man and the Cause*, New York, NY: Random [reprinted London: Paladin, 1987].

Donn, L. (1988). *Freud and Jung: Years of Friendship, Years of Loss*, New York, NY: Scribner.

Flem, L. (2003). *Freud the Man: An Intellectual Biography*, New York, NY: Other Press.

Freud, S. (1912e), *Recommendations to Physicians Practising Psycho-Analysis*, S.E., 12: 109–120, London: Hogarth.

Freud, S. (1914d), *On the History of the Psycho-Analytic Movement*, S.E., 14: 7–66, London: Hogarth.

Freud, S. (1925d), *An Autobiographical Study*, 20 S.E., 20: 3–70, London: Hogarth.

Freud, S. (1908d), *'Civilised' Sexual Morality and Modern Nervous Illness*, S.E., IX, 179–204.

Freud, S. (1930a), *Civilization and Its Discontents*, S.E., 21: 59–151, London: Hogarth.

Gay, P. (1987). *A Godless Jew. Freud, Atheism and the Making of Psychoanalysis*, New Haven, CT: Yale University Press.
Gay, P. (1998). *Freud: A Life for Our Time*, New York, NY: Norton.
Groddeck, G. W. (1921). *Der Seelensucher – Ein psychoanalytischer Roman, Part I*, Leipzig: Internationalen Psychoanalytischen Verlag.
Jaspers, K. (1998). *Die geistige Situation der Zeit*, Berlin: de Gruyter.
Jones, E. (1953–1955–1957). *Sigmund Freud: Life and Work, Volume 1–3*. New York, NY: Basic Books.
Jung, C. G. (1916). *Psychology of the Unconscious: A Study of the Transformations and Symbolisms of the Libido, a Contribution to the History of the Evolution of Thought*, London: Kegan Paul, Trench, Trubner.
Jung, C. G. (1962), *Memories, Dreams, Reflections*, Revised Edition, New York, NY: Vintage Books.
Mannoni, O. (1971). *Freud, The Theory of the Unconscious*, London: Random House [reprinted New York, NY: Verso, 2015].
Marcuse, L. (1969). *Freud*, Madrid: Alianza.
Masson, J. M. (Ed.) (1985). *The Complete Letters of Sigmund Freud to Wilhelm Fliess, 1887–1904*, Cambridge, MA: Harvard University Press.
McGuire, W. (Ed.) (1974). *The Correspondence Between Sigmund Freud and C. G. Jung*, Princeton, NJ: Princeton University Press.
Meng, H. & Freud, E. (Eds.) (1963). *Psychoanalysis and Faith: The Letters of Sigmund Freud and Oskar Pfister*, New York, NY: Basic Books. (1) (2)
Nachmannshon, M. (1915). Freuds Libidotheorie verglichen mit der Eroslehre Platos: *Internationale Zeitschrift für ärztliche Psychoanalyse III.*
Pfister, O. (1922). *Die Liebe des Kindes und Ihre Fehlentwicklungen*, Bern: Bircher.
Pfister, O. (1923). *Some Applications of Psychoanalysis*, London: George Allen & Unwin.
Pfister, O. (1931). "What transformation does psychoanalysis require in ethics and moral education?" *Psychiatric Quarterly*, *5*: 407–422.
Pfister, O. (1934a). *Zur Psychologie des philosophischen Denkens*, Bern-Leipzig: Bircher Verlag.
Pfister, O. (1949). "Die Rolle des Unbewussten im philosophischen Denken". *Dialectica*, *3*: 254–271.
Pfister, O. (1952). Jaspers als Sigmund Freuds Widersacher. *Psyche*, *6*: 241–275.
Putnam, J. J. (1911). A plea for the study of philosophic methods in preparation for psychoanalytic work. *The Journal of Abnormal Psychology*, *6* (4): 249–264.
Robert, M. (1964), *La révolution psychanalytique. La vie et œuvre de Freud*, Vol. 2, Paris: Payot.
Rodrigué, E. (1996), *Sigmund Freud. El siglo del psicoanálisis*, Vol. 2, Buenos Aires: Ed. Sudamericana.
Roudinesco, E. & Plon, M. (1997). Quoted in *Pfister entry, Dictionnaire de la Psychanalyse*, Paris: Fayard.
Schjelderup, H. & Schjelderup, K. (1932). *Über drei Haupttypen der religiösen Erlebnisformen und ihre psychologische Untersuchung*, Berlin: Walter de Gruyter.
Stettner, J. (1973). Pfister as Pastoral Theologian. *Journal of Religion and Health, 12 (3)*: 211–222.
Widlöcher, D. (1966), Quoted by him in *Préface à l'edition française de la Correspondence avec le pasteur Pfister 1909–1939*. Heinrich Meng (Ed.), Paris: Gallimard.
Zulliger, H. (1966). Oskar Pfister, Psychoanalysis and Faith. In: F. Alexandre, S. Eisenstein & M. Gotjahn (Eds.) *Psychoanalytic Pioneers* (pp. 169–179), New York, NY: Basic Books.

3

MUTUAL CONTRIBUTIONS

The contributions of psychoanalysis to Oskar Pfister

Psychoanalysis and "cure of souls" (Seelsorge)

The first interest and the first benefit that Oskar Pfister pursued with his approach to psychoanalysis was, no doubt, the one of deepening the understanding of pastoral action, "cure of souls" (*Seelsorge*) in the German terminology of the time, which was the object of his radical consecration. The liberal theology, to which Pfister felt he belonged since the earliest times, comprehensively conceived the "cure of souls" as a global search for the parishioners' spiritual, psychic, and human good. His father's model, in his aspiration to become a physician for the body and a pastor for the soul, also pulsed certainly in this conception of his own pastoral, to the point that Oskar Pfister, once he was introduced in the psychoanalytic field, glimpsed the possibility of undertaking the study of medicine. But Freud discouraged him from such purpose, thus keeping him one of the first lay analysts, whom he would later vehemently defend.

Pfister's interest in psychology or medicine underscores his comprehensive understanding of pastoral action and its theology. Theologians Karl Barth and Leonard Ragaz shared Pfister's negative judgement on theological thought. They too, found it old, abstract, scholastic, and disoriented. However, for Barth or Ragaz, the problem lay in theology's dependency on the romantic and positivist culture. Pfister, on the contrary, considered that theology should urgently confront the results obtained by modern science. The moral degradation that industrialisation had so strongly stepped up drives him in this direction. The full casuistry before his eyes: conjugal difficulties, the growth of falsehood, cruelty, vandalism, kleptomania, etc.......is what makes him feel the need to find support

DOI: 10.4324/9781003389804-4

in the findings of psychology. He is convinced that it is the resource to see some of the best possibilities to get beyond the incapacity of the old, abstract, and scholastic theology and give an answer to the anxiety of modern man (Pfister, 1912). From that conviction, Pfister criticises without mercy the ineffectiveness of the traditional pastoral methods, not only the Catholic ones but also, and perhaps even more, the Protestant tones, for their lack of sensitivity and their lack of psychological, historical, and critical approach.

H. W. Kienast (Kienast, 1974a, p. 83), a friend of the Pfister family since 1949, established as a psychiatrist and neurologist in Chicago, studied the pastor's work in depth. (His global judgment looks excessively determined by his friendship and admiration. As Kienast affirms, it isn't easy to accept that Pfister should be considered a theologian and philosopher at the level of R. Bultmann or K. Barth. Even more daring is his assertion that Psychoanalysis would have amounted to just an esoteric method, restricted to the Jewish circle of its founder, were it not for the depth conferred by Pfister's solid theological and philosophical knowledge.) Kienast summarises the analyst-pastor's fundamental aim of all his *work* as the will to intervene most effectively in crises for human beings and, at the same time, be able to offer them moral-religious freedom. Or, in Pfister's terms, how to accomplish the reintegration of love, removing unconscious tendencies and releasing repressed psychic energies (Ellenberger, 1970, pp. 67–71). (H. E. Ellenberger, in his analysis of the relationship between the cure of souls and psychoanalysis, pays attention to the therapeutic dimension of confession in the Roman Catholic world and the "cure of souls" in the Protestant one. The release of the so-called "pathogenic secret" plays a therapeutic role in them. He mentions on this point C. G. Jung and Oskar Pfister, whom we know was his psychoanalyst.)

Coming back to Oskar Pfister, it is in that release of the subject's capacity for love that he finds the closest analogy or coincidence between the Gospel's proposals and those of psychoanalysis. In one of his most interesting works, entitled *New Testamental Cure of Souls and Psychoanalytic Therapy* (Pfister, 1934b), and read at the Lucerne Psychoanalytic Congress on the 30th August 1930, Oskar Pfister tried to accomplish an organic justification of his reflections on this matter. Schematically, this is his approach:

1. Neo-testamentary cure of souls and psychoanalysis are born from the need to eliminate the anxiety from the sense of fault.
2. In both cases, psychic suffering is seen as punishment for a transgression against authority, conceived as absolute.
3. As much in the cure of souls as in psychoanalytic therapy, that absolute and overwhelming instance is replaced by another one, a higher, warm, and welcoming one, in better correspondence with the requirements of autonomy existing in the person.

4. As a result, both in Jesus' conception (not so much though in those of Paul, John, and others) and in analytic therapy, a regression takes place from what we can consider an authoritarian father figure to that of a naturally good father and a mother who loves without limits.
5. In Jesus' conception, the release from the feeling of guilt and the restoration of the capacity to love to lead to a transformation in the person's behaviour that we call "conversion". The intervention of divine grace is decisive. In psychotherapy, it is up to the patient to draw the ethical consequences of his transformation.
6. Also, in both cases, positive transference plays a fundamental role: in both is necessary the presence of a mediator possessing at the same time the repressive traits and the more human ones.
7. Finally, in both situations, recovery of childhood is not achieved without a comprehensive correction and renewed workout.

These are the essential analogies registered by Pfister. He does not ignore the notable differences between the Gospel and the psychoanalysis proposals. Among them, he points to four:

1. The first concerns the primary aim: the love for God and for the neighbour as the final and fundamental goal of the New Testament proposal versus simple healing in the psychotherapy project.
2. The second difference relates to the points of view to consider and elaborate on each case. The first comes from a religious perspective, and the second from a strictly scientific one.
3. In the third place, the treatment method employed in each case: religiously based on general observations versus rigorous analysis of the particular determinant factors on each subject.
4. Lastly, regarding personality structure or, in psychoanalytical terms, regarding its topographical location, we should consider that the Gospel proposal occurs at the conscious level, while the analytical work is done from the unconscious perspective.

Pfister finishes his study with the following conclusion: "Since the analyst is required to follow up and examine, first of all with his own unconscious, the hidden journey of his patient's unconscious, Freud has made his therapy mirror New Testamentary pastoral care, which takes place, regardless of all rationalisations, essentially in irrational grounds (...) Psychoanalytic therapy is a secularised and scientifically based cure of souls, concurring on enough points with Jesus's. In any case, despite the fundamental differences between New Testamentary pastoral care of souls and psychoanalytic therapy, both aspiring to free men by truth and the restoration of love, they present such strong affinities that they should not fight each other as adversaries (as has happened until now) but rather see each other as allies. In so far as both seek to free and heal the individual and society through truth and love, they combine, despite all the differences, towards the same result" (Pfister, 1934b, p. 443) [translated for this edition].

Kienast reports about a work (Pfister, 1931b) written by Pfister during his stay in the United States in 1920 for the first Congress on Mental Hygiene. In it, Pfister insists on the unconscious dimension of the religious experience and the connection between a religiousness tied to fear, anxiety, and guilt and the darkest forces of the unconscious. That type of religious experience fatally ends as a cause of illness. Only through the release from such tyranny is it at all possible to access a religious experience that, through love, brings liberation. Then, it is necessary to replace the control of unconscious judgment with the power of God's love. Pfister points up that pastoral care generally addresses just the conscious issues, while the enemy of the authentic Christian experience is placed in that unconscious threat and judgment (in earlier work, he had laid out the possibilities of psychoanalysis in front of neurosis and other emotional disturbances; Pfister, 1918). This way, the liberation of the capacity for love is present throughout Pfister's work as the fundamental principle of his pastoral and psychoanalytic practice. *Only love can lead to love* (Pfister, 1922b). Pfister is conscious that liberation for love implies processes that sometimes can be very costly and complicated. The investigation into the very own personality structures, the identifications of the factors that block the subject himself, the anxiety generated in the demolition of the own defences, the perverse satisfaction that ties oneself to structures from the past, etc... make up complex elements in the analytic process that Pfister does not try to disregard or underestimate. But, at the same time, he points up the diversity of ways along which, throughout history, and not just in the Gospel, the capacity to love has been glimpsed and practised. These would be historical experiences of pastoral care of souls, somehow precursory of the analytical work discovered and deepened by Freud.

So, for instance, in a suggestive study entitled *Psychoanalyse und Weltanschauung* (Pfister, 1922b), Pfister draws a parallel between Socrates and Freud. In his view, after the idealism of Pythagoras and after the sophists with their purely negative connotations, their barren scepticism and their brutal selfishness, Socrates appears and speaks of the daemon, linked to the subject's unconscious. In his proposal, Socrates sought to increase the person's command over his contradictory internal currents using a deep knowledge of the self. He provides the maieutic method and successfully extracts their very best from his disciples through precise induction. This way, he made a greater and free ethical concept possible as the highest duty in existence. Oskar Pfister finds here the essential elements of Freud's thinking. Again, psychoanalysis aims to give back dignity and relevance to the unconscious and, from the basis of self-knowledge, move on to overcome internal resistances. Thanks to specific induction, psychoanalysis brings psychic forces to light and achieves through sublimation a moral affirmation. Pfister thinks the analogy is truly remarkable, despite obvious differences in the working methods. Plato, Pfister asserts in another work, can also be considered a precursor of psychoanalysis when, in the Eryximachus speech in the *Symposium*, he puts medical work forward precisely as "restoration of love". "I have made a wonderful discovery in Plato which will give you pleasure", he comments to Freud when he probably was working on this book–. "Plato wrote the following: 'For the art of healing … is knowledge of the body's loves … and he who is able to distinguish between the good and the bad kinds, and is able to bring about a change, so that the body acquires a kind of love instead of the other and is able to impart love to those in whom there is none … is the best physician'. Plato traces back all art, religion, morality, to love and he also has an admirable knowledge of the unconscious, the conflicting aspirations of the mind …" (Meng & Freud, 1961, p. 80).

However, Pfister's attempt to intimately relate the cure of souls practice and analytic therapy was not exempt from problems both at the theoretical and practical levels. As we already saw, Pfister was prone to be more sensible to catch the analogous points existing in both processes than to perceive the notable differences between one and the other. And he did not always avoid methodological mistakes on this matter. The subject was discussed more than once among the pioneering analysts and came up in correspondence with Freud as a point for debate. But the problems with Pfister's effort to relate the cure of souls and psychoanalysis did not come only from what psychoanalytical theory or praxis required. Also, from the side of pastoral care, the attempt was frequently questioned for what was considered a perversion in the ways and ends of this pastoral work or the danger of the cure of souls becoming just a psychoanalytic by-product. Soon Oskar Pfister felt like an object of distrust, if not of open questioning and condemnation. All of that forced him to keep a difficult equilibrium from which he did not always come out unbeaten. For example, self-censorship was the only option when he was trying to present his ideas in the ecclesiastic world, as shown in a text on a psychoanalytic cure of souls case. "That is always as painful to the author as it is to the understanding reader". Freud writes to him in this connection. And he adds: "The censor cuts into the flesh; what he cuts out is always 'the best thing', as the mocker Heine remarks" (Meng & Freud, 1961, p. 20).

Psychoanalysis and education

It is only fair to confer upon Oskar Pfister the honour of being the pioneer in applying psychoanalysis in the field of education, an area so obviously close to pastoral care, especially considering Pfister's integral view on that practice. His *Was bietet die Psychoanalyse dem Erzieher?* (Pfister, 1917) had one of the broadest outreaches, translated soon into French, English, Italian, Polish, Greek, and Danish. Freud sent him this comment: "It has a gladdening warmth and demonstrates all the fine qualities which we so value in you; your enthusiasm, your integrity, and love of humanity, your courage and candour, your understanding and also – your optimism" (Meng & Freud, 1961, p. 61).

Unlike in other theological fields, Oskar Pfister was received with open arms by the pedagogues, finding soon acceptance and friendship among the teachers. And, during the periods of higher persecution and need, when his theologian friends and his parishioners started to doubt and judge him, the teachers were the ones who kept their doors open and encouraged him in his effort to develop the method he called paedoanalysis. "I address myself to parents and teachers, because my faith in the pundits has notably shrunk", somewhat disappointed he tells Freud, referring to the work he has just published (Pfister, 1922b; Meng & Freud, 1961, p. 84). Very soon, he started to do child analysis, so he is also honoured to have pioneered a field that would become fundamental in subsequent psychoanalysis.

The ultimate motivations for this passionate dedication to educational tasks are found by his disciple and friend H. Zulliger in some events that marked his childhood in the area of education. After his father's death, three years old Pfister moves with his family to the Black Forest, and lives an experience that will remain forever in his memory. One of his kindergarten friends fell asleep in the classroom and was brutally punished by the teacher for it: "I could never forget – he says as per Zulliger's account – the painful expression of the sick child as he vomited on the severe teacher's dress. A few days later, while we intoned songs of sorrow and mourning at the open grave of my little friend, I felt I wanted to keep the teacher well away from the child's white face" [translated for this edition]. A desire is born at that moment to become one day a teacher and a pedagogue, precisely to be so very differently from the way he had been forced to witness (Zulliger, 1968, p. 28).

Later, in 1880, when he returned with his mother and siblings to his home in Zurich, he attended public school and lived another traumatic experience with an alcoholic teacher who found his best educational resource in physical punishment. So he did with two mentally disabled girls, whom he punished daily, bent on forcing them into learning to read. All of that marked a strong contrast with his experience when he was moved with another teacher whom Oskar later considered a "benefactor and spiritual conductor" [translated for this edition] and of whom he grew exceptionally fond. This teacher taught him always to maintain a critical attitude towards everything he received (Zulliger, 1968, pp. 28–29).

Besides his interest in all pastoral implications, Pfister's dedication to education shows his optimism and faith in the possibilities of change and personal transformation. It points then to one of the facets he was most sharply different from Freud, who was so sceptical in this field. We do not know how certain it is, but it has been said that, on one occasion, faced with an anxious question from a mother about her son's education, Freud replied: "Please yourself. Whatever you do will be bad" (Robert, 1966, p. 200).

In his work mentioned above (Pfister, 1917), he first shows the need for the educator to mind psychoanalysis as the ground where he will be able to properly understand children's behaviour, sometimes so puzzling. He also clearly and easily explains the scientific basis of psychoanalysis and the fundamental theoretical principles of psychoanalytic pedagogy. The last part of the work deals with the specific practice of that psychoanalytic education, looking at some particular problems such as children's information on sex matters, aggressiveness from the children towards parents, or the roles of frustration, effort and responsibility in the educational development.

Pfister reveals from the beginning of his work what will become a guiding idea of all his pedagogic, analytical and even theological "Loveless life is bound to founder in anxiety and fear". Education then will have to become conscious that its whole project should somehow be presided by the purpose of liberating the capacities for love in the subjects. Because "In the light of psychoanalytic investigation the art of life is in good part the art of loving". It follows then, from this perspective, that the primary task of the pedagogue will be that of trying for the replacement of the more selfish drives with those of "an altruistic and idealistic love, reaching even to the heights of the Christian love of God" (Pfister, 1922a, pp. 3–4). In conclusion, Pfister formulates this basic principle in education: "Love alone can lead to love" and only love "the passage of the individual from animality to humanity" (Pfister, 1922a, p. 153).

But reaching there requires knowledge of the unconscious mechanisms that move the person and have been the most crucial target of psychoanalytic research. Their knowledge supposes the possibility of their control to place them in favour of education and development. For the educator, psychoanalysis becomes thus an opportunity to destroy harmful inhibitions and develop an autonomous personality with a sense of love and devotion to duty. Summing up his basic ideas, Pfister concludes that psychoanalytic education is the pedagogy that "traces back to their meaning and origin the harmful inhibitions brought about by unconscious mental forces, undertaking to overcome the discovered unconscious forces by rendering them accessible to the will of the moral personality" (Pfister, 1922a, p. 14).

One of the most critical problems noted by our author is that of many children who find themselves unable to properly work along what is expected of them, and even what they would consciously wish because they suffer a split personality in which their original conscious thrusts are controlled or corrupted by unconscious opposite wishes. Therefore, no punishment or threat will remedy these difficulties. Complete investigation work on the possible causes is needed. To do that, the pedagogue will need information about the theory of instincts, repression, and its unconscious outgrowths. In effect, when those inhibitions' true motives are found, the gaps opened between the conscious and the unconscious are closed, offering the possibility of true freedom, of integration of all the soul's forces under the proposed ideal, be it moral or spiritual. The Gospel formulation "The truth shall make you free" (Jn. 8:32) becomes thus, for Pfister, "the Magna Charta of educative analysis" (Pfister, 1922a, p. 61).

At one point, Pfister admits that he, as a teacher and minister, had paid in the past scarce attention to religious and moral complications coming from the unconscious of his pupils. Later, however, he found that many character faults eased up with analytic treatment and that certain moral flaws should be understood as neurotic symptoms in healthy and sick individuals. From this discovery came his belief that ethics should consider as much spiritual health as moral one (Pfister, 1931a).

In the education field and for traditional morality, shaping moral conscience was always one of his first concerns, always insisting on paying greater attention to psychoanalytical contributions. The science founded by Freud – Pfister thinks – can render an invaluable service to ethics and moral education. It is true – he recognises – that the assessment and moral judgement do not properly belong in the analytical task itself. Still, psychoanalysis can help design the ethical requirements that rule any education.

Psychoanalysis and religious experience

If the education circles paid attention soon to Pfister's ideas, nothing similar happened in the field of theology, even if this was the field to which Pfister dedicated more attention and interest. "It is a great grief to me that the theologians are so backwards and wanting. I have now been at work for eighteen years. The educationists have accepted a great deal, and I hear on all sides that analysis engages more and more of their interests. But the theologians are too involved in stupid squabbles about principles to care very much about the mental well-being of the laity – or their own. All the same, it has not been all in vain. I am writing an article for 'Sigmund Freud' in the great encyclopaedia *Die Religion in Geschichte und Gegenwart* ..." (Meng & Freud, 1961, p. 104). The assertion is not too compatible with that of Peter Gay, saying "Even in his lifetime (Freud's), the tribe of Freud's sympathisers among the theologians had been growing" and that "schools of divinity were eager to have Pfister lecture on the religious implications of psychoanalysis for the cure of souls" (Gay, 1987, pp. 86–87).

The attention of Pfister to dogmatics was inexcusable from many points of view. As we already saw, theology was an object of permanent care and questioning since the beginning of his education. On the other hand, the altruist and humanitarian concern that marked with strong traits his character was directed towards an explicitly religious and Christian option. Belief is always behind pastoral action, and Pfister's belief determined his fundamental choices in life intimately. His contact with psychoanalysis could not fail to affect the actual contents of that faith that dominated his life and his prime dedication.

Many aspects of the religious experience and Christian doctrine were the objects of Pfister's psychoanalytic attention. Going through his extended bibliography, we see that, from very early days, beyond the pure pastoral concern, he looks at different chapters of general religious beliefs and Christian faith in particular: pietism, Marian worship, the relationships between the mystic and the hysterical experiences, glossolalia, the religious personalities of Paul, Luther or Calvin, Catholicism, Judaism, Buddhism, as well as the general relationship between theology and psychoanalysis … all of these themes trace his work from the beginning to the end.

One of the first works by Pfister to earn the consideration of psychoanalysts was the one he dedicated in 1910 to the well-known pietist Count Zinzendorf (Pfister, 1910b). Freud was enthusiastic about the work, even challenging Jung to keep it away from the Jahrbuch, where Jung intended to publish it. "Splendid material", Jung tells Freud in a letter dated 24 May 1910. In the letter dated 17 June 1910, Freud tells Pfister, referring to his refusal to give the work to Jung, "So you will have to tell Jung that for the first time I am refusing him something" (McGuire, 1974, p. 319). And to Pfister himself, he tells in his usual provocative tone that Count Zinzendorf will go to print after his Leonardo (Freud, 1910c) ("It will cause plenty of offence") and that he expects that also the Zinzendorf "will anger a good many good people" (Meng & Freud, 1961, pp. 34–35). P. Gay comments on this point: "That was the kind of psychoanalytic dissection that Freud could applaud – the anticlericalism of the clerical" (Gay, 1987, p. 85).

The study deals with Count Nikolaus Ludwig von Zinzendorf, who lived in the 18th century, theologian and bishop of the Moravian Church, who became the most prominent pietist of the century in the Holy Roman Empire and the American colonies. His preaching emphasised devotion to Christ's wounds and blood, showing at the same time authentic contempt for conjugal love. "This led", Pfister noted severely, to 'the ugliest sexualisation of religion' and to 'religious orgies'" (Gay, 1987, p. 85).

In his interpretation, Pfister illustrates the huge edipic potential of the person he studies. Count Zinzendorf's father, minister of state at Saxony, had died from a haemorrhage due to lung tuberculosis when he was just a few weeks old baby. When he was four years old, his mother, a devout pietist, married again, and he was sent to live with his maternal grandmother, Baroness Henriette Catharina von Gersdorff. She was a well-known religious woman, and her castle had become a meeting place for eminent pietists. Along with his godfather, a man of strong religious feelings, they were, with excessive severity, the Count's educators. He was, for instance, not allowed to enjoy the company of other children from ten to sixteen years of age.

Pietist fervour gained a place in Zinzendorf's heart very soon. Deprived of his father, about whom he had heard frequently and equally deprived of his mother, Zinzendorf found comfort and love in the figure of Jesus, whom he called "creator" or "betrothed of my soul".

After 1750, the Count progressively concentrated on the wounds, the blood and the dead body of Jesus, and, above all, on the side wound, which carried his religious libido towards orgasmic ecstasy. According to Oskar Pfister's interpretation, Zinzendorf describes this side wound unmistakably as female genitals, birth passage and sexual relation organ. But the Count was also fascinated by Jesus' circumcision, about which he created many texts and hymns. The representation of Jesus as an androgynous father-betrothed went along in parallel with the representation of the Holy Spirit as a mother and that of God the Father as a grandfather or even as a Father-in-law.

For Oskar Pfister, Zinzendorf's obvious hyper-sexualisation of religion reflects a tremendous displacement on Jesus of a perverse libido that did not find its normal evolution through opportune parental relationships. In his passion for Jesus, so much encouraged by the family's pietism, Zinzendorf displaced his homosexual, sadistic, masochistic and necrophile components, elements all of them that subsequent generations of Moravian pietists had to expurgate away from their hymns and religious literature. He unconsciously associated the blood-covered dead body of Jesus with that of his father, whose death was described with similar graphic detail when he was a child. At the same time, his androgynous Jesus served as an object of the desire which would have been addressed to his mother and other women he was deprived of. All of it led to the desexualisation of marriage, highly promoted by Zinzendorf among his followers, and to move children away from their parents as early as possible so that their love could concentrate on the spiritual betrothal.

Zinzendorf, then, represented for Pfister the perverse route that the libido could follow across the religious experience instead of taking a road to personal development and fulfilment by way of sublimation, which, as we will later see, constituted for him the great possibility and richness that religion offered.

In the same way he approached pietism as a sample of psychic and religious deviance, he examined the hysterical character latent in some elements of specific modalities of Catholic Marian worship or the mystical experiences of some historical figures (Pfister, 1910d, 1912, 1928a).

Oskar Pfister was convinced he had found an invaluable instrument to purify religious faith in psychoanalysis. He did not hesitate to use it to diagnose certain historical forms of faith aberration. But he was not only concerned with phenomena like pietism in the 17th century or specific aberrant mystical experiences of the past. He also tried to identify in the religious expressions of his own time and place the more problematic aspects, even if that could cause him difficulties. An example of this was the very acid criticism by H. Saalfeld for Pfister's "alliance" with Freud in his interpretation of religion (Saalfeld, 1928).

Another similar problem happened with his *Die Legende Sundar Singhs* (Pfister, 1926), where he analyses with finesse the case of an Indian faquir who, as a Christian holy man, was winning attention and admiration from many believers, fascinated by the miracle-work surrounding the character. In his interpretation, Pfister tears apart the whole supernatural and miraculous components of the case and reduces it to its most primitive psychic elements. The reactions were strong:"

I was attacked", – he tells Freud – "not just as if, like Luther, I had laid hands on the sacred person of the Pope, but as if I had made a bad smell in the Holy of Holies. Now these gentries have got their desserts. The saint is exposed like a prima donna extricated from a stinkbutt and the outcry his fanatical admirers are making is enough to make the devil sick. The freer Protestant circles are delighted at my disclosures. I wanted to strike a blow at superstition, stupidity and goggle-eyed self-abasement, but one should really spend one's time less unprofitably" (Meng & Freud, 1961, p. 102). For his part, Freud replies very much in his style: "The book amused me more that it pleased me. For myself I was glad that I have no religion and therefore do not find myself in the cleft stick which you cannot avoid. So far as you were concerned, I was sorry that you had to busy yourself with such (let us call it) muck. No doubt it will do good in some circles, or you would not have done it" (Meng & Freud, 1961, p. 103).

Psychoanalysis and Judeo-Christianism

Over time, however, Pfister's work in applying psychoanalysis to faith became more profound and broader. Since 1940, the most central aspects of the Judeo-Christian faith captured his attention. The theme of salvation and its possible relations with anxiety and neurotic-compulsive components polarise his watch more and more and gives shape to some of his more fundamental writings.

This theme came up already in the correspondence with Freud in 1930 on the occasion of a conference the New York Psychoanalytic Society was preparing on the origin and the overcoming of anxiety and compulsion in the history of Judeo-Christian religion. "It is a subject which has been on my mind for years", Pfister tells Freud. And he adds: "and it first attracted my attention because it provided such magnificent corroboration of your theories. But then big new problems presented themselves, such, for instance, as the substitution of the doctrine of revenge and sacrifice by the principle of love and forgiveness" (Meng & Freud, 1961, p. 134). Thus Pfister approached one of the fundamental problems of 20th-century theology when it tried to rethink Christology and soteriology. One of the most debated and reworked themes by contemporary theological thought, both Catholic and Protestant, has been how to understand the reconciliation of God with humanity based on Jesus and his death (Vorgrimler & Vander Gucht, 1970). Psychoanalytic deepening into the father-child relationships, affective ambivalence and guilt feelings also contributed to reassessing this central chapter of Christian dogma (I examined these relationships between psychoanalysis and soteriology in an earlier work) (Domínguez-Morano, 1994).

For Oskar Pfister, the problem holds great complexity since certain ways of conceiving God's love and forgiveness could be seen as a simple regression to a kind of God-Mother who does not yet have the requirements of good and evil. A relationship, then, still without the intervention of the paternal function of the law. "In regard to the genuinely Christian conception of forgiveness, as represented, for instance, in the parable of the prodigal son (Luke, xv), there is obviously a regression to the childhood state in which the child is not yet treated by the standard of good and evil, but simply with love and kindness. However, that does not solve the real problem", Pfister concludes. As an educator, he knows very well that the norm, the ethical requirement, must play a fundamental role in personal development, even if the application of forgiveness and atonement constitutes one of the most challenging problems to settle. Finally, however, forgiveness and compassion signify a triumph, after accepting the law and the ethical requirement, precisely of that law and that requirement that was so important for development and maturity. "Is there not analytic action in all acts of grace and forgiveness? …" Pfister asks in his dialogue with Freud (Meng & Freud, 1961, p. 134).

With all these disquisitions, Pfister seems to be conscious of the serious problems implied in the ways of understanding the Christian dogma of redemption. They keep an intimate relationship with God's paternal representation and possible oedipal connotations. Nevertheless, the theme will remain the object of his reflections without reaching a systematic theoretical formulation. Be that as it may, he moved away from the theory of satisfaction, which considered the sacrifice and death of Jesus as necessary for the reconciliation of God with humanity. "God should not be appeased with sacrifices, but instead be loved as one's brother", he asserts emphatically in *The illusion of a future: A friendly disagreement with Prof. Sigmund Freud* (Pfister, 1993, p. 562).

In any case, it also seems evident – as we will see further on – that Oskar Pfister was more sensible to the problem of the protective illusion shown by Freud in *The Future of an Illusion* (Freud, 1927c) than to the ambivalence and guilt marked as the critical point in *Totem and Taboo* (Freud, 1913a), a work that no doubt we have to consider the most important piece in the Freudian psychoanalysis of religion, and which I have studied in earlier work (Domínguez-Morano, 1991, pp. 99–144). Certainly, Pfister kept in mind the close relationship established by Freud between obsessive neurosis and religion but discussed it just at the level of personal experience, paying scarce attention to what that oedipal affective ambivalence could mean at the level of dogma. A higher sensibility to the issues of the age of enlightenment and the relationship between religion and science mainly captured his reflections on psychoanalysis and the Judeo-Christian faith. The most original and specific element in the Freudian interpretation of Judeo-Christianism had, in consequence, a scant echo in the ensemble of the pastor's reflections.

However, the problems of anxiety and compulsion, considered more from the perspective of religious experience than from the dogmatic formulation, took an essential place in Oskar Pfister's thought. Indeed, his *Christianity and Fear* (Pfister, 1948), initially published in German in 1944, must be considered more significant in this respect and one of the broadest impacts among his publications. There, Pfister tries to establish the place and the role that anxiety has played in the history and the praxis of Judeo-Christianism.

In the book's first part, the author presents a series of general considerations about anxiety in normal individuals and neurotic ones. The ideas of Sören Kierkegaard, Martin Heidegger, and Alfred Adler are reviewed alongside Freud's. The defences against anxiety, and its intellectual and emotional impacts, are analysed from a psychoanalytic viewpoint, trying to equally understand the possibilities of success (through sublimation and liberation of the capacity to love) or failure (with the development of neurotic symptoms, particularly the obsessive ones) in the management of anxiety. Finally, the author tries to understand the analogies and differences in personal or collective anxious experiences (Pfister, 1948, pp. 123–124).

In the book's second part, Pfister studies anxiety shaping in Judeo-Christianism. He looks over this at different ages of Judaism, alternating between periods in which solutions to anxiety and fear predominate with others in which these emotions prevail. The liberating action of the prophets is thus followed by opposite movements, which reinforce the mechanisms of anxiety again (Pfister, 1948, pp. 157–175).

Jesus' position on this theme is analysed in more detail. The experience of divinity through love is essential in the teaching of Jesus, who comes to soothe and solve anxiety. The faith in a God felt as a close Father is what drives Jesus to break the Jewish law system and its representation of God as a fearsome, jealous being. As presented by Jesus, salvation does not come from adhesion to a dogma, from the observance of a law or the fulfilment of religious rites. Jesus did not appear as a new legislator or an ascetic.

But the love that the Gospel message puts forward is not a sentimentalist or regressive love, but one that pushed towards an ethical fulfilment beyond mere compliance of a legal code "A joyous love has been restored to its rights, and it puts an end to the traditional compulsive neurosis which had been forced upon the people by the cult of the loveless Law" (Pfister, 1948, p. 191).

Pfister highlights the liberating significance of the Gospel proposal, which invites us to consider only God as a father. The principle of love is thus guaranteed against any temptation of submitting to whatever type of authority hinders the person's ethical autonomy. In this way, he sees Jesus not only as a prophet who denounces the false conceptions of God but also as an effective liberator from anxiety and fear. Somehow, Pfister presents Jesus as a therapist, a precursor of modern psychotherapies. "Jesus wanted to liberate the Jews and mankind in general from the domination of fear caused by guilt, of uncharity, of the spirit of compulsion emanating from the Rabbis and the Pharisees, and of the rule of sin" (Pfister, 1948, pp. 209–210).

But every spiritual innovation brings reaction phases, and Jesus' work did not escape this rule. The freedom-giving work of Jesus, soothing and solving anxiety, was progressively changed through the dogmatic work of Paul, the Catholic Church and most Protestant Reformers. The analysis Pfister performs on the figure of Paul is fascinating. Without any doubt, the apostle solved the anxiety problem in his person. But it does not seem that he managed to express that Christian liberation from anxiety in the ensemble of his ideas. His thought is not free from dark areas and contradictions in this respect. We find texts in which he may appear as a champion of the liberation of the Christian spirit of liberty and others in which he seems to strangle that Christian freedom through dogmatic or ascetic formulations presenting strong resonances with stoicism. In Paul's ethics – he tells us – the way to maintain the spirit of the Gospel was not always found. The shadows of anxiety which Jesus had dispelled came somehow back. Paul's texts (which along dogmatic history have been as a source of authority even more significant than that of the canonical gospels) have worked as a small Bible in which each one, depending on his personal needs, has searched and found in connection with what his unconscious processes required. "Tell me what you derive from reading St. Paul and I will tell you the state of your disposition towards religious fear; in other words, the state of your Christian freedom", Pfister concludes (Pfister, 1948, p. 269).

The analysis of the Swiss pastor becomes particularly critical of the Roman Catholic Church, which he sees as very far from primitive Christianity or Protestantism in managing anxiety. A true neurotic, compulsive character has been born in its bosom, and one has the impression that life itself is no more than an unceasing fight with anxiety. Pfister insists on the multiplication of the symptoms of anxiety and guilt that originate even since childhood in the dogmatic orthodoxy and obsessive praxis of the sacraments and in the dualist morality that represses natural, instinctual life to the limit, placing the life of the monk as the ideal of life in the renunciation of sexuality, of personal independence and the "world". The Catholic priest's very figure appears to Pfister as surrounded by a halo of anguished taboo, in his powers to change bread into Christ's flesh, forgive sins, etc…

Pfister affirms that one of the main reasons for the development of anxiety in Catholicism is the representation of God usually made in its midst. It is not the God of love, the close Father, who gives the gift and the pardon. Catholic dogma, without denying the love of God, makes it very difficult to live the experience of it. The dogmatics about the devil, the purgatory and even the very treatment of the Trinity dogma make for the concealment of the fatherly face of God and for requiring a series of intermediaries, such as the churchly hierarchy of priests, bishops and the Pope, the saints, the angels or the figure of Mary, to have access to that distant and fearsome God. Christ is not the Saviour of sins, but the second person in the Trinity, who can only forgive, not by pure grace and gift, but by paying a fine or satisfaction.

Pfister analyses the Catholic treatment of the figure of Mary as one more dogmatic element, which reveals the essential distortion of the image of God made by Catholicism. Her motherly presence becomes all the more necessary, the more distant the paternal dimension of God. The insistence on her virginity (through actual violence on the texts that seem to mean the opposite) reveals – from Pfister's viewpoint – the problem felt about sexuality and the defence in front of the anxiety that sexuality provokes. Likewise, the Catholic regulation of celibacy, the pre-eminence given to virginity, and the ideals of monasticism show the same anxious and defensive attitude in the face of sexuality. Catholicism is a religion of the "great beyond" and, as such, despises and demonises pleasure.

Not far from the cliché, Pfister goes on to revise the meaning of the Church hierarchy, the Popes, the Inquisition, etc...as elements that show a religiosity impregnated by fear and anxiety. The obsessive-compulsive character prevails in Catholic thought and praxis. Irrationality, magic, scrupulousness, and the compulsive trends characteristic of the dogmatic and sacramental Catholic theology are thoroughly reviewed and illustrated with examples, such as those of Saint Alphonsus Liguori, who was unable to drink a drop of water without his confessor's permission. All of that speaks of a kind of spirituality, very far from that of Jesus, in which the Gospel proposal of love comes second.

However, the protection obtained in the bosom of the Roman Catholic Church itself, using the subordination to authority and the institution, plays a powerful lenitive against anxiety. But while love was for Jesus the fundamental principle that should rule his disciples' lives, Catholicism dethroned love through the dominance of dogmatic thought and ritual action. ".and instead (of love) an unconditional subordination to a Church claiming pre-eminence in every religious and moral action was made man's highest duty and the sole condition of salvation" (Pfister, 1924). That is the measure set up as the fundamental defence against anxiety, which Pfister feels able to confirm based on his clinical experience in the analysis of many Catholic persons (Pfister, 1948, p. 314). These measures turned out to be "effective" in many cases but not free of important dangers for the mental life of the subjects and, indeed, very far from the intentions and propositions of Christianity's founder. Pfister dedicates several pages to illustrate with a clinical case his view of Catholicism and how he handles anxiety through subordination to the Church authority.

Having so treated Catholicism as a monolithic block, although with a certain cliché-ish, even caricature-like, character (although less than what we could think today considering the state of the Church and Catholic thought in those years, well before the new approaches brought forth by the Second Vatican Council) Pfister goes on to analyse the various Protestant reforms. He will not be more indulgent with his own religious affiliation propositions.

Protestantism willed to be a different way to face the problem of anxiety. Unbearably overwhelmed, Luther tried to find relief from anxiety and better treatment of the problem in his deep revision of Christian faith. Significantly, anxiety was an essential element in the motivations of the Lutheran Reform. Pfister, like E.H. Erikson (Erikson, 1962) and R. Dalbiez (Dalbiez, 1974) later, does not forget to consider this factor as one of the most determinants in the upheaval of the Augustinian monk. The most revolutionary element in his theological reform, justification by faith alone, besides other scriptural motivations that Pfister questions, responds primarily to an interior psychic urge (Particularly, he criticises how Luther understood Paul on this point of justification by faith) (Pfister, 1948, pp. 351–353). But, through his own anxiety, Luther, rediscovers an essential aspect of Christian faith, that of the grace and the love of God, which had been dethroned from Catholic thought (Pfister remarks that Luther's religious reform brought a different view on sexuality. The introduction of clerical marriage was a big step in the new consideration of sexuality and exposed that "the greatest religious reform in Christianity was contemporary with a sexual reform". Luther himself, though, according to Pfister, "married from duty more than from inclination") (Pfister, 1948, pp. 366–367). However, this rediscovery of God's grace and love was not sufficient to fully calm down anxiety in the theological vision of the reformer. Other sinister traits remained in the Lutheran representation of God and salvation: predestination, the small number of the elect, horror in front of the final judgment, the devil's power ... Not surprisingly, his teachings considered anxiety a common and even necessary element. So, Pfister concludes that even if his doctrine of grace meant a vital step in confronting religious anxiety, Luther failed to restore the full sense of love as the centre of the whole life, just as Jesus teaches.

After Luther, Pfister analyses the figure of the Zurich reformer Zwingli. The most humanist among the reformers and the most "human among humanists". It is not fear and guilt, as was Luther's case, that drives his reform but a deep sensibility in the face of human suffering, which he saw as originating in Catholic propositions. If Luther was the defender of Paul, Zwingli was the defender of the Gospel of Jesus. If the forgiveness of sins was essentially what drove Luther, Zwingli was directly moved by love in its fulfilment in the present world. And if Luther, in his confrontation with the Catholic Church, persisted in divesting Christianism of its Judaizing elements, Zwingli did so to strip it of the pagan elements adhered along with history.

Pfister's liking for Zwingli is palpable. He finds in the reformer his own insistence on placing love at the very core of Christian life and moral freedom, as well as having Jesus and the Gospel as the basis of his whole doctrine, instead of through Paul or other prominent figures in the ecclesial history. Faith centred on God's love liberated Zwingli "from the neurotic and mass-neurotic effects of fear, from Catholic orthodoxy, and from the magical fear-mechanism manifested in the prevailing sacramentalism" (Pfister, 1948, p. 387).

But despite reaching further than any other reformer, Pfister acknowledges that Zwingli's doctrine was not entirely consequent with the fundamental principle of love. Having decidedly opposed the burning of witches, he accepted the execution of four Anabaptists because of their positions against state laws and let the shadow of anxiety show in his conception of the afterlife as a space for eternal reward or eternal punishment. He went beyond any other reformer but did not reach Jesus' radical conception of God and love. "But has any man succeeded in this?" (Pfister, 1948, p. 389), says Pfister concluding his reflection on the Zurich reformer.

The analysis of the anxiety problem in Calvin is more complex than with any other reformer. There are substantial gaps in the knowledge of this figure, regardless of his biographers' efforts. And although his prominence is unquestionable, the assessment of his significance in the religious sphere is very controversial. For some, Calvin is no more than a schizoid psychopath; for others, a typical fanatic. For Erich Fromm, he "belonged to the ranks of the greatest haters among the leading figures of history, certainly among religious leaders" (Fromm, 1942, p. 82); for others, Calvin is one of the greatest religious geniuses.

The Calvinist representation of God is essentially that of supreme majesty and power. An omnipotent and sovereign God rather than a merciful Father. And it seems undeniable that his doctrine on predestination induced high anxiety levels in many of his followers. This helped bring about that sort of demonisation of the image of God that many see in Calvinism.

Calvin's doctrine reveals a personality marked by profound conflict and terrible ambivalence towards the tyrannical father of his childhood. That paternal representation was projected into his image of God and gave room to religiousness marked by guilt, self-hate (in fundamental contradiction with the Gospel's command, Pfister notes), strong sadomasochistic tendencies, and a desperate and failed attempt to manage anxiety. In Pfister's eyes, Calvin, paradoxically, created a new sort of Catholicism dominated by anxiety and compulsion. Quoting Freud, the Swiss pastor saw all obsessive character traits in the reformer. The internal dynamics of these subjects – Freud said – are "distinguished by the predominance of the super-ego, ... the fear of their conscience .... They develop a high degree of self reliance ... they are the true, pre-eminently conservative vehicles of civilisation" (Freud, 1931a, p. 218).

Despite so critical a view on Calvin, Pfister does not envisage using it to efface the admirable dimensions of the personality and the achievements of the reformer. Calvin is a genius personality – he tells us – which forcefully reveals the divine and the diabolical, the *fascinosum* and the *tremendum* of the sacred (Pfister, 1948, p. 449).

As an appendix to the chapters dedicated to the three great reformers, Pfister summarises the essential characteristics of their ways of treating anxiety. The three insist on the exclusive effectiveness of the grace and gift of God, apart from good works, rituals, and charity. The gratitude for the received gift so replaces the anxiety for salvation. One of the fundamental aspects of Jesus' teachings is thus restored under his point of view. Only through Christ do we become children of God. Hence, mediation by Mary or another authority in heaven or earth is considered superfluous. The reformers "put an end to the Catholic fear-compulsion neurosis" (Pfister, 1948, p. 450).

But the limitations were also significant. They remained far from admitting freedom of faith and conscience. "The Reformation was an act of liberation, but it was relative and narrowly limited" (Pfister, 1948, p. 451). The reason was that the reformers themselves were subject to repression and suffered a lack of real love. They were far from fully restoring the Christian love that Jesus postulated as the essence of all religiousness, from giving love the central power as much in faith as in life. That is why they failed to find a satisfactory solution to the anxiety problem.

Pfister analyses the post-Reformation era as another age dominated by a new collective obsessive neurosis, which has replaced the Catholic one but presents the same traits and occasionally with greater harshness and virulence. In the same way that sometimes the mere disappearance of the neurotic symptoms is falsely taken as the disappearance of the neurosis, the same mistake can be made with religious reforms.

Some years before, in a suggestive work (Pfister, 1940), *"Loesung und Bindung von Angst und Zwang in der israelitisch-christlichen Religionsgeschichte"*, Pfister looked at the repression-liberation dialectic that he believed could be noticed throughout the different religious movements within Judeo-Christianism. In his view, the periods in which anxiety and compulsion intensified through rigid orthodoxy were always followed by other reforming movements bringing rest and relief measures, always undertaken by those with a strong experience of God's love, trying to convey it to humanity. Yet, at once, a new process in the opposite direction was set in motion. The explanation by Pfister was that the reaction towards the collective neurosis of orthodoxy comes from the fact that repressed forces are never fully solved during the reform periods. A review of the religiousness of Protestant movements such as Baptists, Quakers, or Pietists (in the style of the one seen in the Zinzendorf case) eloquently shows that the Protestant Reform stood far from reaching its first liberating purpose.

The Enlightenment entailed a process of emancipation from any ecclesiastical tutelage, which, in parallel, brought a dynamic of liberation from the irrational tendencies which generated religious anxiety. The restoration of love in its broadest sense is one of the aspects which Pfister highlights in the enlightened movement. A deed – he tells us – that should provoke in the Christian a feeling of shame since irreligious men were effectively the most outstanding in the effort to emphasise the force of love and to fight against the elements generating fear and anxiety. During this period, in the field of belief, the image of God appears with the most positive and encouraging traits, expressing the characteristic optimism of believers. It is neither the *tremendum* nor the *fascinosum* nor even that of Trinity, but, essentially, the one ready to help. Jesus is not so much an incarnate divine essence but a kind master of wisdom. There is no room otherwise for the Devil in the religious temple of the Enlightenment.

Pfister does not hesitate to consider the effects of the Enlightenment on theological thought as essentially healthy. A positive idea of the human being, a critical attitude in the study of the Bible, and separation of Church and State are some of the elements which, determined by the new culture, had a positive influence on Christianism. In a way, the Enlightenment embodied the Christian ideal of eliminating religious anxiety and can therefore be considered a step in the

"Christianisation" of religious faith. Pfister's identification with the Enlightenment movement is patent in these pages. From them, we can even better understand how his debate with Freud apropos *The Future of an Illusion*, on which we shall come later, is, despite everything, a typical discussion between two enlightened thinkers.

Notwithstanding their arguable absolutisation of reason, the Enlightenment contributed to a sanitary restructuring of Christian thought, whose best expression became the new Protestantism. This new Protestant theology, in which Pfister feels fully incorporated, tried to take on the challenge of the Enlightenment and modernity seriously, denounced the grave distortions suffered by the Gospel principle of love, and sought to encourage in pastoral action new representations of God and an active work to relieve human suffering. Starting from this healthy new ethical-religious approach, the new Protestantism was able to work in unison with what, from a scientific perspective, the psychoanalyst tries to achieve.

The third and last part of the book receives the title "The Hygiene of Religion" from Pfister. Despite the dreadful tendencies that historical Christianity presented in the growth of anxiety, Pfister was convinced of the possibility of a religious faith that not only avoids the traps of fear and anxiety-generating guilt but works actively to relieve suffering and improve psychic health among humans. The sole condition is to place the Gospel principle of love, "There is no fear in love" (1 John 4:18), as the centre of all the theology and Christian ethics. Pfister is also convinced that the religious experience can favour the personal evolution processes and even better development of the analytic experience. In this same direction, he writes elsewhere:" The domain of religious ideals offers admirable opportunities of sublimation which do not avoid reality, but on the contrary bring back to it purified energies in rich measure" (Pfister, 1922a, pp. 146–147).

The whole historical study in the book tried to detect the periods in which Christianity turned off its original purpose, helping develop fear, anxiety, and guilt. At the time, the psychoanalytic theory appears to Pfister as a unique opportunity to better understand the actions of these factors that trigger anxiety and unhappiness in human beings. The cooperation between theology and psychoanalysis can render an unbeatable effect on fostering psychic and moral well-being in people. Letting once again his fairly concordist positions and his tendency to confer a moralising character to analytic work be revealed, Pfister affirms that the psychotherapist and the Christian are engaged in the fight against the same foe: the neurotic tendency towards anxiety. Nobody will find a solution to this problem without tolerant love. It then seems due to conclude that the most necessary hygiene in our time is active faith in love (Pfister examines the Nygren distinction between the Eros and Agape concepts, which produced such a strong echo in the Protestant world) (Pfister, 1948, pp. 516–518). Pfister reviews all aspects of Christian dogma in the book's last chapter (Christology, eschatology, the Bible, theological anthropology, morals, sacramental life, ecclesiology, etc.) together in that essential core of the Gospels message, the love that frees from anxiety.

The contributions of Oskar Pfister to psychoanalysis

A non-medical and Christian adept: the question of lay analysis

Even though it proves difficult to accept Kienast's assertion (Kienast, 1974a, p. 84) that psychoanalysis would have remained a simple esoteric method, limited to his founder Jewish circle, were it not for the depth given by Pfister's solid philosophical and theological knowledge, it is also true that the role that the Swiss pastor played on the initial stages of psychoanalysis was not negligible at all and probably was more significant than the one acknowledged up to now.

In the first place, it should be considered what Pfister's presence meant in the initial stages of the psychoanalytic movement as an opening towards non-Jewish worlds and, above all, towards not strictly medical spaces.

We know Freud's concern at the beginning about the possibility that psychoanalysis could evolve while remaining excessively limited to an exclusively Jewish environment. Psychoanalysis was, for him, one more expression of scientific work that should not have any surname. There was no sense in talking of a Jew or Aryan science. And, as he tells Sandor Ferenczi, "If the results reached by a Jewish and a gentile scientist differ, there must be something wrong somewhere" (Gay, 1987, p. 121). He felt he belonged to the Jewish people and was proud of it, but he did not consider himself a Jewish scientist. On the other hand, Freud rightly feared that the identification of psychoanalysis with Judaism would load the movement with all the existing antagonism against his people. In fact, opposition to psychoanalysis grew the more the opposition against Jews grew.

Oskar Pfister, like C. G. Jung, through whom he discovered psychoanalysis, was a Christian and even a son of a Protestant pastor, as C. G. Jung was too. Freud's interest in keeping the bonds with the Swiss group was very much linked to this issue. He also writes to Ferenczi that his objective in strengthening the relationship with the Swiss was "to amalgamate Jews and goyim in the service of Psa (psychoanalysis)" (Gay, 1987, p. 120).

But still more important was that Pfister widened the psychoanalysis circle, reaching non-medical areas. This matter of lay analysis, which, as we know, gained in time an intense virulence, constituted for Freud a capital fight. Specifically, in Pfister's case, it meant a double possibility: on the one side, the opening to psychoanalysis of the "cure of souls" circles and, on the other side, of the world of pedagogues and educators in general. Pfister was so one "colonists in other fields" (McGuire, 1974, p. 276). (Freud added, "I long for mythologists, linguists, and historians of religions".) In addition, given his enthusiasm for the cause, Pfister was thus assessed by Freud: "He could still become one of the most capable men" (Brabant et al., 1933, p. 151).

The first of these possibilities, introduction in the field of cure of souls, could not but cause a certain odd ambivalence in Freud. In a letter to Jung (McGuire, 1974, p. 196), for example, as he comments on specific work sent by Pfister, he says: "your courageous friend Pfister has sent me a paper for which I shall thank him at length. It's really too nice of him – a Protestant clergyman – though rather upsetting to me to see psychoanalysis enlisted on the fight against 'sin'". (The paper in question is the one we saw earlier on delirious representation and the suicide of a scholar.) And at another moment, quoted and praised by Pfister in work published in a Protestant publication, he exclaims: "Think of it, me and the *Protestantischen Monatshefte*!. But it's all right with me. In some respects, a psychoanalyst who is also a clergyman works under better conditions, and besides, he will not be concerned with money". And immediately after, he refers to a course on psychoanalysis that Pfister gives to a group of teachers: "Actually all teachers ought to be familiar with our subject, if only for the sake of the healthy children. For this reason, I give a joyful prosit to your course for teachers" (McGuire, 1974, p. 203).

There were reasons for the toast. It was undoubtedly one of Pfister's main contributions to the psychoanalytic movement: to have been a pioneer in its opening and extension to the field of pedagogy. His characteristic enthusiasm took him to deploy an intense activity in spreading psychoanalytic ideas in pedagogic spaces. "I have now spoken in public about psychoanalysis four times in succession in various places, and each time with great outward success. The teachers of a large part of the canton of Zurich have placed themselves solidly behind me and are calling on the highest authorities to give teachers the opportunity of being acquainted with pedagogic psychoanalysis (paedoanalysis)" (Meng & Freud, 1961, p. 78).

On the other hand, the opening of psychoanalysis to the field of education meant something quite decisive in the build-up of the psychoanalytic movement: access to a world of youth and, at the same time, to areas out of the clinical field. In this way, psychoanalysis was not merely a mere technical health procedure (Freud's aspiration from the very beginning) to produce results as well in its application to mentally healthy persons. Thus, as Freud comments to Pfister, "the optimum conditions for it exist where it is not needed – i.e., among the healthy. Now it seems to me that this optimum exists in the conditions in which you work" (Meng & Freud, 1961, p. 15).

The resistance to psychoanalysis by doctors was high from the beginning, probably the highest of all. Therefore Freud looked to the area of human sciences with the conviction that he would find a better audience. "I am attracted by the prospect of gaining a new and not yet opened-up circle of readers in the field of education", – he writes to Pfister – "Our capacity for expansion in the medical profession is unfortunately very limited, and it is important to secure a footing elsewhere where we can" (Meng & Freud, 1961, pp. 55–56). Later, he comments to Pfister: "Of all the applications of psychoanalysis the only one that is really flourishing is that initiated by you in the field of education. It gives me great pleasure that my daughter is beginning to do good work in that field" (Meng & Freud, 1961, p. 106).

The publication of Pfister's *The psychoanalytic Method* (Pfister, 1915), a comprehensive and clarifying introduction to psychoanalysis mainly intended for pedagogues, was seen as an important contribution by the Swiss pastor to the expansion of the psychoanalytic movement. In the work's introduction (Freud, 1913b), Freud reports on the essentially medical character that psychoanalysis had initially. But at the same time he reveals that, because of its formation process, it was forced to grow beyond the medical field. One of the first and most important applications of psychoanalysis – Freud points out – is precisely in the field of education, which maintains a deep relationship with that of therapy. The priest, he says, who in Protestant countries occupies a place similar to that of the pedagogue, can profit from the results of psychoanalytic research and even reach, in some circumstances, to make the medical intervention unnecessary.

The question then comes – Freud sets out – in terms of the medical training which should be required from the pedagogue or priest to perform psychoanalysis. His answer (ahead of the one he will give in the future controversy originating in the Swiss Society for Psychoanalysis) appears clear already: he sees no obstacle to the practice of psychoanalysis by specialists unconnected with the world of medicine. Psychoanalysis requires not so much medical training as psychological one, while most doctors, according to Freud, are not prepared for the practice of psychoanalysis and have even failed in its appraisal. What is more, Freud considers that pedagogues and priests can be ahead of doctors when it comes to valuing the psychoanalytic method rightly: They "are bound by the standards of their professions to exercise the same consideration, care and restraint as are usually practised by the doctor, and apart from this their association with young people perhaps makes them better fitted to understand these young people's mental life" (Freud, 1913b, p. 331). The only point important for applying analysis without damage will have to be placed in the practitioner's personality.

In fact, the only non-medical analyst who practised the profession before the First World War were Hermine von Hug-Hellmuth in Vienna (She held a doctorate in philosophy and made significant contributions to child analysis, using play for the first time as a technical tool) and Oskar Pfister in Zurich (Jones, 1957, vol. 3, p. 290). Freud always defended them with energy, mainly when controversy arose in the Swiss group, of which Oskar Pfister was a member. As we know, the controversy made way for an important work by Freud titled *The Question of Lay Analysis* (Freud, 1926e), which intended to contain the issue firmly.

It all came from the complaint to justice for the practice of analyst Th. Reik did not have a medical degree. Even if the issue was addressed without difficulty at the court level, it raised a sharp controversy in the analytic circles, which, despite Freud's intervention, is still unsolved today. As we have seen, Freud's position was clear and convincing from the start: psychoanalysis should not be locked up in the realm of medicine. Lay analysis, that is, performed by non-medical analysts, as in Pfister's case, had his decisive support from the beginning. Anthropology, mythology, folklore, history of religions, art or politics all could share a psychoanalysis perspective as a notable contribution to their respective fields. At the same time, the practice of analysis would require extensive training in anatomy, physiology or biology, and, perhaps more importantly, in mythology and psychology of religion. "Unless he is well at home in these subjects, an analyst can make nothing of a large amount of his material (...) For we do not consider at all desirable – Freud concludes – for psychoanalysis to be swallowed up by medicine (...) It deserves a better fate" (Freud, 1926e, pp. 246–248).

Naturally, Pfister felt delighted with Freud's response to a controversy that concerned him. About *The Question of Lay Analysis,* he comments to Freud: "I read through your kind gift at one sitting and with great admiration ... As one of your first lay pupils, the book gave me unspeakable pleasure". However, Pfister misses something, and he does not hesitate to express reproach: "Only one *lacuna* struck me. You mention educational cases, but not the enormous number of adults who are not ill in the medical sense but are nevertheless in extreme need of analysis; I am thinking of alcoholics, people with warped lives, those whose love life has gone astray, frustrated artists, etc. As all these come into the field of the cure of souls, I have a great deal to do with them, and I earnestly appeal to you to cast a benevolent glance at the analytic cure of souls, which is, after all, another of your children. Undoubtedly the cure of souls will one day be a recognised non-ecclesiastical and even non-religious calling. If only men can be made good and happy, with religion or without it, the Lord will assuredly smile approvingly at the work ..." (Meng & Freud, 1961, p. 104).

Freud apologised for the omission, pointing up at the same time that *The Question of Lay Analysis* was essentially "a piece of polemics written for a special occasion, "one which tried to respond to the very specific problem of the practice of analysis by non-medical analysts. And, going on: "Otherwise I should certainly not have omitted the application of analysis to the cure of souls. I considered doing so, but in Catholic Austria the idea of a 'churchman's' (*Geistlicher*) working with analysis is totally unconceivable and I did not wish further to complicate the issue. Besides, my argument would not have benefited; the answer would have been that, if these spiritual gentlemen wished to use analysis, that was no affair of ours, they should apply for permission to their bishop. I am well aware that Catholic analysis exists in Germany, but it would hardly be possible in Austria" (Meng & Freud, 1961, p. 105).

Nevertheless, one year later, in a Postscript, Freud repairs the omission and refers to the cure of souls: "Indeed, the words, 'secular pastoral worker' (*Weltliche Seelsorger*), might well serve as a general formula for describing the function which the analyst, whether he is a doctor or a layman, has to perform in his relation to the public" (Freud, 1927a, pp. 255–256).

The case of Pfister played, no doubt, a significant role in the whole question of lay analysis. Not only as one of the earlier practitioners, not even the fact that Freud took his position on the issue already in 1913 (so before writing his text on the subject), but above all, because Pfister's case compels us to conceive laity on new foundations as an essential attribute to analytic discipline as such. A complex attribute with multiple meanings simultaneously: a high degree of rationality, accessibility for a significant number of persons, and the quality of being transmissible. From the historical point of view, the laity of psychoanalysis generates a break with traditional intellectual contexts, whether medical or religious (Bori, 1990).

An enthusiastic collaborator

One of Jung's first pieces of information to Freud about Pfister is that he is a "redoubtable champion of our cause with a powerful intelligence. He will make something of it. What? I don't know yet" (McGuire, 1974, p. 197).

Indeed, Oskar Pfister did many things for the cause. Some that Jung could not imagine; in a not-so-distant future, and in favour of that cause, he would abandon Jung's psychological conceptions to remain loyal to those of Freud, to whom he was presented at the time.

We saw that Pfister was enthusiastic, passionate, and energetic, with a bursting capacity to work. He gave all of that to the psychoanalytic cause, to which he devoted himself after finding so much clarity for his ideas in it. "He is feverishly busy" – Jung wrote to Freud in the same letter – And a few days before, the first time he mentioned him, he wrote:" has started a big propaganda campaign for your ideas" (McGuire, 1974, p. 196). He tirelessly kept that activity until his final days. Indeed, very few among the psychoanalytic pioneers dedicated themselves to the growth of the psychoanalytic movement and its ideas with the zeal and passion he invested and set in motion.

Pfister developed fundamental work, giving courses and talks in which he fervently tried to show the interest that psychoanalysis offered for diverse fields of thought, particularly pedagogy and theology. During the 1920s, as P. Gay reports, Pfister gave many lectures in Germany and England to persuade influential professors of the wealth of ideas they could find in psychoanalytic theory and the benefit of spreading those ideas among their students. Specifically in Berlin, an early relevant psychoanalytical centre, where many talks on psychoanalysis were given to the general public, Pfister also has a place. In the Society for the Scientific Study of Religion, he lectures, and his ideas "received a friendly reception before an audience of 150 persons, mainly theologians" (Gay, 1998, p. 461). P. Gay also tells us about a non-published letter in which Pfister reports to Freud on one of his activities in favour of analysis: "Today I participated in a meeting in which two professors of theology warmly championed the indispensability of psychoanalysis for historical-critical theology" (Gay, 1987, p. 87). "In Koblenz and Nürnberg I gave lectures to pastors about psychoanalysis and encountered as much interest as ignorance" (Gay, 1987, p. 87).

In 1927, Pfister retook a tour of Europe to spread psychoanalytic ideas. He visits the Nordic countries, where he thinks the results are satisfactory for psychoanalysis, despite, he says, the "especially rooted" resistance against it on these latitudes. In England, likewise, "he was asked to lecture to the theological faculty at Birmingham" (Gay, 1987, p. 87). In 1930, during a visit to the United States of America, he also gives lectures, including one at the New York Psychoanalytic Society on anxiety in Judeo-Christian religious history (Meng & Freud, 1961, p. 134).

Pfister's cooperation in expanding the psychoanalytic movement played a central role in his activity as a prolific writer. We know that his publications were close to three hundred throughout his life. Many were brief, but many had a significant extension, such as *The Psychoanalytic Method* or *Christianity and Fear.* In general, as P. Gay acknowledges, his texts are reliable and readable, always driven by the attempt to make the psychoanalytic doctrine understood. That is his fundamental goal in *The Psychoanalytic Method*, an exhaustive work in which he offers an illuminating exposition of the evolution of psychoanalytic technique, with the honour of being the first systematic presentation of psychoanalysis with Freud himself writing its preface. This exposition of the changes in the method shows the parallel evolution which Pfister points out concerning the psychoanalytic concept of sexuality. Perhaps it should have been better considered, even by Freud himself.

His humanistic education and his particular sensibility made him better understand the profound implications and difficulties that were latent in that Freudian concept. Initially, Pfister explains, Freud attributed the neurotic symptoms to the repression of painful memories, mainly of a sexual nature in the most common and usual sense. Healing was then attempted through catharsis or abreaction. Later, psychoanalysis brought in the repression of phantasies and memories and progressively placed the origin of neurosis in the Oedipal complex. Healing then began to be seen through the analysis of transference and resistance. About this time appears the concept of "psychosexuality", which was intended to account for a broader and more complex reality, comprehending everything contained under the term *Liebe* (love).

In Pfister's opinion, at that moment, the usual concept of sexuality should have been left aside and replaced permanently by the one mentioned above, which would better reflect the vast and complex area that psychoanalysis wanted to contemplate. This would have prevented the hackneyed accusation of pansexualism, which fell from then on over Freudian theory. However, this change was opposed by critics who thought that the concept of "psychosexuality" would hinder the understanding of the theory of the libido and especially that of sublimation. "!How much indignation and animosity would have been avoided if that explanation had been given earlier!", Oskar Pfister commented (Pfister, 1915, p. 63). In his own texts, therefore, he did not hesitate to keep using the term "psychosexuality" to remark on the connections between what is sexual and what is affective, an essential element in his general theory on love. This is shown, for instance, when he writes:" We speak, therefore, preferably psychosexuality, putting emphasis on the fact that one should not overlook nor undervalue the mental factor of the sexual life. We use the word 'sexuality' in the same comprehensive sense as the German language does the word 'love'" (Pfister, 1922a, pp. 50–51).

Pfister's body of written word is not only vast for its extension but also for the diversity of aspects and themes it addresses. The problems of education, cure of souls, and theology are its fundamental axes. However, Pfister's subjects of concern and interest reached further away, and he tried to make psychoanalytic incursions in many other fields. Thus, for instance, the areas of philosophy, and art, where Pfister showed an interest that set him apart from Freud, were objects of his attention in diverse writings (Pfister, 1921a, 1928b, 1934c, 1949). Social and anthropological problems also came under his analysis and interpretation (Pfister, 1920).

Freud knew Pfister's capacity for writing and, above all, his availability to cooperate. Hence, he did not hesitate to ask him for some tasks. So, for instance, about the death of the reputed Swiss doctor, philosopher, and psychologist Théodore Flournoy (1854–1920), he asks for an article underlining his relationship with psychoanalysis (Pfister, 1910e, 1950, 1932). Also, on the decease of Herman Rorschach, with whom Pfister cooperated and held in higher esteem than Freud did, he was invited to write an obituary (Pfister, 1921b; Meng & Freud, 1961, p. 78).

The contribution of Pfister was not limited to the propagation of Freudian theory beyond the psychoanalytic field. Inside the movement itself, he carried out essential tasks and duties. He soon was a member of the Swiss Society for Psychoanalysts, first founded as the Freud Society by twenty doctors on 27th September 1907. He played there a critical role, notwithstanding Freud's wish for him to occupy the presidency ("Too bad that you couldn't put through Pfister as chairman!" Freud wrote to Jung) (McGuire, 1974, p. 320). Later, in 1919, he founded, with Binswanger, Morel, Oberholzer, Rorschach, and Walser, the Swiss Society for Psychoanalysis, which replaced the old one led by Jung. Training analyst of figures such as Henri F. Ellenberger or Hans Zulliger, he would become the most important name of psychoanalysis in Switzerland. He was Freud's man in Zurich (Jones, 1957, vol. 3, pp. 13–14; Roudinesco & Plon, 1997).

A questioning interlocutor

If Freud and psychoanalysis's influence was decisive in Pfister's life and work, it is right to question the role Pfister played in the development of Freud's ideas. Generally, there is a tendency to forget that many concepts and ideas usually taken as Freudian came originally from some psychoanalysis pioneers: Jung, Adler, Ferenczi, Abraham ... above all. It is also true that perhaps Oskar Pfister's most important contribution, as H. Zulliger, his disciple and admirer, acknowledges, would not be in scientific contributions but in the opening of psychoanalysis to other areas in his dissemination ability and incontestable devotion to Freud. However, it would not hurt to examine the possible influence that this long and profound relationship might have had in developing the ideas of the founder of psychoanalysis.

As H. Meng and H. E. Ellenberger told us, we know well that, on themes such as those concerning childhood and puberty, Freud picked up ideas and suggestions from studies by Pfister, whom he quotes on many occasions (Meng & Freud, 1961, p. 10; Ellenberger, 1970, p. 544). We also know that Freud used to keep Pfister informed of his publications and to say that he valued the opinions he received on them from him [see, for instance (Meng & Freud, 1961, p. 82) how he thanked him for his opinion on *Beyond the Pleasure Principle* (Freud, 1920g) and announces the publication of *Group Psychology and the Analysis of the Ego* (Freud, 1921c). Pfister's very idiosyncratic idea that religiousness could also be a defence against neurosis was never objected to by Freud. He even defended it at some point (see, for instance, *The Future Prospects ...* (Freud, 1910d), where he affirms that the loss of religions can bring a considerable increase in neurosis).

On some points, intuitions from Pfister were finally accepted after initial resistances from Freud and other pioneers of psychoanalysis. The idea, for instance, of a kind of repression not only instinctual but also with ethical contents was advocated by Pfister very early on but accepted only when the knowledge of the unconscious dimensions of the super-ego became unquestionable. It had to be assumed that not only "the lowest" but also "the highest" could be objects of repression. In his *Psycho-analysis in the Service of Education*, Pfister recalls how he had referred to the possibility of repression of a moral object some years before Freud did. The admission of possible intellectual, moral and religious content in the unconscious met great resistance in analytic circles, Pfister refers, but it was generally accepted when the work was published.

Likely, Oskar Pfister would sometimes portray for Freud ways he believed he could or should not follow, but that nevertheless activated in him nuclei of ambivalence less resolved than he could, or preferred to, think. The themes of sublimation and religious faith were undoubtedly the ones that could highlight Freud's possible unresolved ambivalence, paradigmatically expressed in the relation with the Swiss pastor. Let's look at it closely.

The subject of sublimation appears from the beginning as Pfister's fundamental interest and concern in his approach to psychoanalytic theory. [Sublimation, as we know, is traditionally defined (Laplanche & Pontalis, 1973) in psychoanalysis as a change in the object and the aim of the instinctual process. This assumes the possibility of a transformation (*Umsetzung*) of the instinctual force that opens up the way of cultural values.] In the letter of presentation, Jung comments to Freud: "His present aim is naturally sublimation, permissible enough in a man of his intelligence" (McGuire, 1974, p. 197).

Since the early days, sublimation has appeared in the correspondence as a subject for reflection and dialogue. Generally, it does as a path in which Pfister finds an excellent possibility for his particular work area. For Freud, it was instead a track that used to be obstructed in his therapeutic practice. Freud's feeling of envy emerges spontaneously: "As for the possibility of sublimation to religion, therapeutically I can only envy you", he commented to Pfister in 1918 (Meng & Freud, 1961, p. 62).

Freud did not believe that in the analytic work he or other analysts carried out, it would be possible to use the patients' sublimatory possibilities, as Pfister hoped. "For us this way of disposing of the matter does not exist. Our public, no matter of what racial origin, is irreligious, we are generally thoroughly irreligious ourselves and, as the other ways of sublimation which *we* substitute for religion are too difficult for most patients, our treatment generally results in the seeking out of satisfaction" (Meng & Freud, 1961, p. 16).

So, the path of sublimation seemed blocked, or at least hindered, by the irreligious character of his patients or his own personal ungodliness. In his view, sublimations different from those following the religious path presented greater difficulty. Therefore, he would feel forced to adopt the way of satisfaction. The idea is worth a more detailed analysis.

Among the patients with whom Pfister worked, there was a higher predisposition for sublimation since they were generally younger persons with more recent conflicts and that, through the trust placed in the pastor, were "ready for sublimation, and to sublimation in its most comfortable form, namely the religious" (Meng & Freud, 1961, p. 16). In Pfister's case, success in the task would be easier in the same way as for Freud and the other analysts, that is, by way of the erotic transfer (*erotische Übertragung*). Religious sublimation looks to Freud as "the most comfortable". In another place, he says, "... you can sublimate the transference on to religion and ethics, which is not easy for the invalids of life" (Meng & Freud, 1961, p. 40).

The texts demand attention, especially if we consider the complex, indeed not easy, relationships that Feud always laid down between religiousness and sublimation. He instead declared as impossible the sublimation path in the religious field, which he mostly placed on the area of repression and, hence, neurosis. For him, the prototype activities in the exercise of sublimation were always artistic or scientific. The text on Leonardo (Freud, 1910c), stands out in this respect as the best Freudian document on both types of sublimatory activities. Religion, on the contrary, always becomes clear – from his point of view – with the neurosis reference: trauma, latency period, and return of the repressed are the fundamental stages of both neurosis and religion. This point is most evident in the text of *Moses and Monotheism* (Freud, 1939a).

But as Freud, in his publications, tends almost totally to relate religion with repression and neurosis and not with sublimation, we see that one of the very few texts (I refer to these in an earlier work (Domínguez-Morano, 1991, pp. 359–364.)) in which religion and sublimation are related is precisely about Pfister. This is *An Autobiographical Study* (Freud, 1925d, pp. 69–70), where, describing the Swiss pastor's activity, Freud writes: "nor did he find the practice of analysis incompatible with the retention of his religion, though it is true that this was of a sublimated kind".

So the impossibility of a healthy sublimation on the religious path seemed clear enough to Freud at a theoretical level. Still, it was not so clear when judging and valuing Oskar Pfister's activity and, probably, his personal reality.

Of course, it can be considered that the attitude of polite tolerance he always kept with the pastor may be one of the fundamental reasons to explain the benevolent position of granting the religious experience the possibility of offering a good path of sublimation. However, he did not do so in other issues, such as the idea of sexuality that Pfister tended to develop in his effort to make it compatible with the Christian ideal of love. Let us not forget, a concept of sexuality intimately linked to sublimation. On this point, Freud argued, punctuated, and expressed disagreement in a straightforward, sometimes blunt and expedient, way. Let us recall the words he used concerning Pfister's *Psycho-analysis in the Service of Education:* "Why on earth do you dispute the splitting up of the sex instinct into its component parts which analysis imposes on us every day? Your arguments against this are really not very strong … in your little book you do not deal quite correctly with the sexual instincts … I think that the relics of your resistance to sexuality must have crept into this. Try and revise that part of yourself". Freud did not hesitate to elaborate, clarifying his theory on the component instincts and the erogenous zones. However, when he touches the sublimation theme in the same letter, he limits himself, as we saw earlier, to express his envy: "As for the possibility of sublimation to religion, therapeutically I can only envy you" (Meng & Freud, 1961, pp. 62–63).

Thus, a concept as complex but crucial in psychoanalytic theory as sublimation does not require clarification from Freud. And, in the background, Pfister's tendency, sometimes a bit sanguine, to draw on this concept to justify his peculiar way of applying psychoanalysis.

It is difficult to avoid the impression that, in the face of what Pfister represented, Freud confronted his own personal difficulties, which prevented him from clarifying the sublimation processes. It seems he could only envy …

The concept of sublimation, in a certain way, defeated him. His project to complete the metapsychological studies with a book on the theme was never achieved. Moreover, it is assumed that it was written and destroyed. The inherent relationship between sublimation and values, sexuality and culture, instinct and ideal, made understanding the phenomenon difficult for him. Confronting the concept of sublimation, which Pfister had put before him in so many ways, would have meant revising many other fundamental concepts of metapsychology, such as drive, libido, sexuality, pleasure, culture, etc. The task must have appeared to him as excessive to undertake successfully, even more so if we consider that his previous positivist notions and an excessively psychopathological perspective did not facilitate the task. [So has been shown by A. Vergote in *Guilt and Desire* (Vergote, 1978), and more recently in an excellent study entitled *La psychanalyse à l'épreuve de la sublimation* (Vergote, 1997), where he undertakes a detailed critical balance of sublimation in the Freudian text, underlining the contradictions, unresolved points and lacunae in the ensemble of Freud's work.] As P. Ricoeur pertinently remarked, the concept of sublimation produces Freud's more significant difficulties, contradictions, and aporias in his understanding of culture in general and religion in particular (Ricoeur, 1970). A series of clearly utilitarian and rationalist prejudices determine his views on the objects that promote sublimation and those that led him to sideline the religious experience from that possibility.

Then, the envy that Freud felt before Pfister because of the possibilities the latter used to guide the subjects in the path of sublimation could very well be caused not only by the unbelief of his patients or his own one but also by his internal contradictions that hindered the understanding of the sublimation process and what it entails. Pfister could appear as the beneficiary of something forbidden to him because of his inner bonds.

It is rather curious that it was precisely at the moment this envy appeared when Freud asked Pfister why psychoanalysis had to wait for an unbelieving Jew to be founded. Let us recall the text: "As for the possibility of sublimation to religion, therapeutically I can only envy you. But the beauty of religion certainly does not belong to psychoanalysis. It is natural that at this point in therapy our ways should part, and so it can remain. Incidentally, why was it that none of the pious ever discovered psychoanalysis? Why did it have to wait for a completely godless Jew? With cordial greeting from your old friend, Freud" (Meng & Freud, 1961, p. 63).

It should be asked: "Incidentally?". Perhaps the question would not be so "incidental" as Freud pretends ..., maybe it was related to that envy of Oskar Pfister he had just mentioned and which, reviving his impotence, could very well generate an aggressiveness that finally discharges. Just to send at once "cordial greetings from your old friend". The remedial action came fast, as we see.

The sublimation problems send us back to the religious experience that Pfister laid before Freud in an exceedingly vivid way over a long and deep relationship of friendship. A religious experience that he, more with his person than with his ideas, revealed as compatible with psychoanalysis, against Freud's predictions, till his final days: "Whether he will be able to preserve his residue of faith – Freud comments to Jung – for long strikes me as doubtful; he is only at the beginning of a far-reaching development, and the bad company he keeps is bound to have its effect" (McGuire, 1974, p. 223). The same assuredness appears in a letter to Ferenczi. He speaks of Pfister's enthusiasm for what psychoanalysis could offer to theology: "He doesn't yet suspect that the analytical conception *carried through to its conclusion* does away with theology. He has yet to come to that" (Brabant et al., 1933, p. 153).

Nothing of the kind happened. The man Pfister that Freud knew until the end of his life kept being the man of faith, the tireless fighter and the committed pastor of souls he always was. Thus, Oskar Pfister stood in his person as the guarantor of the coexistence of Christian faith with an unwavering adhesion to psychoanalytic theory. A position, indeed, hardly understandable for Freud and which at the same time aroused his perplexity, suspicion, and undeniable interest (Widlöcher, 1966).

Somehow, Pfister was on to revive Freud's old feelings concerning his attitude towards religious belief. Allegedly similar sentiments to those activated while young in his academic contacts with Franz Brentano when he attended the courses given by the famous philosopher as a nineteen-year-old student. As Peter Gay reminds us, that ex-priest, who believed in God and respected Darwin, removed and intensely questioned the atheism about which Freud felt so sure. As revealed in his correspondence (Boelich, 1990) with his friend at that time, Eduard Silberstein, Brentano appeared to him as an authentic genius who, with his dialectical wit, made him even consider the possibility of a belief in God. But, as Freud comments to his friend, "I have no intention of surrendering so quickly or completely" (Boelich, 1990, p. 104). "The godless medical man, "as he named himself (Boelich, 1990, p. 70), was forced to pit his strength with some difficulty against that believer he profoundly admired.

Many years later, when he felt obliged to publish his most virulent attack against religion, he had to place himself in front of an interlocutor he could also defeat. And who, at the same time, he admired. In the Future of an illusion, Freud dreamed up a dialogue with an illustrated intellectual of high moral standing, accessible to reason, erudite, cultivated, and even mundane. However, Theodor Reik, not at all suspect of trying to glimpse religious nostalgia in Freud, remarks that the dialogue seemed to come close to an agreement between them at certain moments. As if the antagonism would have almost disappeared. Reik misses a more powerful adversary like, he says, a scholastically trained Catholic priest:

> "I could, for example, conceive as a really competent opponent one of those subtle Catholic priests with whom it is a delight to debate. These are men full of life's wisdom and gifted with a remarkable intellectual sensitivity. They have been pupils of the stern logic that derives from Thomas Aquinas.
>
> At one point in Freud's debate there is no longer any basic cleavage between the two opponents. Suddenly Freud writes that their disagreement is not irreconcilable; it will vanish with time. He could never have forced such a conclusion in a dispute with a priest trained in the dogma".
>
> (Reik, 1940, p. 121)

But it is possible that Freud needed a less radical opposition to represent his own internal debate. Many wanted to see the figure of Oskar Pfister as the imaginary interlocutor in *The Future of an Illusion* (Schur, 1972, p. 399; Meissner, 1984, p. 82; Rodrigué, 1996, p. 420). A voice that would be expressing, partially, the same thought of Freud, a denied thought, the part which he fights off and at the same time causes anxiety in him. A part which he, ambivalently, brings close and sends off time and time again. Let us, then, draw near to that debate that was internal and external at the same time.

References

Boelich, W. (Ed.) (1990). *Sigmund Freud, the Letters of Sigmund Freud to Eduard Silberstein, 1871–1881*, Cambridge, MA: Harvard University Press.

Bori, P. C. (1990). Oskar Pfister, "Pfarrer in Zurich" e analista laico. *Psicoterapia e Scienze Unmane 2*: 33–57.

Brabant, E., Falzeder, E. & Giampieri-Deutsch, P. (Eds.) (1993). *The Correspondence of Sigmund Freud and Sándor Ferenczi, Volume I, 1908–1914*, Cambridge, MA: Harvard University Press.

Dalbiez, R. (1974). *L'angoisse de Luther*, Paris: Téqui.

Domínguez-Morano, C. (1991). *El psicoanálisis freudiano de la religión*, Madrid: Paulinas.

Domínguez-Morano, C. (1994). Teología y psicoanálisis, *Cristianismo y Justicia*, Barcelona, 39–50.

Ellenberger, H. F. (1970). *The Discovery of the Unconscious: The History and Evolution of Dynamic Psychiatry*, New York, NY: Basic Books.

Erikson, E. H. (1962). *Young Man Luther*, New York, NY: W.W. Norton.

Freud, S. (1910c). *Leonardo da Vinci and a Memory of his Childhood*, S.E., 11: 59–137, London: Hogarth.

Freud, S. (1910d). *The Future Prospects of Psycho-Analytic Therapy*, S.E., 11: 139–151, London: Hogarth.

Freud, S. (1913a). *Totem and Taboo*, S.E., 13: 1–162, London: Hogarth.

Freud, S. (1913b). *Introduction to Pfister's The Psychoanalytic Method*, S.E., 1 2: 327–331, London: Hogarth.

Freud, S. (1920g). *Beyond the Pleasure Principle*, S.E. 18:7–64, London: Hogarth.

Freud, S. (1921c). *Group Psychology and the Analysis of the Ego*, S.E., 18: 69–133, London: Hogarth.

Freud, S. (1925d). *An Autobiographical Study*, 20 S.E., 20: 3–70, London: Hogarth.

Freud, S. (1926e). *The Question of Lay Analysis*, S.E., 20: 183–250, London: Hogarth.

Freud, S. (1927a). *Postscript to the Question of Lay Analysis*, S.E., 20: 251–258, London: Hogarth.

Freud, S. (1927c). *The Future of an Illusion*, S.E., 21: 5–56, London: Hogarth.

Freud, S. (1931a). *Libidinal Types*, S.E., 21: 217–220, London: Hogarth.

Freud, S. (1939a). *Moses and Monotheism: Three Essays*, S.E., 23:73–80, London: Hogarth.

Fromm, E. (1942). *The Fear of Freedom*, London: Kegan Paul, Trench, Trubner.

Gay, P. (1987). *A Godless Jew, Freud, Atheism, and the Making of Psychoanalysis*, New Haven, CT: Yale University Press.

Gay, P. (1998). *Freud: A Life for Our Time*, New York, NY: W.W. Norton.

Jones, E. (1953–1957). *The Life and Work of Sigmund Freud, Volume 1–3*, New York, NY: Basic Books.

Kienast, H. W. (1974a). "The significance of Oskar Pfister's in depth pastoral care". *Journal of Religion and Health, 13 (1974)*: 83–95.

Laplanche, J. & Pontalis, J.-B. (1973). *The Language of Psycho-Analysis*, London: Karnac.

McGuire, W. (Ed.) (1974). *The Correspondence Between Sigmund Freud and C. G. Jung*, Princeton, NJ: Princeton University Press.

Meissner, W. W. (1984). *Psychoanalysis and Religious Experience*, New Haven, CT: Yale University Press.

Meng, H. & Freud, E. L. (Eds.) (1961). *Psychoanalysis and Faith: The Letters of S. Freud & O. Pfister*, London: Hogarth [reprinted New York, NY: Basic Books, 1963].

Pfister, O. (1910b). *Die Frömmigkeit des Grafen Ludwig von Zinzendorf: Ein psychoanalytischer Beitrag zur Kenntnis der religiösen Sublimierungsprozesse und zur Erklärung des Pietismus*, Leipzig/Vienna: Deutike.

Pfister, O. (1910d). "Hysterie und Mystik bei Margareta Ebner, 1291–1351". *Zentralblatt Für Psychoanalyse*, *1*: 468–485.

Pfister, O. (1910e). "Analytische Untersuchung über die Psychologie des Hasses und de Versöhnung". *Jahrbuch für psychoanalytische und psychopathologische Forschungen*, *2*: 134–178.

Pfister, O. (1912). "Anwendung der Psychoanalyse in der Pädagogik und Seelsorge". *Imago*, *1*: 56–82.

Pfister, O. (1913). *Die Psychoanalytische Methode*, Leipzig: Julius Klinkhardt.

Pfister, O. (1915). *The Psychoanalytic Method*, London: Kegan Paul, Trench, Trubner.

Pfister, O. (1917). *Was bietet die Psychoanalyse dem Erzieher?* Leipzig: Julius Klinkhardt.

Pfister, O. (1918). *Ein neuer Zugang zum alten Evangelium*, Zurich: Bertelsmann.

Pfister, O. (1920). *Der psychologische und biologische Untergrund Expressionistischer Bilder*, Bern/Leipzig: Bircher.

Pfister, O. (1921a). "Plato als Vorläufer der Psychoanalyse". *Zentralblatt Für Psychotherapie*, *7*: 264–269.

Pfister, O. (1921b). "Théodore Flournoy". *Internationale Zeitschrift für Psychoanalyse VII*, *VII*, 101–106.

Pfister, O. (1922a). *Psycho-Analysis in the Service of Education*, London: Henry Kimpton.

Pfister, O. (1922b). *Die Liebe des Kindes und Ihre Fehlentwicklungen*, Bern: Bircher.

Pfister, O. (1924). "Katholizismus and Psychanalyse". *Kirchenblatt für die reformierte Schweiz*, *39*: 15–16.

Pfister, O. (1926). *Die Legende Sundar Singhs*, Bern: Bircher.

Pfister, O. (1928a). *Religiosität und Hysterie*, Leipzig: Bircher.

Pfister, O. (1928b). *Psychoalnalyse und Weltanschauung*, Leipzig: Bircher Verlag.

Pfister, O. (1931a). "What transformation does psychoanalysis require in ethics and moral education?". *Psychiatric Quarterly*, *5*: 407–422.

Pfister, O. (1931b). *Der innerste Richter und seine seelsolgerliche Behandlun*, Leipzig (Pfeiffer) (unveröff.). Der Verlag ging Konkurs. Vgl. Nasc (1993), S.594.

Pfister, O. (1932). "Instinktive Psychoanalyse unter den Navaho-Indianern". *Imago*, *XVIII/1*: 81–109.

Pfister, O. (1934b). "Neutestamentliche Seelsorge und psychoanalytische Therapie". *Imago*, *20*: 425–443.

Pfister, O. (1934c). *Zur Psychologie des philosophischen Denkens*, Bern/Leipzig: Bircher.

Pfister, O. (1940). "Loesung und Bindung von Angst und Zwang in der israelitisch-christlichen Religionsgeschichte". *Imago*, *25*: 206–213.

Pfister, O. (1948). *Christianity and Fear: A Study in History and in the Psychology and Hygiene of Religion*, London: Allen & Unwin.

Pfister, O. (1949). "Die Rolle des Unbeswuste im philosophischen Denken". *Dialectica*, *3*: 254–271.

Pfister, O. (1950). "War and peace as a psychoanalytic problem". *International Journal of Psycho-Analysis* *31*: 150–151.

Pfister, O. (1993). "The illusion of a future: A friendly disagreement with Prof. Sigmund Freud". *The International Journal of Psychoanalysis*, *74* (*3*): 557–579.

Reik, T. (1940). *From Thirty Years with Freud*, New York, NY: Farrar & Rinehart.

Ricoeur, P. (1970/1977). *Freud: una interpretación de la cultura*, Mexico, F.C.E. [*Freud and Philosophy: An Essay on Interpretation*, New Haven, CT, Yale University Press].

Robert, M. (1966). *The Psychoanalytic Revolution: Sigmund Freud's Life and Achievement*, London: Allen & Unwin.

Rodrigué, E. (1996). *Sigmund Freud. El siglo del psicoanálisis, Volume 2*, Buenos Aires: Ed. Sudamericana.

Roudinesco, E. & Plon, M. (1997). Quoted in Pfister entry, *Dictionnaire de la Psychanalyse*, Paris: Fayard.

Saalfeld, H. (1928). *Das Christentum in der Beleuchtung der Psychoanalyse*, Gütersloh: Beterlsmann.

Schur, M. (1972). *Freud: Living and Dying*, New York, NY: International Universities Press.

Vergote, A. (1978). Dette et désir, Paris, Seuil, *Guilt and Desire. Religious Attitudes and Their Pathological Derivations* (1988), New Haven, CT: Yale University Press.

Vergote, A. (1997). *La psychanalyse à l'épreuve de la sublimation*, Paris: Cerf.

Vorgrimler, H. & Vander Gucht, R. (Eds.) (1970). Bilanz der Theologie im 20. Jahrhundert, *Bd. 4. Bahnbrechende Theologen*, Freiburg: Herder.

Widlöcher, D. (1966). Quoted by him in *Préface à l'edition française de la Correspondence avec le pasteur Pfister 1909–1939.* Heinrich Meng (Ed.). Paris: Gallimard.

Zulliger, H. (1968). *Oskar Pfister*, in: *Historia del psicoanálisis* III, 22–36, Buenos Aires: Paidós.

PART II

An Interminable Dialogue

4

THE GREAT DEBATE

The Future of an Illusion and the Illusion of a Future

The Future of an Illusion[1]

The general framing of the text

On 16th October 1927, Freud announced to pastor O. Pfister the publication of *The Future of an Illusion*: "In the next few weeks a pamphlet of mine will be appearing which has a great deal to do with you. I had been wanting to write it for a long time, and postponed it out of regard for you, but the impulse became too strong. The subject-matter – as you will easily guess – is my completely negative attitude to religion, in any form and however attenuated, and, though there can be nothing new to you on this, I feared, and still fear, that such a public profession of my attitude will be painful to you. When you have read it you must let me know what measure of tolerance and understanding you are able to preserve for the hopeless pagan" (Meng & Freud, 1961, pp. 109–110).

He was sending to print the proofs of the work he began in the spring of that same year, without any doubt one of the most questionable and controversial he had written until then. He dialectically expresses his position regarding religious beliefs, their nature, and expected social functions by resorting to dialogue with an imaginary interlocutor. He does it thinking of the religious system he best knows and whose environment he happens to be living in. He, therefore, dispenses with any attempt (so awkward always for him otherwise) to mark the stages and the evolution of those beliefs, to concentrate on "the final form taken by our present-day white Christian civilisation" (Freud, 1927c, p. 20).

As we shall see, the text's tone is markedly combative, impregnated with that atheist militancy halo that Freud exhibited on certain occasions. He also hopes to be popular and reach the public at large, not only a narrow circle of specialists.

DOI: 10.4324/9781003389804-6

E. Jones and P. Gay tell us that such a position and aggressive attitude stirred up one of Freud's most virulent controversies (Gay, 1988, pp. 523–525; Jones, 1957, vol. 3, p. 138). He foresaw it from the start, and, in the book, he confesses that he was ready to take the attacks which he was accustomed to. He tells us that the attacks do not matter much when one is close to death. He continues with evident irony: "In former times, it was different. Then utterances such as mine brought with them a sure curtailment of one's earthly existence and an effective speeding-up of the opportunity for gaining a personal experience of the after life". On the other hand, fitting the work's militant character, he concludes with a certain heroic tone: "But if one puts in any plea at all for the renunciation of wishes and for acquiescence in Fate, one must be able to tolerate this kind of injury too" (Freud, 1927c, p. 36).

Diverting from his purpose for *Totem and Taboo*, his interest when approaching *The Future of an Illusion* is not so much the problem of the faith's origin but rather what he would later call "what the common man understands by his religion" (Freud, 1930a, p. 74), the doctrines and promises system that explains the world for him and ensure him of supreme protection.

The withdrawal from the problem of the origin, and the educational intent of the project, resulted in the absence from the book of the more specifically psychoanalytic character we find in other of his works on the same theme. Freud was conscious of this. In *The future of an illusion*, he puts forth his more personal positions regarding religious belief, knowing very well that there is no reason those positions should coincide with what would strictly derive from the fundamental psychoanalytic postulates. He thus shows clearly in another letter to Pfister around the date the work was published: "Let us be quite clear on the point that the views expressed in my book form no part of analytic theory. They are my personal views, which coincide with those of many non-analysts and pre-analysts, but there are certainly many excellent analysts who do not share them. If I drew on analysis for certain arguments – in reality only one argument – that need deter no-one from using the non-partisan method of analysis for arguing the opposite view".

As we shall verify, the only properly analytic argument in the book is the one derived from the concept of illusion. No more, but we should say no less, either. However, an illusion, which, as Freud himself remarks, can appear in any sphere of life besides religion, even in those which can seem better equipped against it, including the very future of scientific reason he champions. The opportunity was thus open to Oskar Pfister for what would be his response in *The Illusion of a Future*.

A significant fact in the assessment of the Freudian analysis of religion, not often taken into account, is that *The Future of an Illusion* was not precisely the most valued by his author among his interpretations of religious phenomena. Freud's opinion on this work was never very favourable. But in this case, his low esteem did not come, as on other occasions, from the depressive condition which often invaded him after writing his great works. For instance, it had happened with

Totem and Taboo, undoubtedly the most representative and psychoanalytic of all he wrote on religion. This time Freud's judgment was negative from the beginning and kept so until the end. Already with the proofs, he sends a letter to Eitingon saying that the book has little value but would serve to bring some income to the psychoanalytic publishing firm. And on the same days, even more explicitly, he writes to Ferenczi: "Now it already seems to me childish; fundamentally I think otherwise; I regard it as weak analytically and inadequate as a self-confession" (Jones, 1957, p. 138).

His self-criticism is not limited to epistolary comments. Three years later, in *Civilization and its Discontents,* he confesses his omission in *The Future of an Illusion* of a crucial piece of information: the guilt feelings (which had played so essential a part in his interpretation of religion in *Totem and Taboo* and later on in *Moses and Monotheism: Three Essays*) (Freud, 1930a, p. 136). Equally, in the 1935 *Postscript* to *An Autobiographical Study,* he avows that in *The Future of an Illusion,* he did not give its due to religion. He forgot there (something not really true) that its power lies not in its material truth but its historical one; in other words, not in the contents of its beliefs but the historic fact supporting it: the primal horde drama described in *Totem and Taboo* (Freud, 1935a, p. 72).

But there is more on this same line. We should not forget (as E. Jones seems to do intentionally) the comments made by Freud in 1929 to René Laforgue, his friend and former analysand when the latter visited him in Schneewinkel. Laforgue had read the book "with a novice's fervour" and reports that, when they met, Freud immediately took up the subject of his last book: "He confessed that it was always a pleasure for an author to be complimented about one of his works, but he then poured cold water on my enthusiasm. 'This is my worst book!' he said, 'It isn't a book of Freud'. Can you imagine my utter surprise? How I protested! He continued talking. 'It's the book of an old man'. Well, I nearly fainted. He added, laying stress on each word. 'Besides, Freud is dead now, and believe me, the genuine Freud was really a great man: I am particularly sorry for you that you didn't know him better'. I stammered something like, 'But Herr Professor, what makes you say that?' So, he answered, '*Die Durchschlagskraft ist verloren gegangen* (The punch is lost)'" (Clark, 1980, p. 471). Laforgue later told the story to one of the most notable disciples of the master and the answer was "Freud was right. It is his worst book" (Choisy, 1979, pp. 22–24).

Indeed, even if the assertion is exaggerated (since we recognise much authentically psychoanalytic there is in the essay), most of the experts consider that the work represents, in psychoanalytic terms, a scarcely specific position towards religion and that very similar opinions and criticisms had been voiced before. The echoes of Feuerbach's thesis ("Religion the dream of waking consciousness", he said) (Feuerbach, 1890, p. 141) are evident and have been frequently exposed, by Oskar Pfister too.

In the same text, as he already did in the mentioned letter to the Swiss pastor, Freud insists that psychoanalysis is a method of investigation, an impartial instrument like the infinitesimal calculus. Strictly speaking, no pronouncement can derive from it on the truth or falsehood of religion. In fact, Freud tells us that many psychoanalysts do not share his attitude on religious problems at all (Freud, 1927c, pp. 36–37).

The question of how much specifically psychoanalytic this work contains can only be answered by just the problem of illusion, as it derives from dream analysis and, to a lesser degree, from neurosis. It is about showing the illusory structure and its functions in the cultural process, whether religious or not. In other words, as P. Ricoeur proposes, Freud has added something new and specifically psychoanalytic to the theme of illusion: deciphering the hidden relations between belief and desire. In this sense, P. Ricoeur affirms that psychoanalytic criticism of religion aims to point out the strategies of desire (Ricoeur, 1970, pp. 198–219). Let us come nearer to the text and discover Freud's analysis of the nature and the functions of illusion.

Religion as the protective illusion

To introduce the protective function of the religious illusion, Freud makes a series of general declarations on the nature of civilisation, which will fully develop in Civilization and its Discontents just three years later. In his attempt to mark off what is cultural, Freud refuses to accept the classic distinction between civilisation (as valuable dominion over the forces of nature) and culture (as unselfish, idealistic development of values). From the psychoanalytic perspective, everything is just a simple question of libidinal cathexis; that is, of the doses of energy dedicated to a representation or an object; in other words, and metapsychological terms, an economic question (these are Freudian metapsychology's terms for the relationship between the psyche and the circulation and distribution of instinctual energy). Culture, all of it, including values, implies an eminently utilitarian character. Like Ludwig Marcuse graphically expressed, culture after Freud cannot be still considered a kind of luxury but rather an imperative necessity. Culture is no longer the sacred temple for the seventh day of the week but the inescapable need for the day's 24 hours (Marcuse, 1969).

In this context, culture is for Freud everything that tells the man from the animal, entailing on one side, all the power and knowledge conquered by man in his command of nature and, on the other side, all the necessary organisation to regulate human relations. But, along with this, something essential from the psychoanalytic perspective must be added: culture relies on the repression of the drives, sometimes even to the point of imposing such a sacrifice in the instinctual renouncement that that very culture becomes something unbearable for many of the members. Hence, it can be said that there is a virtual enemy of civilisation in every individual. From this point of view, culture is forced to undertake a significant activity to keep away the continuous threat of destruction weighing on it.

Freud's position on this point is highly pessimistic. It represents one more contrast with Pfister, who, as seen in his review of *Civilization and its Discontents*, considered it unfair to evaluate civilisation just from its urgencies and conflicts, losing sight of what she offers in her successes and "magnificent achievements" (Meng & Freud, 1961, p. 131). He will return to it in response to *The Future of an Illusion*.

For Freud, however, the social institutions are primarily there to exercise coercion since the masses will never willingly renounce the permanent instinctual limitation they are forced to suffer for the sake of civilisation. Not even in the case of attaining a fair distribution of wealth. And in that Freud shows his scepticism on what any type of revolution, including the Russian one, might obtain in terms of increasing the amount of happiness of men since, from his point of view, it is essentially a psychological rather than a strictly economic matter (Freud, 1927c, p. 10).

Culture is, in other words, another name for the Super-Ego in its progressive internalisation in the subjects. That is the prohibition of an ensemble of sexual and destructive wishes; and, in parallel, the protection from the supremacy of nature. To perform that unpleasant task, Freud adds, culture needs gratifying mechanisms to alleviate the heavy burden it imposes on the backs of the subjects. The group ideals on one side, and the artistic type of satisfaction, on the other constitute those important gratification mechanisms.

Ideals contribute to the defence of culture against the hostility which opposes it, providing a narcissistic type of satisfaction. Additionally, through this satisfaction, an important social aim is achieved: the identification of the oppressed with the oppressor, which becomes thus an ideal for the community. Artistic type satisfactions, on their side, turn into substitutes for those drives that the cultural process forces the subjects to renounce. But even so, Freud concludes, the most essential psychical inventory of a civilisation is the ensemble of its religious representations (Freud, 1927c, p. 14). This is where we will identify the illusion process.

Man, despite the sacrifice he makes for the sake of civilisation, feels defenceless too frequently in front of the power of nature. Hurt this way in his narcissism and feeling gravely threatened, he demands comfort and asks for knowledge. Culture tries to provide both. For the first, it invites man to personalise nature's forces and make suffering more bearable. "We are still defenceless", Freud says, "perhaps, but we are no longer helplessly paralysed; we can at least react. Perhaps, indeed, we are not even defenceless. We can apply the same methods against these violent supermen outside that we employ in our own society; we can try to adjure them, to appease them, to bribe them, and, by so influencing them, we may rob them of a part of their power" (Freud, 1927c, p. 17).

But if Freud is in this way referring – without making it explicit as in *Totem and Taboo* – to the animist position in front of the world and magic as the corresponding technical means, he goes immediately on signalling religion as the best-suited way to dominate the threatening situation. The parental figures offer the link for that decisive step from the animist attitude to the religious one.

During our childhood, we have all gone through a period of defencelessness concerning our parents – mainly our father, Freud insists –; but, at the same time, we felt sure of their protection. Desire comes in, like in dreams, to assimilate both situations and recompose things at its measure. So, by the force of desire and with this type of strategy, religion is borne: man not only personifies the forces of nature but also "gives them the character of a father. He turns them into gods, following in this (...) not only an infantile prototype but a phylogenetic one" (Freud, 1927c, p. 17). These gods, whose creation is now represented by Freud preferentially under the oneiric model rather than the neurotic one, play a triple function in its help against helplessness (*Hilflosigkeit*): scare away the terrors of nature, reconcile man with fate's cruelty (especially death) and compensate him for the pains and privations that community's civilised life imposes. *Ananké* (nature and destiny) and society are the two cardinal directions taken by the protection the religious representations intend to offer.

But Freud (who seems unable to avoid the evolutionary approach he shall assume in *Totem and Taboo*) says a progressive displacement occurs in the accent of these functions. As nature becomes better known, the gods are growingly apart from it. On the other hand, life is making more apparent that defencelessness and abandonment do not have many remedies... And so, we reach a situation in which morals become the fundamental element entrusted to the gods. The precepts which constantly force the instinctual renouncement for the sake of culture are more and more based on the will of the gods, who, in their turn, will find a way to compensate without limits that renouncement.

So far, Freud has kept at the level of animism, first, and then of religion, taking all gods in general. The next step, almost unavoidable, is the presentation of the monotheist God. The attributes of supreme wisdom, goodness, and justice concentrate in the figure of the single God, built up from the father's image. From His supreme intelligence, He guides everything towards the good in ways hardly perceptible to human eyes; He also watches benevolently over humanity to protect it from the danger of becoming a toy of natural forces. Death itself does not mean annihilation but only the crossing to a definitive existence. Lastly, this God the Father becomes at the same time an instance of justice that rewards all the good and punishes all the bad, if not in this life, in the future one. Without explicitly mentioning Judaism, Freud tells us: "The people who first succeeded in thus concentrating the divine attributes was not a little proud of the advance. It had laid open to view the father who had all along been hidden behind every divine figure as its nucleus" (Freud, 1927c, p. 19).

These are the most relevant religious representations. They pass for the most precious treasure of civilisation. They even become more appreciated than science and technology, which feed men and cure their illnesses. Even more, many don't believe they can stand life if they do not confer to these religious representations the full worth they themselves claim to have. Therefore, we should analyse where they get their force from and what their value is.

At this moment, Freud brings to the scene an imaginary interlocutor who, before him, like Pfister, plays the role of religion's defender. Through this rhetorical artifice, Freud easily argues on themes such as the alleged revelation of religious contents that his partner brings in. Of higher interest is the issue of the possible link between *Totem and Taboo* and the work we analyse now. The imaginary interlocutor also poses this question.

After reasserting the *Totem and Taboo* theses, Freud explains he wants to position himself at a different level, in which the elements play in a less unconscious mode. Still, their connection with the more hidden factors shown there is easily proven. There is a connection between deep and manifest motivation, between the paternal complex (*Totem and Taboo*'s central core) and the impotence and need for protection of man: "These connections are not hard to find. They consist in the relation of the child's helplessness to the helplessness of the adult which continues it. So that, as was to be expected, the motives for the formation of religion which psychoanalysis revealed now turn out to be the same as the infantile contribution to the manifest motives" (Freud, 1927c, p. 23).

The first object of love is the mother. Following narcissistic interests, the libido sticks to the objects that ensure satisfaction. The "mother, who satisfies the child's hunger, becomes its first love-object and certainly also its first protection against all the undefined dangers which threaten it in the external world – its first protection against anxiety" (*Angstschutz*) (Freud, 1927c, p. 24).

So, the mother appears as the first model from the protection perspective adopted in *The Future of an Illusion*. She is, we have been told, the first *Angstschutz*. However, in Freud's eyes, this first protection model does not seem to have much value when he thinks of protective religious representations. He goes on immediately to the father's register (the father soon replaces the mother, he tells us), who becomes the quintessential protector and therefore the only model to build up the illusory image of the provident and protector God. Like many times in Freudian texts, the mother is also pushed into the background in the order of illusion.

In the fatherly ground, as was to be expected, the affective ambivalence will be the key to explaining the whole process that generates religiousness. The protection against the feeling of impotence, analysed precisely at that moment, has the virtuality of reviving the regression that leads to the father. The protective instance adopts the traits of the father figure. So, Freud concludes, "Thus his longing for a father is a motive identical with his need for protection against the consequences of his human weakness. The defence against childish helplessness is what lends its characteristic features to the adult's reaction to the helplessness he has to acknowledge – a reaction that is precisely the formation of religion" (Freud, 1927c, p. 24).

From now on, Freud gets into the actual analysis of the illusion, a term he used from the beginning to designate religious representations. He begins with a critique of the religious concept of belief, along with those made during the

Enlightenment. All this takes away from the text the touch of geniality that generally is present in his writings.

Religious ideas are defined as "teachings and assertions about facts and conditions of external (or internal) reality which tell one something one has not discovered for oneself and which lay claim to one's belief" (Freud, 1927c, p. 25). Their most relevant characteristic is their total lack of supporting ground. The ensemble of these reflections reveals the utmost positivist scientism. The lack of verifiability is essential in the critical analysis of the alleged justifications of belief. Neither tradition nor the proofs transmitted by the classics are sufficient warranties to support religious beliefs. The interdiction to question their foundations is of course unacceptable and has caused many conflicts and psychic trauma in the course of history. Doubts on faith have been thus choked but at a high price. In sum, religious beliefs have been removed from rational judgment and are understood just through the lens of desire: "we turn our attention to the psychical origin of religious ideas. These, which are given out as teachings, are not precipitates of experience or end-results of thinking: they are illusions, fulfilments of the oldest, strongest and most urgent wishes of mankind. The secret of their strength lies in the strength of those wishes" (Freud, 1927c, p. 30).

Desire is, therefore, the engine of illusion. A desire which prefers to ignore reality. Because, as Freud takes care to highlight, an illusion is not formed against reality but rather outside reality. "An illusion is not the same thing as an error; nor is it necessarily an error", he tells us (Freud, 1927c, pp. 30–31). Its essential characteristic is to have desire as the only starting point. Thus, its closest clinical analogue would be the psychiatric delusions, even though they differ precisely because the psychiatric delusion is in open contradiction with reality. By contrast, Freud insists, "illusions need not necessarily be false – that is to say, unrealizable or in contradiction to reality. For instance, a middle-class girl may have the illusion that a prince will come and marry her. This is possible; and a few such cases have occurred".

Here the problem arises to determine when we face an illusion and when an authentic delirium also born from desire but openly against reality. That the Messiah will come and set up a golden age seems to Freud closer to delusion than to illusion. Now, the measure by which human expectations come close to or move away from reality is difficult to determine. Conscious of that, Freud confesses that, in the end, it will depend on "our personal attitude" to judge a belief as an illusion or a delusion.

For instance, all religious dogmata are unprovable illusions. Still, some are so implausible and so opposed to everything that so laboriously we have discovered in the world's reality that, in essence, we can compare them with delusions. Ultimately, an equation could be established in which the more human desire intervenes, and the less known reality is respected, the higher the risk of leaving illusion towards delusion. In any case, either in the case of illusion or in that of delusion, the price is insincerity and impurity of intelligence. Freud tells us,

"Where questions of religion are concerned, people are guilty of every possible sort of dishonesty and intellectual misdemeanour" (Freud, 1927c, p. 32).

However, it is remarkable that Freud would prefer religion's insincerity to the philosophers when they try to make God justifiable. That God of the philosophers hardly deserves the name; it is a vague abstraction deprived of the dreadful but fascinating greatness of the God of the religions. "That comes from the most varied drinks being offered under the name of 'religion' – he comments on a letter to Marie Bonaparte – with a minimal percentage of alcohol – really nonalcoholic; but they still get drunk on it. The old drinkers were a respectable body, but getting tipsy on pomerit (apple juice) is ridiculous" (Jones, 1957, vol. 3, p. 447). In *Civilization and its Discontents* (Freud, 1930a) and in *Moses and Monotheism: Three Essays* (Freud, 1939a), he expresses the same opinion on the God of the philosophers again.

However, illusion goes across any human activity. Religion has by no means exclusivity. So, Freud asks himself whether the same illusion structure also impregnates political institutions and whether sexuality is not also a significant source of illusion interfering in the erotic relations between the sexes. So, since he is on the road to suspicion, he does not want to evade interrogating how much illusion hides in the very foundations of scientific thought, which he is embracing so rigidly on this issue. Pfister will pick up the question.

Now, if illusion feeds on desire, it does not seem logical that Freud, who always emphasised the primacy of drive over thought, and the great difficulties which follow the rejection of the desires expressing the drive, appears now as the defender of reality and reason. The question is set by Freud in the voice of the imaginary interlocutor, turning him so in a bad connoisseur of his doctrine. These data certainly raise doubts about Freud having thought of Oskar Pfister when conceiving his interlocutor.

In the face of the opposition between drive and culture, Freud avoids a pronouncement. The issue seems superfluous to him since culture is there as a fact, independent of our desire and our will. It is unavoidable. However, there are more or less adequate ways for cultural adaptation. Of course, the religious illusion is not one of the best ways for him. It calls for control of the drives and the desires, but by the more dangerous road: that of repression, regression, and deception, as opposed to the possibility of a more rational, lucid, and adult control that needed to adapt to reality and, from that reality, have access to all possible enjoyment.

Religion has lent excellent services to the human community. Freud acknowledges that. Nevertheless, it has failed to make people happier or even more ethical. Through its priests, religion has carried out a kind of "traffic" with commandments and sins, using penitence and other redemption modes that have facilitated rather than prevented a situation of appreciable immorality. "In every age immorality has found no less support in religion than morality has" (Freud, 1927c, p. 38).

Hence, looking for a non-religious foundation for the necessary regulation of civilisation will be much preferable. More than any other instance, science offers itself to Freud to fulfil the vital function of healthy and rational control of the instinctual world. That will mean, in parallel, the ousting of the whole religious belief system, an essential and indeed not easy task since the expectations of a vast majority of persons are put in the trust of that system. However, it is worth trying; Freud is sure.

In sum, it is a stand for a secularised society in which the aura of the sacred does not spread like an infection from the most solemn spheres to the most marginal and miserly elements. A society without institutions, laws and regulations is not dressed up with a sanctity halo, which is quite bizarre for some of them: "It would be an undoubted advantage if we were to leave God out altogether and honestly admit the purely human origin of all the regulations and precepts of civilisation. These commandments and laws would also lose their rigidity and unchangeableness along with their pretended sanctity. People could understand that they were made not so much to rule them as, on the contrary, to serve their interests. They would adopt a more friendly attitude toward them. Instead of aiming at their abolition, they would aim only at their improvement: This would be an important advance along the road, leading to becoming reconciled to the burden of civilisation" (Freud, 1927c, p. 41).

Reconciliation between the individual and culture would be thus achieved and, in parallel, a higher grade of adulthood and emotional maturity with the renouncement to found morality on the will of an imaginary father, a king of primal proto-father, since, in the end, it is that will that lends the sacred character claimed for the commandments.

The religious illusion, a theme to which Pfister will not pay excessive attention, is deeply linked to the oedipal question, as explained in *Totem and Taboo*. Its great strength comes from that. The belief of the present is tied with a long-time past content, hidden but acting from the unconscious. This gives religion "a truly incomparable wealth of power" (Freud, 1927c, p. 42), against which reasons hardly serve. Hence, the question of what future waits for that illusion.

Without a doubt, no other text from Freud reveals a more optimistic attitude about the future of civilisation. Later on (Freud, 1928b, 1933a), we will find relevant precisions that tempered the significant optimism he now shows. As Max Schur remarks, the years after *The Future of an Illusion* "they taxed to the utmost his belief in the future victory of Logos and Reason" (Schur, 1972, p. 405). Also, from the perspective of this manifest optimism, we can affirm that the book is not too Freudian. But let us see the propositions Freud offers at this time.

Neurosis is unavoidable during specific periods of the child's development when the need to cut off the instinctual demands overflows the Ego's capacity. However, this type of childhood neurosis vanishes with growth. It is possible to think of a similar path at the collective level. The human community has also gone through a period of childhood neurosis, which is religion. Like in the child, its origin is found in the oedipal situation. According to this theory, abandonment of religion will come with the inevitable necessity of a growth process. Even more, Freud thinks we are now inside that stage of evolution.

On the other hand, the interest to undertake actions to make us wake up from the dream of the religious illusion is still higher since it contains not only neurotic elements (especially of the obsessive kind) but sometimes traits close (saving distances) to psychosis; as he tells us: "a system of wishful illusions together with a disavowal of reality, such as we find in an isolated form nowhere else but in amentia, in a state of blissful hallucinatory confusion" (Freud, 1927c, p. 43). Furthermore, we should not forget that if believers, thanks to religion, have been saved from an individual neurosis, it has happened at the expense of their adaptation to a general neurosis.

Everything points then to the convenience of retiring the religious support present in cultural precepts. Only so, replacing repression with a healthy rational control of the instincts to adjust to reality the development and maturity of civilisation will occur. Freud devotes the book's last pages to presenting what could be called an education project for reality.

A genuine apology of reason appears in these last pages. Intelligence is the only means we have to control the instinctual world rightly. Everything contributing to subjugate drives should be considered harmful and should be dismissed. Hence, while religious coercion is present, we will ignore what intelligence can deliver. The proposal is then neat: to get rid of religious education to verify the invigorating effect it brings. If this fails, we will have to recognise that man is a being with weak intelligence, dominated by his instinctual desires.

When, on occasion, interchanging ideas on *The Future of an Illusion*, Lou Andreas-Salomé indicated that perhaps religion should be considered as the expression (epistemologically mistaken) of basic and innate confidence in life, Freud, in his rationalist ardour, replied that he did not run after any illusion, but – in his words – "why should one cling precisely to the one which makes such mock of reason?" (Pfeiffer, 1972, p. 172).

Freud advocates thus an education to reality, an education that, no doubt, would entail a hard ascesis in so far as it leads the individual inevitably to abandon the paternal house, where he feels warm and comfortable. "But – he tells us – surely infantilism is destined to be surmounted: Men cannot remain children for ever; they must in the end go out into 'hostile life'. We may call this '*education to reality*'. Need I confess to you that the sole purpose of my book is to point out the necessity for this forward step?" (Freud, 1927c, p. 49).

We shall have to follow the poet's saying and "leave Heaven to the angels and the sparrows" (Freud, 1927c, p. 50, Heine's quote). Modestly and patiently, hope will be placed on the achievements science will develop. Meanwhile, we should learn to accept without rebellion the inexorable fate. This proposal is, otherwise – unlike the religious one – amendable and modifiable in the part of illusion possibly impregnating it.

A song to the god "Logos" closes the work: his voice is still weak and muted but will not stop until heard. He also aspires to love, to eliminate suffering and to the truth, although in a more realistic, modest and patient way. In sum, only in him do we have a solid ground for hope: "No, our science is not illusion: But an illusion it would be to suppose that what science cannot give us we can get elsewhere" (Freud, 1927c, p. 56). These are the final words of the book.

The illusion of a future

First reactions

The theses maintained by Freud in *The Future of an Illusion* were, of course, no surprise for Oskar Pfister. He knew well that they followed decidedly diverse, if not opposite, paths in religion, philosophy and music. But his open and tolerant position was patent even before the work's publication. When Freud announced to him the public appearance of the opuscule, Pfister advanced his willingness to receive it: he awaited it with "eager curiosity". And he also said: "A powerful-minded opponent of religion is certainly of more service to it than a thousand useless supporters" (Meng & Freud, 1961, p. 110). From his deepest pedagogic convictions, he had always defended the freedom of each person to express their sincere opinion freely. "You have always been tolerant towards me, and am I to be intolerant of your atheism?" he said. But from the same conviction on the need to respect freedom of expression for others, he intended to express his own opinion with the same freedom: "If I frankly air my differences from you, you will surely not take it amiss" (Meng & Freud, 1961, p. 110)

Neither Freud was surprised by Pfister's tolerant and receptive attitude at what he called his "declaration of war" (Meng & Freud, 1961, p. 112) and welcomed the idea of having a public and divergent response from the pastor. After all, he knew very well that what he could get from his friend would be incomparably more benevolent than what he could receive from others. However, after having received and read *The Future of an Illusion*, a more combative attitude can be detected in Pfister. The tone hardens patently. All, naturally, after leaving clear that it will not change his relations with Freud nor with psychoanalysis: "You have the right to expect complete frankness from me, and you know that neither my attitude to you nor my pleasure in psychoanalysis is in the slightest degree diminished by your rejection of religion" (Meng & Freud, 1961, p. 114). He knows that the psychoanalysis he enthusiastically embraced from the beginning is just one part of science and by no means an idea of life and the world. Psychoanalysis offers just what it can offer.

On the other hand, Pfister realises the difficulty in establishing a dialogue with Freud. The philosophic, moral, and aesthetic positions divide them in a probably insurmountable way: "I cannot have things out with you properly on the subject of religion because you completely reject philosophy, approach art in a way that differs from mine, and regard morality as something self-evident" (Meng & Freud, 1961, p. 114). In any case, he will not shy away from giving a public response. Pfister thinks this should appear in *Imago*, the academic journal dedicated to applying psychoanalysis to the sciences of nature and spirit. He believes this action could prevent the public from identifying Freud's personal position with psychoanalysis itself with consequential damage to the psychoanalytic movement.

But in the same long letter in November 1927, he starts an openly critical review, advancing ideas of his future response in *The Illusion of a Future*. The undeniable aggressive load it implies leads him to make sure of Freud's readiness to receive it, writing: "Have you as much tolerance for this frank confession of faith as I have for your long-familiar heresies?" (Meng & Freud, 1961, p. 116). And, as if revealing a reparatory inclination after the aggression, Pfister finishes the letter by saying that he writes with Freud's picture in front of him as if listening with attention and friendliness. There remains a residue of doubt and fear about what could happen in their relationship, which makes him unsure: "I hope that speaking out like this has only strengthened our friendship. It has, has it not?".

Freud is also tempted to join the discussion wielding aggression-filled arguments, preferring to leave it aside for the time being and stick to practical matters. He sees no difficulty in letting Pfister, if he so wishes, publish his work in *Imago*, leaving the record of "our undisturbed friendship and your unshaken loyalty to psychoanalysis". Another issue he clarifies is the difference between his more personal positions on ethics or religion and what would intrinsically derive from psychoanalysis as a scientific discipline. "Let us be quite clear on the point that the views expressed in my book form no part of analytic theory. They are my personal views, which coincide with those of many non-analysts and pre-analysts, but there are certainly many excellent analysts who do not share them. If I drew on analysis for certain arguments – in reality only one argument –, that need deter no-one from using the non-partisan method of analysis for arguing the opposite view" (Meng & Freud, 1961, p. 117).

The clarification given by such assertions becomes, no doubt, an incentive to value still more the friendship between these two men and what their full dialogue on religion and psychoanalysis meant. Thanks to this relationship and the ensuing debate, we dispose, from psychoanalysis' founder, of these elucidation principles, which, for those who wish to notice them, contribute to shedding light on relevant questions along with the debate which took place afterwards and, with other references, continues now.

Three months later, phlebitis kept Pfister in bed for three weeks, allowing him to move forward in *The Illusion of a Future* draft. Freud comments that the Imago journal eagerly awaited the text, adding: "Men's real allegiance is shown in difficult times" (Meng & Freud, 1961, p. 119). Pfister writes with satisfaction because, as he tells Freud, he battles "for a cause that is dear to me with an opponent who is the same. There is not much danger of your turning up for baptism or of my descending from the pulpit". While he writes, he also seems to become conscious that the abyss between them is not so deep: "when I reflect that you are much better and deeper than your disbelief, and that I am much worse and more superficial than my faith, I conclude that the abyss between us cannot yawn so grimly". The suspicion that he is in this way trying to soothe the guilt that his rejoinder causes is revealed at once when he writes: "I very much hope that you will not take amiss what I have to say; I even hope that in spite of my friendly attack on you you will derive a tiny little bit of pleasure from it". Since in his text, he will directly address Freud (something absent in The Future of an Illusion about him), Pfister sends the manuscript to him, asking him if there is anything unfair or inappropriate in it. In the same letter, he refers to what, in his view, is the main difference between the appreciation each one of them has for religion: "Our difference derives chiefly from the fact that you grew up in proximity to pathological forms of religion and regard these as 'religion', while I had the good fortune of being able to turn to a free form of religion which to you seems to be an emptying of Christianity of its content, while I regard it as the core and substance of evangelism..." (Meng & Freud, 1961, pp. 121–122).

Freud did not show any annoyance or discomfort with Pfister's reply. On 24 February 1928, he writes: "(*The illusion of a future*) has already gone to the editorial office. It was very necessary that my *Illusion* should be answered from within our own circle, and it is very satisfactory that it should be done in such a worthy and friendly fashion" (Meng & Freud, 1961, p. 122). We will never know well the motive for Freud seeing as "very necessary" that the challenge to his book would come from within the psychoanalytic movement. It is possible to think of the reason that Pfister had put forward to him: publication in a journal of the Association prevented the identification of psychoanalysis itself with an anti-religious or atheist position. It is also possible to wonder if Freud, in a more or less unconscious manner, found thus a way to counter himself. After all, his identification with the text of *The Future of an Illusion* was not too high, as we saw. Furthermore, Pfister, who was writing now, probably represented Freud's other side, his own imaginary interlocutor, now entirely free to take a stance.

Science and illusion

Pfister's text appeared in booklet 2–3, 1928 of the journal *Imago* (Pfister, 1993 [*1928*]), preceded by a letter addressed to Freud (*Dear Professor!*), full of admiration, praise and gratitude, very much in his style. Interestingly, he presents his work as his answer to a desire of Freud himself, as if the latter would have invited him to publicly express his opposition and criticism of *The Future of an Illusion*. We know, however, that the first idea to reply came from Pfister himself (Meng & Freud, 1961, p. 116).

Immediately comes up, in the same introductory letter, the essential point of view of the author in his consideration of the psychoanalysis-religion relations: even if Freud would smile at it, psychoanalysis is for Pfister a powerful instrument for faith purification, which can wonderfully contribute to its development and maturity. Even more, Pfister is convinced Freud himself battles against religion from a religious basis since he does it in an honest attempt to fight for Truth and the liberation of Love; and whoever does that, want it or not, is a true servant of God according to the Gospel's precept. He who works to relieve human suffering is not far from the Kingdom of God. So, Pfister's permanent commitment to dilute the emergent conflict between psychoanalysis and faith, using visible violence to make purposes meet, manifests itself in this occasion with resounding clarity. With his best intention, Pfister places Freud by God's throne without thinking whether that was where the psychoanalysis founder wished to be.

With this, Pfister ends his open letter by expressing his hope that psychoanalysis abandons the disaffection towards religious belief and reconciles with it as far as method and empirical knowledge are concerned.

The first part of the essay centres on '*Freud's Criticism of Religion*'. It goes over all the drawbacks Freud observes in religious belief, starting with the concept of 'illusion'. Pfister's point of view, always from a psychoanalytic perspective, notably differs from Freud's, and it is striking that he came significantly close to future psychoanalytic approaches to the issue. That had to wait for the psychoanalytic theory to dissociate itself from the epistemological assumptions common in the Age of Enlightenment, to which Freud was so closely attached. As we shall later underline, the resonance of Pfister's proposals is remarkable with those derived from Winnicott's theory and his concept of 'transitional object', which ascribes positive value to illusion in the never-ending task of keeping the interrelation between internal and external realities (Winnicott, 1971, 1986, 1988). For Pfister, illusion can coexist with excellent thoughts well-grounded in reality. The very example that Freud presented to illustrate illusion, the discovery of the Indies by Christopher Columbus, excellently reveals such coexistence. Columbus's illusion was compatible with his precise geographical knowledge and intimately woven with a project that opened a new future. Desire and realistic thought – Pfister insists – can live together and are forced to do so in many dimensions of life, including science itself.

Religion as a neurotic compulsion is the second aspect Pfister addresses in his reply to Freud. He does not question that the religious experience has often appeared intimately linked with obsessive neurosis. However, from Pfister's point of view, that did happen only in the first stages of religious development and at times when, regressively, religious orthodoxy became too intensely present in the life of individuals or communities. But that does not correspond with the essence of religion, according to the Swiss pastor. Like Freud, with a very evolutionary mindset, Pfister thinks that religion, from its very dynamics, goes forward, progressively shedding its less maturative elements. In an evolved religiousness, obsessive compulsivity is manifestly outgrown by the dynamics of love, which overcomes those of law and guilt. Thus, Pfister affirms, Jesus leads over the collective neurosis of his people with his new religious approach based on freedom and love. The fatherly representation is freed from any oedipal fixation through a proposal above any heteronomy. It requires the person to be faithful to his own essence and true determination in a spirit of liberty. That prevents looking with a Mosaic Law spirit (misunderstood so frequently) at Jesus' maxim to love your neighbour as yourself.

All the above comes together, Pfister thinks, in transcending the representation of God determined by oedipal fixations, which, because of the power of emotional ambivalence, would fatally have to end in the father's or the son's denial. "God shouldn't be appeased with sacrifices, but instead be loved as one's brother" (Pfister, 1993 [*1928*], p. 562). This way, Pfister deals with one of the essential aspects denounced by Freud in his analysis of religion without otherwise lingering on them further than this assertion. Neither mention is made of either of the problems that Freud signs about sacrifice in Totem and Taboo as the expression of the eternal ambivalence towards the father, briefly taken up in *The Future of an Illusion.* Pfister makes do by insisting Freud has ignored the more thorough religious expressions because the pre-religious stages create the neurotic obsessions, leading to rites and manifestations with that character. Religious development, particularly the Judeo-Christian one, progressively drives through a process of humanisation in an all-out fight against primal obsessive representations.

Pfister does not forget that the history of Christendom also contains situations of such brutality that they would question the humanisation process he defends. However, in his view, those would be only moments of regression that taint the essence and the natural dynamics of authentic Christian spirituality.

Pfister gives the third section in this first part to the problems of religion as a "wishful construct". He says: "It (is) completely impossible to deny the presence of wishes in the development of religion". And a bit later on:" That ideas of God and the beyond are often painted with colours from a wish-palette is something I have always known" (Pfister, 1993 [*1928*], p. 563). But that is not enough to account for what religion is. "But can all of religious thinking be explained this way? And is this mistaken exchange of wishes and essence a property peculiar to religion? Or shouldn't in religion and science, and even finally in art and morality, the repression of wishful thinking through real thinking and the mobilisation of real thinking through wishful thinking create the ideal toward which intellectual development strives – panting, hoping, and painfully disappointed again and again?" (Pfister, 1993 [*1928*], p. 563).

Pfister has no qualms about referring now, as he will do again at other times, to his own reality as a believer. Remembering the day he first met Freud, he confesses he was ready to abandon his mission as a pastor if the truth required it. Because "One doesn't risk one's soul for an illusion", he solemnly affirms (Pfister, 1993 [*1928*], p. 563).

Whether he was thinking of the *Schreber Case* (Freud, 1911c), analysed by Freud years before, or just of his own *The Psychoanalytic Method* (Pfister, 1915), Pfister reminds the reader how psychoanalysis has unequivocally shown there are ways in which the father's image, vested with a feeling of love but also of hate, is hallucinatorily projected into the relationship with God. But the desire of the creative person is also reflected in his work. And we should ignore even less that the arguments used by God's detractors are also very frequently taken from their own desires, with their atheism being often a disguised mode of father's assassination. We neither know if Pfister had in his mind a short but relevant work (generally not much held in consideration) that Freud had just published in the previous issue of the journal *Imago*. The text, *A Religious Experience*, tells us about a case in which the denial of God is unconsciously motivated by the wish for the father's death. However, that negation of God generates such intense guilt that it sets in motion psychotic mechanisms that try the restoration of that father, unconsciously murdered (Freud, 1928a).

Desire, thus, is present in any human creation, imaginary or not. Also, in the science that Freud tends to place on the outside of the world of desires, assigning it a role as an incorruptible judge of them. Desires initially are egotistical and self-interested, but after a healthy maturation, they learn to shed their egocentric character. The same happens in the Judeo-Christian religious evolution even to the point that, for Pfister, "What Jesus commanded in the name of his religion is, to a great extent, directly opposed to egoism" (Pfister, 1993 [*1928*], p. 564). In the image he presents of his supreme ideal, the Kingdom of God, the religious and moral values do not appear as a disguised and regressive replacement of sexual and selfish unsatisfied desires, as can be seen, for instance, in the Islamic paradise, reward of the earthly renouncement to instincts. Even less, as in hallucination, where desire emerges beside and against reality. However, nobody will ever dare to ban and damn desire as illegitimate by nature.

"One can aim at the gratification of wishes in a way very much in keeping with reality" (Pfister, 1993 [*1928*], p. 564). And that possibility to wisely articulate desire and reality is a sign of personal maturity. That is what Pfister finds in the figure of Jesus when he articulates the representations expressing a spiritual intimacy (the beatitudes and love) with the commandments of Moses (*Matthew 5:17–22*). Therefore, a desire that structures and organises itself to accommodate the demands and requirements of reality.

If Jesus breaks the image of the Old Testament's severe and jealous God to avoid obsessive religiousness and instead presents the God of love, it will not be to find an excuse for wish fulfilment. Christian dogma – Pfister finds in an interesting consideration – cannot be understood as the fulfilment of desires made real but as acknowledging a series of realities that call for recognition. Everything draws from a properly human feature, a calling for love of the fellow man, concluding on the existence of an absolute, original source of being, duty, and values. Christian dogma, in the end, is nothing else than the dogma of love.

On another side, the problem lies in knowing whether the symbolic imagination (*die sinnbildliche Phantasie*) is not at the heart of science itself as the engine of its own development. Its fundamental concepts (cause, action, force, law…), in effect, are filled with a necessary anthropomorphism. Then, why is it – asks

Pfister – that theology would be an exception to this rule? More so when this theology has exemplarily undergone "sacrifices that were of the most uncompromising and most painful sort in regard to wishing" (Pfister, 1993 [*1928*], p. 566). It has digested, not without difficulty, Copernicus, Galileo, and Darwin. And if it maintains a series of contradictions, it may be questioned if science does not, as can be questioned why that science has to be considered the essential guide and primary judge of life. (The contradictions of religious thought, Pfister tells Freud in their correspondence, have been a well-known theme for many years. The defenders of religion have not hidden it and have courageously confronted them, trying to find a solution in a higher philosophical and theological analysis. As an example, he quotes R. Eucken (Eucken, 1912). And on this occasion, once again, Pfister has no qualms about honestly referring to his own reality as a believer: "I believe that I have attained a piety that has mastered the contradictions, even if, as in any other area of human thought, unsolved riddles have remained at every step" (Pfister, 1993 [*1928*], p. 566).

One of Freud's main reproaches to religion is that it performs like an enemy of thought. Pfister devotes the next section in his reply to this issue. The Swiss pastor does not see motives specifically in protestant theology to fit in that type of Freudian judgement. After Luther, Zwingli, and Calvin, the new evangelical theology demanded critical and free thought and an adult religious attitude (*Religion der Erwachsenen*). Many thinkers found no incompatibility between their faith and their scientific work. Pfister shows this with a long list of physicians, mathematicians, chemists, physicists, historians, philosophers, and poets who knew how to combine their thoughts and beliefs. Like Einstein, Becher, or Driesch, many even reached the great religious questions through their intellectual work. However, Pfister recognises that faith will only find its support in personal experience, not in the authority of such figures. That experience has to give testimony to the compatibility of faith and free thought. Again, Pfister did not hesitate to offer his witness: "I myself remember how my own thinking was richly enhanced by religion" (Pfister, 1993 [*1928*], p. 568).

The pastor-analyst argues that no higher intellectual wealth can be found in those persons who have grown and developed outside of any religious belief. The praised education for reality, removed from any religious approach, has not either obtained better results in experiences such as those undertaken by communist sectors of society. Nor clinical experience, at least his own, shows that subjects educated apart from religious belief present richer or more creative thought. Pfister finds that history concludes otherwise.

Religion as civilisation's custodian is the theme of the last section in the first part of the text. It does not seem that Pfister is ready to assign religion the police function that Freud tries to attribute to it in his analysis of civilisation, nor to think of it as the muzzle of instincts or the comforting resource for the many renouncements required by civilisation to hold itself up. Religion has a better task to do. Against injustice, cruelty, savagery, and the nonsense so often present in social life, against oppression and exploitation, the Christian task is to devote oneself to the transformation of human beings and try to make them sensitive to the fact that civilisation is threatened. Therefore, religion is not the conservative guardian but rather the guide that directs towards another type of civilisation through a faith that inspires love. From this Pfister's perspective, religion is called to be the founding element of a critical view of culture, becoming a critical principle of the existing social conditions. A function of ideal, not of coercion or cultural control. Neither heaven is the substitute for earthly frustrations, nor is the Kingdom of God something for the afterlife. That Kingdom, as the Lord's Prayer teaches, should come to us to make possible another kind of human relations.

Pfister gives the title of *Freud's Scientism* to the second part of the work and begins with the critical analysis of Freud's belief in science as a saviour of humanity. By proposing to replace the religious illusion with another type of illusion, Freud offers a new messianism. The deified Logos dethrones the God of religion and governs the kingdom of necessity with power. "Your substitute for religion – Pfister writes to Freud – is basically the idea of the eighteenth-century Enlightenment in proud modern guise" (Meng & Freud, 1961, p. 115).

After comparing Freud's analogies and differences with other thinkers (Comte, Stuart Mill, D. F. Strauss or the baron d'Holbach), Pfister thoroughly criticises their scientific optimism in its positivist frame. It is an illusion to think there is pure science far from any metaphysics like it is to believe in a "pure experience". Our mental categories are always present, impregnating any experience. As he said in a letter collecting these ideas: "'Pure' experience is in my view a fiction in any event, and if we look at the story of the sciences we see how doubtful is the reality hidden behind our so-called experience" (Meng & Freud, 1961, p. 114).

Furthermore, it is highly uncertain for Pfister that science would bring a higher degree of happiness to human beings. Many think it brings unhappiness, and Pfister quotes E. von Hartmann (Hartmann, 1884; Pfister, 1993 [*1928*], p. 573), the German philosopher who identifies logical thought and illogical will in an unconscious spirit that animates the world. "I must confess that, with all my pleasure in the advance of science and technique, I do not believe in the adequacy and sufficiency of that solution of the problem of life. It is very doubtful whether, taking everything into account, scientific progress has made men happier or better" (Meng & Freud, 1961, p. 115). At least it does not contribute to more social justice for the workers, artisans or peasants in as much as science places itself at the service of money and its causes, and serves, when deemed necessary, any passion or cruelty.

It would be then a matter of guesswork to know the wishes concealed behind Freud's belief in the final victory of the intellect. If what he predicts about the end of the illusion is not the beginning of another one, the scientific illusion. Since what Freud shows in defending there is nothing better than science is also a belief. When, in the final words of *The Future of an Illusion*, Freud affirms: "No, our science is no illusion. But an illusion it would be to suppose that what science cannot give us we can get elsewhere" (Freud, 1927c, p. 56), those precise words are, according to Pfister, the very confession of a belief. The whole text of *The Future of an Illusion* reveals an underlying conception of science as a possible substitute for what religion offers the faithful. Pfister confesses he cannot follow Freud in that fascination with scientific reason since he is convinced that man is not just a thinking machine.

"I do not properly understand your outlook on life" – he writes to Freud after reading *The Future of an Illusion* –. "It is impossible that what you reject as the end of an illusion and value as the sole truth can be all. A world without temples, the fine arts, poetry, religion, would in my view be a devil's island to which men could have been banished, not by blind chance, but only by Satan. In that case your pessimism about the wickedness of mankind would be much too mild; you would have to follow it through to its logical conclusion. If it were part of psycho-analytic treatment to present that despoiled universe to our patients as the truth, I should well understand it if the poor devils preferred remaining shut up in their illness to entering that dreadful icy desolation" (Meng & Freud, 1961, pp. 115–116).

Significantly, Pfister seems unable to forgive Freud for a vision of life in which art does not seem to have any relevant place. In another work, he criticised Freud's narrow scientism and tried to find space for art, philosophy and religion (Pfister, 1923). Music, for instance, that expression in which their sensibilities diverged so much, could never be understood by pure science. "The sharpest intelligence cannot state whether a symphony by Mahler or a painting by Hodler is beautiful. (…) Oh! How I dread a scholars' state emptied of art!" (Pfister, 1993 [*1928*], pp. 574–575). In the same regard, in one of his letters, he said to Freud: "Forgive a long-standing enthusiast for art and humanitarianism and an old servant of God. (…) At school my cleverest master used to say that music was a pitiful row. I did not try to convert him but took refuge in Beethoven or Schubert" (Meng & Freud, 1961, p. 127). Something similar was probably the only solution left to Pfister in front of Freud's incorrigible opinion on religion: to benefit from and enjoy something his friend seemed not to understand.

Ethics, Pfister insisted, regardless of what anyone can think, is not neutral nor can be based on scientific thought. Many of his best achievements came from religion, performing primary educational functions. It could hardly be replaced in this area by science. Religion, for its symbols, its poetic value and its emotional sense of reality, is also an educating factor that science, for all its theories, cannot replace at all. Pfister closes the work, insisting on one of his central ideas: an illusion can be valid. The question, for religion, will be to free itself from any magic, or anthropomorphic thought and develop an adult thought fit to represent God as the very incarnation of love. "A balanced religion can result only from the harmonious combination of belief and knowledge, from the interpenetration of wishful and realistic thinking, yet whereby the content of real thinking may not, through wishful thinking, be falsified in its facts or relationships" (Pfister, 1993

[*1928*], p. 577). To that end, the views from the past will need to be submitted to a critical examination. The Bible itself will not be understood as an infallible oracle and will have to suffer a thorough critical analysis. Only so will it regain a priceless value. Lastly, morality will not be conceivable as founded by a heteronomous authority but by the proper autonomy of the individual and society. Reason, in the end, will have considerable work to perform. But precisely, it will not be to void or kill desire.

Pfister seeks reconciliation and bonding bridges in the last paragraphs to save the clear distance separating him from Freud. The Freudian god Logos also shares the loving aim of alleviating human suffering. Like Saint John's, Pfister's Logos is one of "wisdom and love of God". Even though the verification criteria, in each case, are diverse (knowledge or love), both coincide in the end on a common and fundamental basis. Pfister is convinced: "And thus *The Future of an Illusion* and *The Illusion of a Future* unite in the strong belief whose credo is: 'The truth shall make you free!'". These are the final words in the work (Pfister, 1993 [*1928*], p. 578).

Echoes and resonances: Psychoanalysis and ecclesiastic institution

"What the effect on me was of what you have to say you have no need to ask – Freud writes to Pfister after reading The Illusion of a Future – What is to be expected if one is judge in one's own cause? Some of your arguments seem to me to be poetical effusion, others, such as the enumeration of great minds who have believed in God, too cheap" (Meng & Freud, 1961, pp. 122–123).

Pfister's idealism in the treatment of many matters, particularly in his sublime vision of the functions assigned to religion, could appear to Freud, in effect, only as pure lyricism. The fact that many intellectuals were believers was not either a surprise or an argument for Freud. He knew well that religiousness operates in registers that are easily superposed and prevail over the views of reason. The cases he analysed at that time, such as Dostoevsky and the young American physician who recounted his religious experience, let him see well the processes and mechanisms which could occur and the difficulties which could be felt to reach a position of unbelief, even if it was desired and required by the logic of the subjects themselves (Freud, 1928a, 1928b).

Freud, however, does not answer Pfister's criticism of his concept of illusion that, as we saw, was the only properly psychoanalytic argument in his *The Future of an Illusion*. The objection most rooted in psychoanalysis of all those that Pfister makes in his work and that even, as we saw, seemed to announce future significant psychoanalytic theories.

In turn, Freud dwells on countering Pfister's positions on the relationship between science and ethics. He is not ready to admit that science needs "to produce a system of ethics – ethics are a kind of highway code for traffic among mankind" and, more cuttingly, reproaches Pfister for trying to make do take advantage in favour of religion of the unavoidable errors that science makes in its progressive discovery of the laws of nature. Finally, in an open challenge, asks Pfister: "And finally – let me be impolite for once – how the devil do you reconcile all that we experience and have to expect in this world with your assumption of a moral world order? I am curious about that, but you have no need to reply" (Meng & Freud, 1961, p. 123). We do not know whether Pfister replied (we should assume he did) or the terms he would have used since the following letter from him available to us dates from November 1928, nine months after Freud's letter.

The question of his scientific optimism and, hence, that *The Future of an Illusion* became really *The Illusion of a Future* is not either dealt with by Freud. We know, however, that it had to be tackled not with Oskar Pfister, but with other analysts, in one of the Wednesday meetings at his home. In one of them, in effect, held in December 1927, *The Future of an Illusion* was debated. Theodor Reik (Roudinesco & Plon, 1997; Reik, 1931) who, because of his childish dependency on Freud, was known among his colleagues as "simili-Freud",[2] raised the question of the illusory character that Freud's approach to the power of science seemed to have. Reik seriously questioned that a time would come when, under the rule of the god Logos, humanity would be completely free from the power of the illusory. Freud did not contradict with a harsh no, but with the soft *Je doute* of Renan, accepting as well that there existed useful illusions which helped the progress of civilisation and that, in the past, religion had been a valuable force for the education and advancement of society.

Much more pessimistic than Freud on this matter, Reik thought religion would disappear, but another illusion would take its place. "The supremacy of the intellect which Freud foresees – Reik affirms – will never be more than superficial; basically men would still be guided by their instinctual desires (…) And men will continue to pray, 'Lord, give us this day our daily illusion'" (Reik, 1940, pp. 130–131). And, in a curious coincidence with pastor Pfister, he who most vehemently opposed that clerics could perform psychoanalysis, also recognised that science "has not made the scientist any better; that they are neither more patient nor happier nor even wiser", and he concludes: "Freud overestimates both the extent and the strength of human intelligence". For all that, Reik opinion on *The Future of an Illusion* was: "We feel inclined to say that in the first part of this essay Freud had imparted knowledge; in the latter part he has made a confession of faith". And he concludes in total coincidence with Pfister's fundamental idea: "Whereas the main section of Freud's essay shows the future of an illusion, we may say with little exaggeration that this last section presents the illusion of a future" (Reik, 1940, p. 135).

In 1934, Oskar Pfister was named Doctor *Honoris Causa* by the University of Geneva's Faculty of Theology. Freud congratulates him without letting Pfister try to let him know the motives for the award: "I congratulate you on your honorary degree, but cannot agree to your passing on to me the honour conferred on you; as the champion of religion against my *Future of an Illusion* you have the sole right to it. The fact that the Geneva theological faculty was not deterred by psychoanalysis is at least worthy of recognition" (Meng & Freud, 1961, p. 141). Thus, Freud believes that the degree is awarded to Pfister for his attack on *The Future of an Illusion* (in the same way he thought that some honours granted to the famous anthropologist W. Schmidt,[3] a declared enemy of psychoanalysis since *Totem and Taboo*'s publication, were due to the latter's fierce and continuous opposition to him.) On the other hand, Freud recognises and rejoices that the Geneva Faculty of Theology has had no problem granting that award to a defender of psychoanalysis; the war between psychoanalysis and theology did not look too hot. However, it did not seem that he desired too friendly a relationship. That shows in the comment that, shortly after the publication of *The Illusion of a Future*, he makes to Pfister about his secret intentions when he wrote *The Future of an Illusion*: "I do not know if you have detected the secret link between the *Lay Analysis* and the *Illusion*. In the former I wish to protect analysis from the doctors and in the latter from the priests (*Priester*). I should like to hand it over to a profession which does not yet exist, a profession of *lay* curers of souls who need not be doctors and should not be priests" (Meng & Freud, 1961, p. 126).

Of course, Pfister thought this observation required an explanation. After all, doctors were present in psychoanalysis from the start; he was the only clergyman. The aggression was manifest. "Please allow me to return to your remark that the analysts you would like to see should not be priests", Pfister writes to argue precisely with the ideas he received from Freud himself apropos the disputed theme of neutrality. "It seems to me that analysis as such must be a purely 'lay' affair. By its very nature it is essentially private and directly yields no higher values. In innumerable cases I have done nothing but this negative work, without ever mentioning a word about religion. The Good Samaritan also preached no sermons, and it would be tasteless to have a successful treatment paid for in retrospect by religious obligations. Just as Protestantism abolished the difference between laity and clergy, so must the cure of souls be laicised and secularised", Pfister argues. Because, taking to the extreme Freud's proposal of excluding priests, "If no priest should analyse, neither should any Christian or any religious or morally deep-thinking individual, and you yourself emphasise that analysis is independent of philosophy of life" (*Weltanschauung*). If any doubt about his thinking was left, Pfister also reminds Freud that "Disbelief is after all nothing but a negative belief" (Meng & Freud, 1961, p. 127), but faith after all.

It dawns on Freud. He acknowledges that his remark that the analysts of his phantasy of a future should not be priests "does not sound very tolerant, I admit"; and he adds: "I was referring to a very distant future. For the present I put up with doctors, so why not priests too?" Nevertheless, he insists on his purpose, showing one of his more intimate convictions: the incompatibility of psychoanalysis and religion. Freud's "other part", the one who cannot forget that Pfister, despite his open and cordial disposition, is a clergyman and hence a representative of that Christianity which causes in him such a profound rejection, emerges again and attacks ruthlessly. "You are quite right to point out that analysis leads to no new philosophy of life, but it has no need to, for it rests in the general scientific outlook, with which the religious outlook is incompatible. (...) Its essence is the pious illusion of providence and a moral world order, which are in conflict with reason. But priests will remain bound to stand for them. It is of course possible to take advantage of the human right to be irrational and go some way with analysis and then stop, rather on the pattern of Charles Darwin, who used to go regularly to church on Sundays". Like on other occasions, Freud tries to use a balm after the aggression. Pfister, he comments, reminds him of "the monk who insisted in regarding Nathan as thoroughly good Christian. I am a long way from being Nathan but of course I cannot help remaining 'good' towards you" (Meng & Freud, 1961, pp. 128–129).

Good with the man Pfister but implacable towards his religious vision on life and his clerical function, the latter tolerated just as something unavoidable at that moment. Seemingly, circumstances require it. However, the acceptance of what Christianity means is intolerable for him. Motives rather than causes determine it. That is why he drags that conviction since childhood, as shown in his early identification with Hannibal in his victory over Rome, the symbol for him of Catholicism and enmity towards Jewishness (Freud, 1900, pp. 196–197). Pfister's distinction between Catholics and Protestants was for him rather irrelevant.

Nor the Church in the Catholic environment of Freud for most of his life helped to modify his opinion in this respect. Instead, the opposite is true. The religious atmosphere was in open opposition to everything associated with the French Revolution. A restoration movement was going on with the sole purpose of recovering the order lost (Congar, 1970, pp. 455–458; Pottmeyer, 1975, pp. 21–60). The Church decisively confronted everything coming from modernity with the Pius IX and Pius X pontificates. The extreme rationalism of Neo-Scholasticism, mainly driven since Leo XIII's pontificate, dominated the whole theological field. We find thus figures such as J. Perrone, Franzelin, Passaglia, or C. Schrader, who mark the theological thought of the time as wholly defensive in front of the new mentality background. Other theological streams, such as those of the Tubingen school, or Scheeben, Newman, and Fr. Pilgram could do nothing against the strong ultramontane current dominating the European theological scene (Castillo, 1987; Thibault, 1972).

The most glaring evidence of that attitude of open opposition between the Catholic institution and the socio-cultural patterns born from the Revolution in which Freudian thought evolved appears in the 1864 *Syllabus*, described by Peter Gay as "that monument of resistance to modernity" (Gay, 1987, p. 10). The document offered no alternative for conciliation; it condemned, in painstaking detail, latitudinarian and liberal positions going all the way to rationalism and communism. Its number eighty error condemns those who defend that the Church comes to terms with progress, liberalism and modern civilisation (*Romanus Pontifex potest ac debet cum progressu, cun liberalismo et cum civilitate se reconciliare et componere*)

(Pope Pius IX, 1864). It was the response to the liberal French Catholics who ventured to instil their religious credo with touches of modern thought or to the positions such as those of l'Abbé de Lammenais, who in 1830 proclaimed in Paris that God and liberty could be united and dared to consider Catholic liberalism as a viable creature (Oldfield, 1969).

The *Lamentabili* decree and the *Pascendi* encyclical, both of 1907, were another attempt by Pius X to finish once and for all with all trace of modernism and meant a clear brake for the development of all Catholic thought. The Pontifical Biblical Commission published in 1906 a document that maintained as the only defensible thesis that Moses was the authentic author of the Pentateuch. We can only imagine Freud's judgment had he known about this assertion when he was engulfed in the exegetical study of Moses and the history of Judaism.

Hostile feelings mark from the start Freud's position towards the Church. From the anthropologic conception born from neurosis and dream interpretation research, the ecclesial institution appears as a harmful social agent because of its inept handling of the instinctual world. It supports sexual repression, the cause of so many psychic conflicts. Therefore, Freud welcomes any lay education which succeeds in taking it away from priests and religious orders (Freud, 1907, p. 139). Sexual repression, besides, usually comes with more general repression, affecting freedom of thought. According to Freud, the best way to forestall such freedom is – deceit in sexual matters and intimidation in religious issues (Freud, 1907, pp. 136–137, 1908, pp. 199–200).

But, in addition, the rejection Freud makes in this connection is not exclusively in the field of psychopathology. It is also made on moral grounds. The Church does not play fairly in the control it tries to carry out in the instinctual world. The Church's ministers have made significant concessions to instinctive human nature to keep people submissive. Also, advocating a loving illusion in its own heart drives violence to the outside to preserve itself from it (Freud, 1921, pp. 98–99). Its repression can, therefore, unchain a high degree of violence. When he considered that psychoanalysis could also be the object of that destructiveness, he affirmed: "Such violent methods of suppression are, indeed, by no means alien to the Church; the fact is rather that it feels it as an invasion of its privileges if someone else makes use of those methods" (Freud, 1939a, p. 55).

Consequently, the relationship between psychoanalysis and the Church always stood in a background of mutual lack of trust. Since the publication of *Totem and Taboo*, the Catholic institution was alert against psychoanalysis through Wilhelm Schmidt. The Rivista Italiana di Psicoanalisi, founded by E. Weiss, was forbidden, apparently at the request of the Vatican and Schmidt's sway.

The last stages of the relationship of Freud with the Catholic institution had to be especially filled with intense ambivalence. The Jewish question was also in the middle (Gay, 1987; Yeruschalmi, 1991). On one side, he cannot ignore that Christianity has been one of the sources of antisemitism in Western culture (Freud, 1939a). But ultimately, the Catholic Church was the only institution he could trust as protection and defence against Nazism. "…strange to say, – he writes – it is precisely the institution of the Catholic Church which puts up a powerful defence against the spread of this danger to civilisation" And, he ends: "The Church which has hitherto been the relentless foe to freedom of thought and to advances towards the discovery of the truth!" (Freud, 1939a, p. 55).

With such an image of the ecclesial institution rooted since his earliest infantile representations, it is understandable that Freud distrusted the idea of his precious psychoanalysis being used in the heart of the Church domain. An intense affective ambivalence also resulted in an enormous theoretical ambiguity to his positions thereon. Pfister was also in good measure a target of that ambivalence and ambiguity. Although the friendship with the pastor probably helped reduce it, it was never fully resolved. So we find on one side that in the *Introduction to Pfister's The psychoanalytic Method* he affirmed, as we saw, that the educator and the priest are perhaps better placed than the doctor for understanding mental life in young people (Freud, 1913, p. 331). And on another occasion, he wrote to the pastor: "If these spiritual gentlemen wished to use analysis, that was no affair of ours, they should apply for permission to their bishop" (Meng & Freud, 1961, p. 105). But at other times, something that, probably doubtful in his thoughts, prevailed on him from the rest of his personality: the impossibility of making faith and analysis compatible and harmonising analytical and pastoral work in the same person.

All this tells us of the difficulties and inevitable setbacks in the hard and complicated dialogue which started when these two men first met. Both were engaged in a passionate search for the truth. But they also represented two different discourses, the one of the unconscious and the one of faith, which for the first time were then explicitly confronted and which until today maintain their mutual questions and suspicions.

Notes

1 In this chapter, I follow the chapter dedicated to this work in my *El psicoanálisis freudiano de la religion* (1991), Madrid, Paulinas, pp. 238–254.

2 Reik dressed like Freud, trimmed his beard like Freud, and smoked the same cigars as Freud. He was marked by an imperative need for a father, which he seemed to satisfy through his relationship with Freud. The latter adopted him as a spiritual son, paid his analysis with Abraham, and took him in analysis himself. Among his works, we should highlight *Ritual: Psycho-Analytic Studies* (Reik, 1931).

3 The Reverend Wilhelm Schmidt was the inaugural director of the Pontificio Museo Missionario-Etnologico del Laterano, integrated now at the Vatican Museums as Missionary Ethnological Museum. Freud feared the influence this man had at the political level in Austria and the ecclesial level at the Vatican. When Schmidt received the decoration of honour from Austria, Freud wrote to Arnold Zweig:

"I count it on my credit that our arch enemy P. Schmidt has just been awarded the Austrian decoration of honour for Art and Science for his pious lies in the field of ethnology. Clearly this is meant to console him for the fact that providence has allowed me to achieve the age of 80" (Freud, 1970, p. 130).

References

Castillo, J. M. (1987). La exaltación del poder magisterial en el siglo XIX, in AA.VV.: *Teología y magisterio*, Salamanca: Sígueme, pp. 139–160.

Choisy, M. (1979/1948). *Psicoanálisis y catolicismo*, Buenos Aires, La pléyade: Quoting Laforgue.

Clark, R. W. (1980). *Freud, the Man and the Cause*, New York, NY: Random [reprinted London: Paladin, 1987].

Congar, Y. (1970). *L'Église de Saint Agustin à l'époque moderne*, Paris: Ed. du Cerf.

Eucken, R. (1912). *Der Wahrheitsgehalt der Religion*, Leipzig: Verlag von Veit, quoted by Pfister (Meng & Freud, 1961, p. 115).

Feuerbach, L. (1890). *The Essence of Christianity*, London: Kegan Paul, Trench, Trubner.

Freud, E. L. (Ed.) (1970). *The Letters of Sigmund Freud and Arnold Zweig*, New York, NY: Harcourt Brace Jovanovich, Inc.

Freud, S. (1900). *The Interpretation of Dreams*, S.E., 4–5, London: Hogarth.

Freud, S. (1907). *The Sexual Enlightenment of Children*, S.E., 9: 131–139, London: Hogarth.

Freud, S. (1908). *'Civilised' Sexual Morality and Modern Nervous Illness*, S.E., 9: 179–204, London: Hogarth.

Freud, S. (1911c). *Psycho-Analytic Notes on an Autobiographical Account of a Case of Paranoia*. S. E., 12: 9–82, London: Hogarth.

Freud, S. (1913). *Introduction to Pfister's The Psychoanalytic Method*, S.E., 12: 327–331, London: Hogarth.

Freud, S. (1921). *Group Psychology and the Analysis of the Ego*, S.E., 18: 69–133, London: Hogarth.

Freud, S. (1925). *An Autobiographical Study*, S.E., 20: 3–70, London: Hogarth.

Freud, S. (1927c),). *The Future of an Illusion*, S.E., 21: 5–56, London: Hogarth.

Freud, S. (1928a). *A Religious Experience*, S.E., 21: 168–172, London: Hogarth.

Freud, S. (1928b). *Dostoevsky and Parricide*, S.E., 21: 175–196, London: Hogarth.

Freud, S. (1930a). *Civilization and its Discontents*, S.E., 21: 59–151, London: Hogarth.

Freud, S. (1933a). The Question of a Weltanschauung, *New Introductory Letters on Psycho-Analysis*, S.E., 22: 158–182, London: Hogarth.

Freud, S. (1935a). Postscript to *An Autobiographical Study*, 20: 71–74.

Freud, S. (1939a). *Moses and Monotheism: Three Essays*, S.E., 23:73–80, London: Hogarth.

Gay, P. (1987). *A Godless Jew, Freud, Atheism, and the Making of Psychoanalysis*, New Haven, CT: Yale University Press.

Gay, P. (1988). *Freud: A Life for Our Time*, New York, NY: W.W. Norton.

Hartmann, Eduard von (1884). *Philosophy of the Unconscious*, London: Trübner.

Jones, E. (1953–1957). *The Life and Work of Sigmund Freud, Volume 1–3*, New York, NY: Basic Books.

Marcuse, L. (1969). *Freud*, Madrid: Alianza.

Meng, H. & Freud, E. L. (Eds.) (1961). *Psychoanalysis and Faith: the Letters of S. Freud & O. Pfister*, London: Hogarth [reprinted New York, NY: Basic Books, 1963].

Oldfield, J. J. (1969). The evolution of Lammenais catholic-liberal synthesis. *Journal for the Scientific Study of Religion, VIII*: 269–288.

Pfeiffer, E. (1972). *Sigmund Freud and Lou Andreas-Salomé, Letters*, New York, NY: Harcourt Brace Jovanovich.

Pfister, O. (1915). *The Psychoanalytic Method*, London: Kegan Paul, Trench, Trubner.

Pfister, O. (1923). *Some Applications of Psycho-Analysis*, London: Allen & Unwin.

Pfister, O. (1993). The illusion of a future: A friendly disagreement with Prof. Sigmund Freud. *The International Journal of Psychoanalysis, 74 (3)*: 557–579 [(1928) Die Illusion einer Zukunft. Eine freundschaftliche Auseinandersetzung mit Prof. Freud. Imago 24:149–184].
Pope Pius IX (1864). *The Syllabus of Errors*, Rome: Holy See.
Pottmeyer, H. J. (1975). *Unfehlbarkeit und Soveranität*, Mainz: Matthias-Grünewald-Verlag.
Reik, T. (1931). *Ritual: Psycho – Analytic Studies*, London: Hogarth.
Reik, T. (1940). *From Thirty Years with Freud*, New York, NY: Farrar & Rinehart.
Ricoeur, P. (1970). *Freud: una interpretación de la cultura*, Mexico: F.C.E. [*Freud and Philosophy: An Essay on Interpretation*, New Haven, CT: Yale University Press].
Roudinesco, E. & Plon, M. (1997). Quoted in *Pfister, Dictionnaire de la Psychanalyse*, Paris: Fayard.
Schur, M. (1972). *Freud: Living and Dying*, New York, NY: Intl. Universities Press.
Thibault, P. (1972). *Savoir et Pouvoir. Philosophie thomiste et politique cléricale au XIX siècle*, Québec: Les Presses de l' Université.
Winnicott, D. W. (1971). *Playing and Reality*, London: Tavistock.
Winnicott, D. W. (1986). *Holding and Interpretation*, London: Hogarth.
Winnicott, D. W. (1988). *Human Nature*, London: Free Association Books.
Yeruschalmi, H. (1991). *Freud's Moses: Judaism Terminable and Interminable*, New Haven, CT: Yale University Press.

5

THE PSYCHOANALYSIS AND FAITH DIALOGUE OVER TIME

The rudimentary dialogue between Pfister and Freud

"In itself psychoanalysis is neither religious nor non-religious, but an impartial tool which both priest and layman (*der Geistliche wie der Laie*) can use in the service of the sufferer" (Meng & Freud, 1961, p. 17). This sentence by Freud in his letter to Pfister in February 1909 has been perhaps the most quoted in all the correspondence between them. It points at the attempt to analytic neutrality towards religion and his position well apart from any pronouncement for or against religious faith. Psychoanalysis is "an impartial tool". Its scope of action is limited to the area of the unconscious, and it aims to seek the liberation of those who suffer and (we would add today) some truths about themselves to those who desire it. No more and no less.

However, this initial proposition by Freud, so transparent, became very soon cloudy. It is clear from the start that for him religion is not simply "another field" (Meng & Freud, 1961, p. 17), alien to psychoanalysis ("But the beauty of religion certainly does not belong to psychoanalysis" (Meng & Freud, 1961, p. 63), he also comments to Pfister), but an "opposite" (Meng & Freud, 1961, p. 117). "A different look" (Meng & Freud, 1961, p. 136) of what psychoanalysis seeks and manages in its work in the realm of the unconscious. In front of the rejected, the impure, the instinctual and the frightening that beats in the dark kingdom of the unconscious, religion aims to show the pure, the ideal, the fascinating ultimate and most decisive pole of attraction for the human being – the kingdom of light. But analysis had to distrust any light, even more, if more intense. Behind the brightness, it often found the horrified flight of darkness, the way to fend off the darkest desire, the terrified escape to an unbearable fascination with the impure. Thus, religion was viewed as part of the unconscious defence that needed to be reduced to make access to the new field just discovered possible.

DOI: 10.4324/9781003389804-7

This conviction is easily noticed in Freud's relationship with Oskar Pfister. We already saw him persuaded that Pfister would find all his world of religious belief crumbling in so far as he would progress in the field of analysis. Let us remember what he wrote to Jung about the pastor: "Whether he will be able to preserve his residue of faith for long strikes me as doubtful; he is only at the beginning of a far-reaching development, and the bad company he keeps is bound to have its effect" (McGuire, 1974, pp. 222–223). And we also saw Ferenczi's comment at seeing Pfister thrilled by what psychoanalysis seems to offer theology: "He doesn't yet suspect that the analytical conception *carried through to its conclusion* does away with theology. He has yet to come to that" (Brabant et al., 1933, p. 153). Freud did not ask himself, however, why, along the thirty years of his relationship with the pastor, these predictions were not fulfilled at all, and Pfister instead seemed to achieve a higher depth in his belief while, with great effort and surmounting many resistances, he also deepened his psychoanalytic knowledge and experience. Freud undoubtedly saw his wish frustrated, which probably played too in the ambivalence his pastor friend raised in him.

That certainty of Freud on the opposition between psychoanalysis and faith, coupled with a dormant aggressiveness at finding it disproven in Pfister's case, was probably the motive for the famous question of why no pious man discovered psychoanalysis and it had to wait for a godless Jew.

The Pfister and Freud encounter and their debates on psychoanalysis and religion appear as the beginning of a dialogue that reaches our days, although significantly changed in its accents and shades. But today's exchange would probably have never existed in the present form without that initial encounter which provided us, among other things, with a rich and ample wealth of ideas and also of doubts and questions by the psychoanalysis founder. Pfister was for him the opportunity to establish a debate. A debate he needed to engage as much with religion as with himself.

Following that initial dialogue between Freud and Pfister, one of the most challenging tasks is establishing a due boundary line between what spoke in Freud as a psychoanalyst and what spoke as the son of his time and his biography. It will also be required to differentiate what came from his cultural and biographical coordinates in Pfister. The task, especially if we consider psychoanalysis light on the building up of the subject, will prove to be practically impossible.

However, it seems possible to isolate a series of easily noticeable elements of that initial dialogue which may contribute to further clarification and a better approach to the perception of the fundamental issues which should stand up to keep the discussion itself in progress.

We shall not enter here into the detailed analysis of the biographical events that, in Freud's case, could determine his position towards religion. Much ink has run on it without contributing substantially to the clarification of the issue (Domínguez-Morano, 1991 pp. 438–446; García Cabero, 1976, pp. 145–297; Plé, 1968; Zilboorg, 1962). Rather the contrary, we think. Psychoanalysis at a distance and, above all, guided by intense counter-transference-loaded questions such as those pulsing in belief or atheism easily lead to really wild interpretations that only increase obscurity and inflame the controversy. Specific mention must be made of the previously quoted work by Ana-Maria Rizzuto, in which she undertakes a brilliant and rigorous psychodynamic interpretation of the motivations of Freud's atheism (Rizzuto, 1998a). She thoroughly analyses the early family life of the psychoanalysis founder (especially the troubled relations with his father) and how that framework of primary bonds somehow made the belief in God impossible.

Nevertheless, let us move to a more limited field, perhaps with a higher probability of making objective judgments. It would be necessary to centre the question on determining how much two fundamental elements influenced the dialogue: on one side, the illustrated, rationalist character of Freud, as an exemplary son of the Age of Enlightenment and, on the other hand, Pfister's concordist disposition, fostered by his connatural idealism. In effect, the enlightened Freud and the concordist Pfister seemed to give that initial dialogue a rudimentary character, even though, without any doubt, they succeeded in raising at that time questions that even today are somehow still outstanding.

Peter Gay is right when in his work on Freud's atheism, he presents him as "the last *philosophe*" and an illustrated atheist (Gay, 1987, p. 35). Early in that embroiled fight between religion and reason, he took sides between laicity and clericalism, which developed from the French Revolution. Voltaire, Diderot or Feuerbach ("Among all philosophers, I worship and admire this man the most", he wrote while he was a student in Vienna to his friend Silberstein) (Boehlich, 1990, p. xxvi) are his true intellectual ancestors.

We cannot forget that as Freud grew up, went to university, started his medical practice, or developed psychoanalysis, the tensions over God and the Church's power spread everywhere. He did not hesitate to engage soon in the fight, armed with the belligerent language characterising the contest. Like Thomas Huxley, he did not believe in a possible conciliation between free thought and traditional authority, particularly the religious one. Like socialist Leon Gambetta, his foe was also clericalism, and, like young Marx, criticism of religion was for him the first condition for any criticism. As a loyal son of the Enlightenment, he drew a neat distinction between science and religion. Each of them describes, in his view, two incompatible styles of thought about the world: the theological or metaphysical on one side and the scientific one on the other. And at the same time, he was convinced that no mental gymnastics, no effort of will, could ever conciliate them.

Moreover, the impregnation of the medical materialism of the time also left its mark on his position on religion. His idol and master, Ernst Brücke, with whom he worked for almost six years, had introduced the Age of Reason in the laboratory and had no doubts at showing his aversion to Romantic philosophy and, above all, to theology.

This led Freud to see himself as a "destroyer of illusions". And this by the absolute prevalence he, as a son of Enlightenment, wanted to grant reason. Because, as

P. Gay affirms, "… when it comes to reason (…), Freud, the specialist in unreason was a monotheist" (Gay, 1987, p. 65).

That is the mental framework in which psychoanalysis is born, and his dialogue on religion with Oskar Pfister occurs. But it seems evident that while this framework provided a positive and solid basis that made possible the erection of new knowledge, it also impregnated that knowledge with foreign ideological positions, which (like in the case of medical materialism) played even as obstacles to its very development. As an enlightened man, Freud worked to oust God and religion in favour of technical and scientific reason. "Whether this is also essential for psychoanalysis is another matter altogether" [translated for this edition], as A. Barrutia affirms, interrogating, in the introduction to his book, P. Gay, who, as we shall see later on, is convinced of that need to oust God and religion (Barrutia, 1989, pp. 10–14).

That enlightened impregnation, that naïve optimism about the power of reason, that slanted conception of the individual and of culture brought along that, in the initial dialogue between psychoanalysis and religious faith, the questions moved towards a space that was not the most genuinely psychoanalytic. That the great debate between Freud and Pfister centred on the theme of illusion, leaving aside matters which concerned oedipal ambivalence and guilt feelings, shows the degree to which Freud's rationalism impaired that initial dialogue. As we have already noted, it is surprising how little presence works like *Totem and Taboo* and *Moses and Monotheism* have in the interchange of ideas between our two characters. It is also surprising that Oskar Pfister does not even mention *Totem and Taboo* when he goes over the role of anxiety in primitive religions, particularly in the totemic system (Pfister, 1948). The reference to *Moses and Monotheism* is also scarce in this work. It is present only in a brief note on Judaism. Surprising, since it is in these works that the most profound questions can be posed by psychoanalysis to Judeo-Christian beliefs: the most profound and, as we have also noted, the most specifically psychoanalytic. *The Future of an Illusion* is undoubtedly not the best work by Freud on religion nor the most representative of what psychoanalysis means regarding faith. Moreover, from that naïve alignment in the ranks of the Enlightenment, Freud failed to do justice to the intricate opposition between science and religion. As P. Gay affirms, "His stark vista of a historic confrontation in which educated atheists were pitted against unlettered believers lacks the subtlety he lavished on his analysis of the neuroses" (Gay, 1987, pp. 11–12).

Neither Oskar Pfister posed the question on different grounds nor seemed to feel especially implicated in his faith or pastoral work by what those other works, more centred in the oedipal problems, meant. After all, he was also a son of Enlightenment, a liberal cleric who applied his best efforts to respond to modernity's questions on the Christian faith. However, the polarisation in these problems diminished the sensitivity to capture not what the past Enlightenment but what modern psychoanalysis could formulate. As E. Rodrigué notices in the same direction, all his correspondence with Freud seems on both sides to come out of the

Age of Enlightenment (Rodrigué, 1996, p. 419). That is why its high point is the debate about *The Future of an Illusion* and its response, *The Illusion of a Future.*

But if the polarisation initially biased the dialogue between psychoanalysis and religion in problems previous to psychoanalysis, it also suffered from a lack of depth because of the clearly concordist position maintained by Pfister. The Swiss pastor, keen on the light he was receiving from psychoanalysis, plunged into it without grasping sufficiently how much that same psychoanalysis had to question his previous conception of faith and life. His reading, guided by his educational and pastoral interest, was more attentive to the coincidences than to the questioning it could bring. *Mirabilis consensus!* was what Pfister thought he had found between the Gospel proposal of love and the Freudian theory on the libido.

In his evolution about sexual theory, it is true that Freud no longer looked at it as a sum of quantifiable arousal and instead deemed it as an inclination by all living beings to come together in ever-growing units. In this way, he kept integrating the broader dimensions of the affective world into it. In his final idea of Eros, he perceived a fundamental harmony with the same concept by Plato or the Christian idea expressed by Paul in Corinthians. As Freud tells us: "In its origin, function, and relation to sexual love, the 'Eros' of the philosopher Plato coincides exactly with the love-force, the libido of psychoanalysis, and when the apostle Paul, in his famous epistle to the Corinthians, praises love above all else, he certainly understands it in the same 'wider' sense" (Freud, 1921c, p. 91). Naturally, this proposal excited pastor Pfister. However, it seems that his enthusiasm led him to ignore their differences too much. We already saw Pfister's tendency to set aside the problems related to partial instincts and their permanence in imaginary adult life and proceed immediately to a generic conception of love, closer to the Gospel proposal. "Why on earth do you dispute the splitting up of the sex instinct into its component parts which analysis imposes on us every day? (…). It looks to me as if you want a synthesis without a previous analysis", Freud reminded him (Meng & Freud, 1961, p. 62).

For Pfister, Jesus, in proclaiming love as the central principle of his message, would have become close to the first psychoanalyst or at least the predecessor of psychoanalysis. However, he forgot that the psychoanalytic version of love was centred on the analysis of its most primitive roots and its inescapable connections with aggressiveness, hate, and death instincts. Thus, he was less sensible to sufficiently value those dark forces of aggression, of *Thanatos*, which, in its diverse shapes, Freud always saw in blend with *Eros*.

For all these reasons, he tended to underestimate the differences between Freud's proposal and his own. The violence he had to apply to the concepts to make them coincide with the synthetic option he aimed for also took him sometimes to lose the recognition and respect that differences require. In this way, he endeavoured with all his good will to baptise Freud even against the latter's will. So much as even telling him: "A better Christian there never was". And this, in addition, is his reply to Freud's famous question on why it had to wait for a

Godless Jew to discover psychoanalysis. Pfister believes that the best way to reject Freud's malicious question was to deny his condition of atheist and, not content with this, that of Jew as well: "… in the first place you are no Jew, which to me, in view of my unbounded admiration for Amos, Isaiah, Jeremiah, and the author of Job and Ecclesiastes, is a matter of profound regret, and in the second place, you are not godless, for he who lives the truth lives in God, and he who strives for the freeing of love (*Befreiung der Liebe*) 'dwelled in God' (First Epistle of John, iv, 16)" (…) "I should say of you: A better Christian there never was" (*Ein besserer Christ war nie*) (Meng & Freud, 1961, p. 63). Ana Freud rightly expressed displeasure for the lack of respect hidden in the well-meaning words of the pastor. In reading the correspondence of Pfister with her father, she exclaimed in all justice: "What in the world does Pfister mean here, and why does he want to dispute the fact that my father is a Jew, instead of accepting it?" (Gay, 1988, p. 150). The only explanation for his clumsiness on this occasion was the denial of the difference separating him from Freud's unbelief.

So, there was in Freud too much uncritical positivism and too much idealistic optimism in Pfister. And if the latter was right in his criticism of Freudian optimism in *The Future of an Illusion*, he fell himself into the illusion of a kind of "social gospel", which amounted to a reduced Christianity, and reduced psychoanalysis as well. Only this way was he able to reconcile psychoanalytic theory with his moral order and respond to the question one day thrown to him by Freud: "How the devil do you reconcile all that we experience and have to expect in this world with your assumption of a moral world order?" (Meng & Freud, 1961, p. 123).

His ethical objective could fit what was later proposed in America by the mental hygiene movement, even though his broader theoretical references gave him a more profound approach than the pragmatic one of that "counselling" movement (Irwin, 1973a).

So, Freud and Oskar Pfister's debate on religion leaves us somehow unsatisfied. Most of the argumentation on the two sides scarcely relates to what is properly the analytic experience. It is the usual one at the time in intellectual and philosophical circles. But none of the two could or would take any further engagement. Freud should have pointed out more vividly the lack of rigour in Oskar Pfister's psychoanalytic conceptions. The latter should have made Freud feel his insensibility to ethical and philosophical aspects more clearly, negatively affecting his consideration of sublimation. That initial dialogue between psychoanalysis and religion could have gathered more breadth and depth on those premises. It is also true that this first dialogue had essential effects on clarifying many terms, which would later frame any future encounter of the two orders. It forced Freud to think of the limits that psychoanalysis should respect and tell his own positions from those fitly deriving from psychoanalysis. "It remains to be considered whether analysis *in itself* must really lead to the giving up of religion", he wondered out loud to psychoanalyst Max Eitingon (Gay, 1987, p. 12). Oskar Pfister probably contributed, with his reflections and, perhaps more, with his personal relation, to make Freud pose such a question to himself and (even ignoring it on some occasions) give his clarifying answer more than once.

The religious and pastoral experience, represented by Pfister, had to face also very tough questions that, sometimes without pity, Freud raised and that, while addressed to the Swiss pastor, somehow remain there for us all to answer. With its defences and resistances, mutual approaches and interrogations, the psychoanalysis-faith dialogue had a start and, for all that, a fruitful start in this deep friendly and intellectual relationship between a godless Jew and a Christian pastor of souls. And there remained, entirely valid, a series of pertinent questions stirred up in that encounter, such as those in Pfister's critical query about Freud's concepts on illusion and reality, his criticism of Freud's poor idea of sublimation, and the call to a better knowledge of the Christian doctrine on redemption and pardon. The mutual resistances and approaches in the psychoanalysis-faith dialogue after Pfister and Freud would continue for a long time; the mistrust and suspicion and, in parallel, the fascination and the open questions would also have a long road ahead. And there we are even now.

Approaches and resistances

It took a long time until it became possible to establish a genuine dialogue between psychoanalysis and theology. Like J. Scharfenberg affirms, "an iron curtain of malevolent impenetrability" emerged, and a jealously guarded coexistence came, in which the theologian gave a technical pinch to a generally devalued version of psychoanalysis, which was regarded as "an ancillary science"[translated for this edition] (Scharfenberg, 1974, p. 168). The psychoanalyst kept thinking that Church and religion offered little interest or, even worse, represented psychopathogenic factors that should be fought, as Freud did. Perhaps Scharfenberg is somewhat optimistic in seeing that situation as something from the past. After many years, there are significant sectors in the psychoanalytic field with that type of attitude. Similar distrust and malicious oversight, if not disengaged manipulation, can also be found in the theological area.

From the psychoanalytical field

The psychoanalytic interpretation of religion by the first generation of analysts essentially stayed in the paradigm designed by the master (Pruyser, 1973). Most of them were Jewish, and none a believer (Gay, 1987, p. 104). The psychoanalysis-religion tension was taken for granted in the early psychoanalytic scene. E. Jones (Jones, 1953–1957), who stood out among them for his interest in religious themes, shared Freud's views on the matter entirely. When the latter let him know about his *Totem and Taboo* project, Jones tells him: "The most exciting news in your letter was that you had determined to devote yourself to religious problems. Obviously that is the last and firmest stronghold of what may be called the anti-scientific, anti-rational, or anti-objective *Weltanschauung*, and no doubt it is there we may expect the most intense resistance, and the thick of the fight" (Gay, 1987, p. 105). Jones himself, whom Freud saw as the person to complete the analysis of religion in its applications to particular beliefs, devoted many writings to the psychoanalytic interpretation of religion. With an uncommon erudition, his work explored three main directions: the study of the religious symbol, the historical role of the Catholic Church, and the psychology of Christianism. He had the merit of bringing out the role of the feminine in the religious experience, a theme, as we know, so strikingly forgotten by Freud nor especially remarked by Pfister. Jones assigned a capital part to that feminine factor in the inception of primitive Christianism and its victory over the Roman religion of Mithras. The representations, of course, of Mary, but also those of the Holy Spirit, had the role of giving relevance to the maternal dimension of religiousness (Jones, 1951, 1974). Free of the reductionist formulations so explicit in Freud, Jones took, however, the exact position of his master in this respect.

Theodor Reik, whom we know with his designation as "simili-Freud", also paid particular attention to religion due to his infantile imitation of the master. His work was undoubtedly best when dealing with rituals, with specific attention to those of the Jewish world he belonged to. His attitude to religion was, as we can suppose, parallel to that of Freud, despite having made his strong criticism of Freud`s optimism in *The Future of an Illusion*. He was especially intolerant of the possibility of priests performing analysis. Commenting on Freud's assertion that psychoanalysis is a neutral instrument that believers or unbelievers can use, he came out this way: "But analysis depends upon who practices it; and the situation is considerably changed when we are attempting to analyze the content of truth in religion. When a priest practices analysis, he does not cease to be a spiritual shepherd, and gradually the original aims are displaced, the ideational base shifts and contradictory tasks arise. When this happens, psychoanalysis pays the piper. Undeniably, many priests have shown a broad understanding of analysis. But along with this is an inflexible, though cleverly conceived desire to put it to work in the service of the only Holy and Apostolic Church. For the first we thank them; for the second we say, no, thank you. Everyone who has followed the literature knows that the Church is preparing to take over psychoanalysis. But it cannot be denied that the Church is one of the strongest repressive forces in our society. When it utilises analysis, it places it at the service of repression. In our practice we have often noted how an obsessional neurotic not only cleverly weaves newly acquired knowledge into his system but often uses it to enlarge his obsessional pattern. This is precisely what happens to analysis in the service of religion" (Reik, 1940, pp. 126–127). It is difficult not to ask if such ideas were not heard from his master, so closely followed by Reik (Reik, 1946). In any case, they reflect well the intolerant and scarcely "neutral" attitude of his author and the image of the Church prevailing in the psychoanalytic circles at that moment.

Finally, among the first generation of analysts, it is required to name Géza Róheim, credited with the introduction of psychoanalysis in the anthropological field (Dadoun, 1972, 1980; La Barre, 1968). His anthropology, marked by an intransigent and Talmudic Freudianism, was soon rejected despite the conciliatory attempts made by Margaret Mead between Róheim and the rest of her colleagues. Bringing in elements from Sandor Ferenczi (who was his analyst), Karl Abraham and Melanie Klein, Róheim tried to analyse primitive religious rites starting from the different stages of libidinal evolution. Between 1928 and 1931, he did fieldwork in Somalia, central Australia, Melanesia and the Yuma Indians in Arizona. In all this research, he tried to analyse the dreams, religious rituals and beliefs of the so-called primitive people. But, as we see, all in a line of work without the slightest deviation from orthodox Freudianism and, in consequence, equally marked by an essentially reductionist attitude on religious issues (Róheim, 1921, 1925, 1971).

So, only Pfister and Binswanger, in Europe, and J. Putnam, in the United States, showed a differing position regarding religious and philosophical beliefs inside the first generation of the psychoanalytic movement. However, the latter, much more than our Oskar Pfister, moved in the area of moral-theological speculation to draw up an alleged synthesis with psychoanalysis. We know that Freud firmly rejected the attempt, as he dismissed any effort to create any worldview from psychoanalysis. In his *Human Motives* (Putnam, 1915), Putnam tries to amalgamate psychoanalytic elements with moral and theological ones without reaching, obsessed with synthesis, an authentic dialogue, since previously the differences have been pretty much voided for the sake of concordance. We see then that in this first stage of the relationship between psychoanalysis and religion, we move permanently between reductionism and concordism. Authentic dialogue and confrontation were not possible in these first stages.

The second generation of analysts was no longer so definite in its disesteem of religion. Without any doubt, among those who dealt with it, the figure of Erich Fromm stands out. In his works, there is a clear evolution from his first ideas, nearer to Freud's interpretations and hence more critical in front of religion, until later works, where his now well-known distinction between authoritarian and humanistic religion gained ground. In his *Psychoanalysis and Religion,* he insists on the most positive sides of faith and its liberating possibilities. The religious need is envisaged as something connatural and beneficial if the trap of authoritarian religion. Therein, everything is conceived as submission to a power beyond man, which by its dominion demands from him obedience and adoration. In this way, the subject is discouraged about himself since he feels force and ability are out of him; a feeling of impotence hinders his human productivity and, since obedience is the cardinal virtue of that religiousness, the self-destructive feeling of guilt arises immediately. In the humanist religion, however, the concept of God is embedded in the true image of man and his process of liberation. By associating Old Testament ideas with those of the German mystic Meister Eckhart and Marxist philosophy, Fromm develops a proposal of religiousness in which the person is the centre and humanity is its ultimate objective. The essential content of the idea of God would be the denial of idols and the liberation from incestuous links with family, clan and land. That history of freedom leads – not in fact, but as a logical consequence – to a dissolution of theology, since the idea of God remains embodied in man, in the image and likeness of God, and liberated for himself.

It may be questioned, however, if that humanist religiousness is at all religious or if, deprived of the more specifically transcendent dimension, has not been reduced to simple ethics (the question of religion is not the question of God but the question of man, he affirms in his *Psychoanalysis and Religion*). From that position, it becomes easy (perhaps too easy) to harmonise Freudian postulates with those of religion and even consider Freud a defender of it. The values of truth, justice, etc., are the values Freud defends and make him speak in the name of the essence of religion: "Freud opposes religion in the name of ethics – an attitude which can be termed 'religious'" (Fromm, 1950b, p. 20, 1947). The similarity with some of Pfister's postulates is evident. And so is its concordism. Not, of course, its conception of transcendence.

In a similar line in concordism, the figure of V. Frankl should be considered in his attempt to encompass psychoanalysis as part of a broader project he calls "logotherapy" and pleads for the need to include transcendence as an inalienable objective for mental health (Frankl, 1967) Also worth mentioning would be Igor A. Caruso (Caruso, 1946), during his first period (before his remarkable turn towards Marxism), in an attempt to conjugate psychoanalysis with a Christian philosophy of existentialist tone, and the members of the Vienna Working Circle for Depth Psychology (W. Daim, P.R. Hofstäter and others), who tried to develop a synthesis between psychoanalysis and Catholicism (Wyss, 1968, pp. 341–348).

Peter Gay, however, is not fair when in his *A Godless Jew*, he tries to disqualify all attempts after Freud to establish a dialogue between psychoanalysis and religious belief. In this book, which we have quoted repeatedly, Gay attempts to answer Freud's famous question to Pfister on why psychoanalysis had to wait for an unbelieving Jew to come up. In the form of a thesis, his answer is the absolute need for that atheism (not that Jewishness) to make psychoanalysis possible. Peter Gay is an excellent biographer of Freud in his formidable and indispensable *Freud: A Life For Our Time*. He is also a recognised scholar of the Age of Enlightenment and an excellent specialist in the history of ideas. However, he surprises and deceives us in this minor work on Freud's atheism with his questionable claim that atheism is, in essence, intrinsic to psychoanalysis itself. Gay affirms instead of arguing (as shown tangibly in his commentaries on W. Meissner's *Psychoanalysis and Religious Experience*) (Meissner, 1961, 1984, 1987, 1992a). What's more, he does it with his unique sharpness and brilliance (Gay, 1987, pp. 111–112). He also demonstrates a higher capacity for biography and history of the ideas than for capturing the psychoanalytic language, theory and sensitivity. Furthermore, after the rigour he had used on other occasions, it is surprising how he bases his opinions by setting aside a very relevant bibliography, which does not get a single reference from him and could certainly question his thesis on the impossibility of establishing a dialogue between psychoanalysis and faith. Peter Gay simply ignores many attempts at this dialogue, made from entirely different approaches from those criticised by him (At the end of the book, we offer extensive bibliography on the relations between psychoanalysis and religion, where significant contributions ignored by Peter Gay can be found. Outstanding among them are those of French-speaking authors like Antoine Vergote, Louis Beirnaert, André Godin, Françoise Dolto or Jacques Pohier, and also the Spanish ones like Andrés Tornos, Juan Rof Carballo, Enrique Freijó o Pedro Fernández Villamarzo). In this way, it becomes easier for him to make the alleged proof that it was not possible (not because of social and cultural conditions, but by its essence) that a believer would discover psychoanalysis and that it is possible to establish compatibility between psychoanalysis and religious faith. Peter Gay sets aside a broad range of psychoanalysis that, beyond concordist temptations such as Pfister's or Fromm's, undertakes the encounter and confrontation with religious faith from an epistemological position not as narrow as that of Freud (which P. Gay adopts so uncritically) and untangled from the prejudices typical of the Enlightenment and rough positivism.

Gay, like Freud, and Pfister, too, centres the whole debate around the ideas considered in *The Future of an Illusion*. His dedication and knowledge of the Age of Reason (Gay, 1995, 1996, 1999) seem to have led him to an essential identification precisely with the Freud he calls "the last *philosophe*" and not with the Freud who, from the more psychoanalytic, becomes an overcoming of it. Besides that, when he finds assertions by Freud in the line of psychoanalysis being an instrument of search which is neither religious nor contrary to religion, Gay circumvents the issue by saying that Freud did not mind a believer joining psychoanalysis "as long as the believer was someone like Pfister" (Gay, 1987, p. 73).

Not only E. Fromm and his followers with their concordist positions, or W. Meissner from more rigorous and certainly more psychoanalytic approaches, have worked on the great questions that psychoanalysis poses to religious faith. Nor P. Tillich has been the only Christian theologian (next to the only one mentioned by P. Gay) who has examined psychoanalytic theory to elaborate his thought. Many other figures (ignored by P. Gay, centred in the English-speaking world) in France, Belgium, Germany, Switzerland, and other countries in Europe and Latin America, have worked on the relations between psychoanalysis and faith. They have followed a path (not an easy one because of what it requires of dispossession of oneself) which has led them to better understand psychoanalysis as much as religion. They have done this while keeping questions open and assuming dark areas without prematurely rushing to elaborate comforting synthesis. The result has been an increasing focus on where to confront psychoanalysis's questions.

In France, analysts emerged to reflect on what psychoanalysis signifies as a challenge to faith. René Laforgue was followed by others such as Maryse Choisy (Choisy, 1950, 1955), philosopher and writer, analysed first by Freud in 1927 and then analysed again, after meeting Pierre Theilard in 1938 and converting to Catholicism, by René Laforgue. She was a founder of the journal *Psyché*, where she left proof of her interest in the dialogue between psychoanalysis and the Catholic Church's postulates. We should also mention Louis (Beirnaert, 1987), a Jesuit priest who became a close collaborator of Jacques Lacan and a founding member of the International Association for Medical-Psychological and Religious Studies to promote understanding of psychoanalysis in the Catholic Church. In the early sixties, joining Marc Oraison (Oraison 1957) and Albert Plé, he created the Association Médico-Psychologique d'Aide aux Religieux in France, which gave clerics access to psychoanalysis and a better understanding of its possibilities. We find the well-known figure of Françoise Dolto so profoundly and originally combining her religious faith with a worldwide recognised analytic experience (Dolto & Séverin, 1978). She took part with Lacan in creating the École Freudienne de Paris. From her Catholic faith, so perplexing for many, she knew how to read the Gospels under the light of psychoanalysis, with an original and suggestive interpretation underlining Jesus' most human dimensions. So also, Marie Balmary, the disciple of Jacques Lacan, became known in the 1970s for her new reading of the Oedipus complex in her *L'homme aux statues. Freud et la faute cachée du père* (Balmary, 1979). She pursued her work with interdisciplinary studies searching for the meeting points between psychoanalysis, religions, the Bible and mythology. In her defence of the transcendental dimension of the person, she has expressed her convictions in books such as *Freud jusqu'à Dieu* (Balmary, 2010) and one of her best-known books, *Le moine et la psychanalyse* (Balmary, 2005) the fruit of her talks with Marc-François Lacan, Jacques Lacan's brother and a Benedictine monk.

Other outstanding French psychoanalysts also showed interest in religious facts from different non-believing and sometimes clearly reductionist positions. Such are the cases of Octave Mannoni (Mannoni, 1972, 1976) from the Lacan entourage and Istanbul-born Guy Rosolato (Rosolato, 1987), president of the Association Psychoanalytique de France (APF). The latter, a Lacan follower for a time, explored Freud's idea of the dead father of *Totem and Taboo* with intriguing approaches in the field of sacrifice and mystical experience. Also, Didier Anzieu (Anzieu et al., 1976, 1980), with a complex and singular relationship with Lacan, is interested in mysticism as an experience that can occur, as in his case, aside from religious faith. Finally, Daniel Sibony (Sibony, 2001), a philosopher, mathematician, and Lacanian psychoanalyst, because of his Moroccan origin and his belonging to a Jewish family, offered suggestive writings on the idea of God in the three great monotheistic faiths of Judaism, Christianity and Islam.

We can point out other personalities in France, closer to religious and theological circles, but always from their psychoanalytic practice and experience. Denis Vasse (Vasse, 1991), Jesuit, physician and Lacanian psychoanalyst with relevant reflections on psychoanalysis and spiritual life, the mystical experience of Saint Teresa, theology and the Bible. Jean-Daniel Causse (Causse, 1999) has brought significant views on the Jewish and Christian religions and the personal relationship of Lacan with Christianity. René Sublon (Sublon, 1975) physician and medical professor turned theologian and psychoanalyst of L'École Freudienne de Paris who worked creatively from a Lacanian point of view on ethical and theological matters. Also, figures such as Philippe Julien, former Jesuit and member of Lacan's school (Julien, 2008); Dominique Bourdin (Bourdin, 1999) (Bourdin and Souletie, 1999), philosopher and theologian apart of psychoanalyst; Nicole Jeammet (Jeammet, 1993a), psychoanalyst and theologian. Likewise, Jacques Arènes (Arènes, 1999), a psychoanalyst and an expert in the anthropology of religion, has produced leading works on the relations between faith, spirituality and psychoanalysis.

In an area more comprehensive than the relationship between religion and psychoanalysis, it is unavoidable to mention Julia Kristeva (Kristeva, 1987) for her innovative writing on the intersection of linguistics, culture and literature. Her highly complex work shows the light of Claude Lévi-Strauss, Roland Barthes, Michel Foucault, Sigmund Freud and, above all, Jacques Lacan. Starting with an education in a religious environment during her childhood and early youth in Bulgaria, her interest in spirituality and religion is present in several works under her singular point of view and exceptional attention to the feminine dimension of religious feeling.

In Belgium, the works of Antoine Vergote and André Godin represent two honest attempts of psychoanalysts who confront their religious experiences with psychoanalysis. The first one, Antoine Vergote (Vergote, 1988, 1997a) is one of the most outstanding figures in the area of psychoanalysis and religion relationship. Trained by J. Lacan and with a profound philosophical background in phenomenology, he was a co-founder of l'École Belge de Psychanalyse. He was the author of an extensive production covering diverse themes of the religious experience, always from a critical attitude towards religious facts and certain psychoanalytical positions. An excellent study on Antoine Vergote is offered by J. B. Lecuit (Lecuit, 2007).

In turn, André Godin (Godin, 1986), Jesuit and psychoanalyst, analysed by Gregory Zilboorg, strongly contributed to making the psychoanalytical point of view play a decisive part in the contemporary studies on religion done in Belgium. In the same Université Catholique de Louvain, Josef Corveleyn (Corveleyn, 1996) carried out substantial work on the psychology of religion from his expert knowledge of clinical psychoanalysis.

Born in the Netherlands, Paul Wille Pruyser (Pruyser, 1973) moved to the United States after graduation as a clinical psychologist. Following the work of W. James, S Freud, R. Otto and D. Winnicott, he played a decisive role in the psychological theories on religion. He created the Psychology and Culture model, analysing the three "worlds" in which people live: the autistic, the illusionistic and the realistic.

Patrick Vandermeersch (Vandermeersch, 1991b) has also worked in the Netherlands. A Catholic priest, psychoanalyst and professor at Université Catholique de Louvain, he offers interesting studies on very diverse themes in religiousness, always approached from a creative, original, and provocative frame of mind.

Ernest Jones (Jones, 1923) stands as the fundamental figure who paid attention to religion in the first generation of psychoanalysts in the United Kingdom. Always sharing Freud's views, he had the merit of underscoring the essential role of the maternal feminine in religious experience (Domínguez-Morano, 2020a). After this emblematic figure of early psychoanalysis in the United Kingdom, others appeared, outstanding among them that of Harry Guntrip (Guntrip, 1956a), a Methodist pastor well-known for his relevant contributions to object relationships. His work encapsulates Melanie Klein, Ronald Fairbairn, and Donald W. Winnicott, maintaining a critical attitude in front of some of Freud's positions towards religion (Dobbs, 2008, 2009). Then, turning to Scotland, we should mention David M. Black (Black, 2011), the South-Africa-born poet and psychoanalyst. In addition to his considerable poetic work, he has published many papers on psychoanalysis and religion. Interested in Buddhism and Hinduism, he later joined Westminster Pastoral Foundation (WPF) and the British Psychoanalytical Society. Finally, Rachel Blass (Blass, 2003), although born in New York and now living in Israel, is a member of the British Psychoanalytical Society and Israel Psychoanalytical Society. In London, she developed her Kleinian perspective, mainly focusing on truth as a form of lived experience and its relationship with religious experience.

Neville Symington is a remarkable figure in the British scene (Symington, 1994a), born in Portugal, a Catholic priest and then a psychoanalyst. He worked at the Tavistock Clinic and emigrated to Australia, chairing the Australian Psychoanalytical Society between 1999 and 2002. His studies on religion drove him to highlight narcissism's part in personality development, considering the positive role of religious experience from a Winnicott perspective. At the same time, he underlined the moral dimension of psychoanalysis, which brought him criticism for an undue moralisation of the therapy.

In the English-speaking European area, we should note Edward B. Barrett (Barrett, 1924), the Irish Jesuit. Like the already mentioned case of the French Dominican monk Jacques Pohier, he can embody a not-easy, often conflicting dimension in the attempt to reconcile psychoanalysis and faith. Born in 1883 in Ireland, he entered the Society of Jesus in 1904 and studied psychology and psychoanalysis in Belgium and England. He moved to the United States in 1924 after suffering conflicting situations with his superiors because his publications were always critical of Catholic institutions. But the friction did not cease (Pohier, 1986). He finally left the religious order and set up as a psychoanalyst in New York's Village, even if his practice was far from psychoanalytic orthodoxy, mainly about the analyst's neutrality. A controversial figure, always critical of the institutions and perhaps, as in O. Pfister's case, stubbornly committed to reaching a doubtful concordist synthesis between psychoanalytical postulates and those of religious institutions.

Albert Görres (Görres, 1983) stands out in the German area. A philosopher and psychiatrist (disciple of Viktor von Weizsäcker), he completed his psychoanalytic training in Berlin, Heidelberg and Amsterdam. He studied Freud closely and was chosen to take the first German depth psychology chair at the University of Mainz. Throughout his many writings and lessons, Görres repeatedly approached the tension between psychology and theology, particularly concerning moral aspects. He was close friends with the great XX-century Catholic theologian Karl Rahner. He wrote with him: "*Das Böse. Wege zu seiner Bewältigung in Psychotherapie und Christentum*", "*Evil. Ways to cope with it in psychotherapy and Christianity*" (Görres & Rahner, 1982). He was critical of certain postulates of Catholic sexual moral teaching, defending guilt-free sexuality and describing "ecclesiogenic neuroses".

It is worth remembering the honest reply that A. Görres gave Zahrnt (Görres, 1974, p. 97) when asked how to be a Christian and an analyst at the same time: "With the precision you desire, of course, I don't know (...) I see it this way: as a child, I was initiated by my parents on faith. And, with time, I have not found any solid reason to eliminate as something outdated that faith which, at the time, enlightened and convinced me. "[translated for this edition].

Other outstanding German figures include Joaquim Scharfenberg (Scharfenberg, 1988), who, from a protestant perspective, focused most of his research on the relationships between psychoanalysis and some aspects of Christian theology. We also find Eckhard Frick (Frick, 1993), a Jesuit, philosopher, theologian, and psychiatrist. As a psychoanalysis and psychosomatic medicine specialist, he has done interdisciplinary research on diverse aspects of religious experiences and spirituality.

For his part, Hartmut Raguse (Raguse, 1992), of German origin, has carried out a critical mass of work in Switzerland as a theologian and a psychoanalyst, including suggestive psychoanalytical interpretations, particularly from Winnicott's perspective, on biblical hermeneutics and Christology.

In Switzerland, Oskar Pfister's pioneer role in opening the dialogue between psychoanalysis and religion found a following with relevant figures such as Thierry de Saussure (Saussure, 2009), psychoanalyst and theologian, president of de la A.I.E.M.P.R. (International Association for Medical-Psychological and Religious Studies) and professor of psychology at the University of Lausanne. For her part, Isabelle Noth (Noth, 2008), a professor at the University of Berne and the Institut für Praktische Theologie, stands as a great student of Pfister's work. She has published essential studies on the Swiss pastor, jointly with the theologian Christoph Morgenthaler (Noth & Morgenthaler, 2014b).

In Spain, scholars such as Jordi Font i Rodon (Font i Rodon, 1983), a psychiatrist and Jesuit, contributed decisively by introducing the psychoanalytical perspective to analyse the religious experience and spirituality. From the Vidal i Barraquer Foundation in Barcelona, he exercised a significant influence by creating master courses for the study of religious fact and spirituality from a psychodynamic point of view. Especially prominent is the Master's Degree in Transcultural Spirituality, in which psychoanalysis plays a central axis. Pedro Fernández Villamarzo (Villamarzo, 1979) a psychoanalyst and priest, also played a relevant role in psychoanalytical education as a student of Freud's work and as a Professor of Psychology at the Pontifical University of Salamanca. He was founder of the "Oskar Pfister" Psychoanalytical Institute in Madrid. Also, the psychoanalyst Carlos Padrón (Padrón Estarriol, 1997) upheld a psychoanalytic view of religious belief in which the latter can perform a relevant function in personal development.

Freud's impact in the United States was significant since the very beginning of the psychoanalytical movement, with surprising reach and, at the same time, vigorous debate both inside and outside the movement. The rise of psychoanalysis in America struck Freud himself, not without complaining about unjustified attenuations of his theory. As psychoanalysis permeated all strata of North American culture, it did strongly in the religious realm, Christian and Jew and that of the oriental traditions so present in Western spheres. The large production done in the United States is well reflected by Israeli Professor B. Beit-Hallahmi (Beit-Hallahmi, 1992), who, besides his extensive work, offered a priceless bibliographic collection in his *Psychoanalytic Studies of Religion: A Critical Assessment and Annotated Bibliography* (Beit-Hallahmi, 1996).

Many authors either reflect on their psychoanalytic experience and practice or work from studies on Freud's work and their relationships with theology or religion in general, without any psychoanalytic praxis.

In the first group, we should highlight the name of Geza Róheim (Róheim, 1925), a Hungarian who carried out most of his activity in the United States. One of Freud's early disciples, Róheim, made the first attempt to apply the data obtained in psychoanalytic research to cultural anthropology. It was a challenging task, partly because of the haphazard history of agreements and disagreements between Róheim and the leading anthropologists of the time, between anthropology and psychoanalysis. The controversy occurred among G. Róheim, Malinowsky, R. Benedict, M. Mead, Goldenweiser, A. Kardiner, A.L. Kroeber, etc… Nevertheless, the controversy also brought the need to approach a series of methodological questions before applying psychoanalysis to foreign disciplines with methodologies of their own.

The contribution of psychoanalysis to cultural anthropology and specifically to religious phenomena continued with the work done by Weston La Barre (La Barre, 1962) in ground-breaking field studies in South America with anthropology inspired by psychoanalytical principles.

Among the pioneers of psychoanalysis in the United States, we should also mention the Austrian Theodor Reik (Reik, 1931), who did his most important work there, despite the difficulties he faced in psychoanalytical circles for not having a medical degree. In addition to his research on masochism, criminology and literature, he made significant contributions concerning guilt and religious rituals.

One of the first psychoanalytic approaches to mystical experience came from Franz Alexander (Alexander, 1935), a Hungarian who settled in the United States. With the reductive resolve of early psychoanalysis, he established a connection between mysticism and catatonia that would greatly influence future interpretations of religion and, above all, mysticism.

But, after the first reductionist temper of early psychoanalysis, the new clinical and metapsychological rethinking by Donald W. Winnicott (1896–1971), Wilfred R. Bion (1897–1979) or Jacques Lacan (1901–1981), apart from the attention they may have paid to the issue, opened the door to new perspectives and improved consideration of religious experience (Domínguez-Morano, 2020b, pp. 121–130). Also, the specific views of Erich Fromm (Fromm, 1947, 1950b) in his work in the United States and Mexico no doubt helped that new consideration of religion.

These new approaches help us understand proposals such as those of Michael Eigen (Eigen, 1998), inspired by W. R. Bion, D. W. Winnicott, and more distantly, by J. Lacan. From his conviction about the intimate bond between the psychological and spiritual, this author rethinks the relationship between mysticism and psychoanalysis (Domínguez-Morano, 2020a, pp. 128–129), recognising the role of mysticism in the therapeutic process. According to Eigen, faith plays an essential function in the daily experience of human beings because we cannot sustain life on pure knowledge. For all that, he has been described as a psychoanalyst and mystic, perhaps even more mystic than a psychoanalyst.

Taking also a Bion-based point of view, James S. Grotstein (Grotstein, 1997) has brought relevant and suggestive elements to understanding religion and spirituality. In *Who is the Dreamer, Who Dreams the Dream? A Study of Psychic Presences* (Grotstein, 2001) offers a profound search into the nature of human suffering and spirituality. On his part, McDargh (McDargh, 1992) examines the connection of faith with the psychoanalytic theory of object-relationships. In his *Psychoanalytic Object Relations Theory and the Study of Religion: On Faith and the Imaging of God* (McDargh, 1983), through the use of case studies with a combined psychological and theological analysis, the author sustains that the theory of object-relationships offers a robust basis for a fuller understanding of the human construction of the image of God and the psychological dynamics of faith.

In North America, an outstanding, already-mentioned figure in the area of psychoanalysis and religion is, without any doubt, William W. Meissner (Meissner, 1961). A psychiatrist and psychoanalyst, he also did important work as a professor and supervisor at Boston College, with numerous publications throughout his clinical and intellectual career. His *Psychoanalysis and Religious Experience* (Meissner, 1984) should be considered a classic. His rigorous work on the life and the spirituality of the Jesuits' founder, *Ignatius of Loyola: The Psychology of a Saint* (Meissner, 1992a), establishes a courageous example of a psychoanalytic approach to an emblematic religious figure, followed later on the same note by *To the Greater Glory: a Psychological Study of Ignatian Spirituality* (Meissner, 1999). His solid psychoanalytical knowledge and profound Catholic theological scholarship make him a necessary reference in psychoanalysis and religion. Working with him for a long time was Ana María Rizzuto, a psychoanalyst from Argentina, whose name also outstands in this area of work and whom we shall address later on.

Edward Paul Shafranske (Shafranske 1992), close to William W. Meissner and Ana María Rizzuto, should also be noted for his extensive research of the unconscious implications of the religious experience and his analysis of the management of spiritual and religious themes in the context of psychoanalytic therapy.

Stanley A. Leavy (Leavy, 1980), starting from his Jewish faith, became a Christian, led a long medical and psychiatric career and applied psychoanalysis to religion and literature. On their part, Jeanette G. Simmonds (Simmonds, 2006b) and Gerald J. Gargiulo (Gargiulo, 2004) have developed significant research on the relationships between psychotherapy and religion. From Canada, Dan Merkur (Merkur, 1988a) in Toronto has made engaging contributions to the understanding of mystical experience, particularly in his work *Mystical Moments and Unitive Thinking* (Merkur, 1999) and *Explorations of the Psychoanalytic Mystics* (Merkur, 2010). Equally, Randall Lehmann Sorenson (Sorenson, 1990), in his double capacity of analyst and professor, has done multidisciplinary work setting together psychoanalytical history, sociology of religion, comparative theory and clinical interpretation to delve into the intimate relationship between psychoanalysis of religion and spirituality.

Many studies have been done in the United States about Judaism's relationship with psychoanalysis. We shall look further on to those made by theologians. Still, we should first review the contribution made by psychoanalysts who, after Freud, analysed anew the psychoanalytic implications of the Jewish faith. Outstands among them Moshe HaLevi Spero (Spero, 1985). A highlight of his many publications, *Religious Objects as Psychological Structures: A Critical Integration of Object Relations Theory, Psychotherapy, and Judaism* (Spero, 1992), offers an original view relating religious objects and representations of God. Also, Rabbi Yosef Hayim Yerushalmi (Yerushalmi, 1989), a Professor at Columbia University and a great student of Jewish history and historiography, did significant research on Freud's relations with Judaism, notably in *Freud's Moses: Judaism Terminable and Interminable* (Yerushalmi, 1991).

Oriental religions and spirituality have also drawn North American psychoanalysts' attention, as already happened with Franz Alexander, though with a more accommodating attitude than the reductionist one in his case. Special mention is due to Alan Roland (Roland, 1972), a writer and painter and a psychoanalyst with clinical experience in India and Japan. Born into a well-known Jewish family, he developed an interest in Indian philosophy early. He did inter-Asian comparative studies (*In Search of Self in India and Japan: Toward a Crosscultural Psychology*) (Roland, 1988). In the approach to Zen Buddhism also stands Paul C. Cooper (Cooper, 1999a), with many writings inspired by Bion's theory.

In this closer look into oriental spirituality and religions, a required name is Sudhir Kakar (Kakar, 1981), an Indian psychoanalyst, well-trained and working closely with European and North American circles. His remarkable work with Catherine Clément, *La folle et le saint* (Clément & Kakar, 1999) is a comparative analysis of the Madeleine of Pierre Janet and Ramakrishna, the XIX century

Bengali mystic (Domínguez-Morano, 2020a, pp. 128–132, 360–362). Equally, his *The Analyst and the Mystic* (Kakar, 2007) shows an understanding of mysticism exempt from any reductionist trait. On his part, Robert A. Paul (Paul, 1996) made suggestive anthropological and psychoanalytic approximations of Asian religiousness and critical studies on Freud's more anthropological writing. The work of Jeffrey B. Rubin (Rubin, 1992) represents an attempt to integrate Eastern and Western spiritualities; from his experience in clinical psychotherapy and psychoanalysis, he fostered the practice of what he called Meditative Psychotherapy.

Turning to a field apart from psychoanalytic circles, the research on religious fact, particularly from the angle of the psychology of religion, we should list relevant figures in the United States. One of those outstanding is Paul Clayton Vitz (Vitz, 1977), who, born and educated in a Presbyterian environment, later took an atheist position before finally converting to Catholicism. Therefore, from his authority in general psychology, he has approached with relevance an assessment of the tensions and paradoxes of Christian themes in Freud's life and work. His work, *Sigmund Freud's Christian Unconscious* (Vitz, 1988), raised an engaging debate. Worth mentioning is Joel Whitebook (Whitebook, 2017c) and his comments on Freud's interpretations of religion.

William B. Parson (Parsons, 2021) is a relevant figure in the psychoanalysis and faith dialogue. In his work, he points to the evolution he finds in what concerns mysticism. Starting from the interpretations of Freud himself on the oceanic feeling as mere regression to pre-oedipal narcissism, a second phase gave way to the role of mystical experiences in the psychological growth of the ego. It then reached a third position, driven by the rise of non-religious spirituality, that tried to establish an integrating, non-reductionist dialogue between psychology and mysticism. Also worth mentioning are his studies on Saint Augustine (Parsons, 2013). Working often with William B. Parson has been Diane Jonte-Pace (Jonte-Pace, 2001a), a great student of psychoanalysis and religion matters with a particular sensitiveness to feminine angles. And, from the attachment theory, we need to name Lee A. Kirkpatrick, especially in his work *Attachment, Evolution, and the Psychology of Religión* (Kirkpatrick, 2004), a look from that perspective at the evolutionary psychology of religion.

On his part, Kenneth Pargament (Pargament, 2007) has insisted on pointing to the healthy role religious experience can perform in psychotherapeutic processes in general. In the broad field of psychology of religion outstands Ralph W. Hood Jr. (Hood, 2001), a member of the Society for the Scientific Study of Religion and joint editor of The International Journal for the Psychology of Religion and Archiv für Religionpsychologie. With a broader point of view than the psychoanalytic one, he has substantially contributed to the study of religious experience in general and mysticism in particular. Similarly, J. W. Jones (Jones, 1991a), a great student of the religious phenomenon from a psychological, psychoanalytic and psychiatric, but also theological, perspective, offers us an ample production concerning very diverse religious themes, with a particular sensitivity towards psychoanalytical theory. Finally, not from psychology but in sociology and cultural research, Philip Rieff has paid close attention to Freud and his relationships with morality and philosophy. In particular, his *Freud: The Mind of the Moralist* (Rieff, 1961) has been the subject of a significant debate, among other reasons, because presumably his wife, well-known writer Susan Sontag, should be seen as the real author of the work.

In Canada, Don Carveth is a psychoanalyst and professor of sociology and political thought in Toronto and New York. Inspired by Melanie Klein and Donald W. Winnicott, he profoundly reflects on the super-ego, conscience and moral life in his *The Still Small Voice: Psychoanalytic Reflections on Guilt and Conscience* (Carveth, 2013).

The impact of psychoanalysis on Latin American culture has been meaningful, particularly in Argentina, Mexico, Chile, and Brazil. Most of these countries have seen studies of the religious experience as expected from the nuclear role of religiousness in those socio-cultural spaces. Argentina, in particular, brings a line-up of psychoanalysts including Pichon-Rivière, A. Raskovsky, M. Lange... (Roudinesco & Plon, 1997, pp. 57–63) and, although religion would not take a central place in their interests and concerns, there was neither a lack of significant reflections about it. Such was the case of the Spaniard Angel Garma (Garma, 1966), a political exile from Franco's Spain and one of the founders of the Argentine Psychoanalytic Association, who offered interesting thoughts on this issue (Garma, 2013). But, as shown in the bibliography, plenty of works were published in Argentina.

Without any doubt, one of the most relevant scholars in psychoanalysis concerning religion is Ana Ma Rizzuto (Rizzuto, 1974), born in Cordoba, Argentine, but who has done most of her work in the United States (Reineke & Goodman, 2017). As you can see in our bibliographic notes, her work is extensive. We should, above all, point to *The Birth of the Living God: A Psychoanalytic Study* (Rizzuto, 1979) or *Why did Freud reject God? A Psychodynamic Interpretation* (Rizzuto, 1998a). With a Winnicott influence, her search for the shaping of God's images in early childhood and their rework throughout the life cycle is an indispensable contribution to studying the religious experience.

Also, the A.I.E.M.P.R. mentioned above (International Association for Medical-Psychological and Religious Studies) had associates in Buenos Aires, with several studies on psychoanalysis and religion, inspired by Miguel Rodríguez Amenábar (1979, 1995).

In Latin America, Brazil has also seen religious problems treated both by theology and, even more, psychoanalysis. Joel Birman (Birman, 1994), a psychiatrist and psychotherapist of Jewish origin, is a prolific psychoanalytic writer on Judaism and the Freud and Pfister dialogue. Karin Wondracek (Wondracek, 2003a), a psychoanalyst and a theologian, has focused a good part of her work on that initial dialogue between psychoanalysis and faith. Besides Brazil, she has been active also in Germany and Portugal, with numerous, highly valued studies on Pfister.

The Jesuit and psychoanalyst Ricardo Torri (Torri de Araújo, 2015), professor at the Pontifical Catholic University of Rio de Janeiro, has offered influential works on Freud and Catholicism, mystical experience and Ignatian spirituality, always in the light of psychoanalysis. On his part, William Castilho Pereira (Castilho Pereira, 2004) has carried out relevant work applying psychoanalysis in Catholic spaces, with particular attention to consecrated priestly life.

In Mexico, psychoanalysis did get a significant resonance also. Again, we should point to the psychoanalyst, theologian and Anglican presbyter Ricardo Blanco, who, besides his valued publications, has been a prime mover of studies on psychoanalysis and religion in many research seminaries. Another figure is Víctor Hernández Ramírez (Hernández Ramírez, 2020), a psychoanalyst, theologian and Presbyterian pastor who has made profound and suggestive psychoanalytic interpretations of biblical and theological aspects of the Christian faith. He works at present in Barcelona, Spain.

Chile, on its part, under the influence of psychoanalysts Otto Kernberg and Ignacio Matte-Blanco, developed an interest in religious matters, resulting in the "Symposium on Psychoanalysis and Religious Faith" in 1995. The participants, Ana Ma Rizzuto, Juan Pablo Jiménez, José A. Infante (Infante, 1996), myself and others, shared productive exchanges. Ignacio Matte-Blanco (Matte-Blanco, 1975a), the founder of the first psychoanalytic institutions in Chile, before carrying out notable activities in Rome, Italy, introduced substantial original concepts in the psychoanalytical field with significant impact on philosophy and theology.

In Italy, we find Mario Aletti (Aletti, 1992a), psychoanalyst and professor at Catholic University of the Sacred Heart, Milan (UNICATT) and founder with J. Milanesi of Società Italiana di Psicologia della Religione. Also noteworthy is Leonardo Ancona (Ancona, 2006), doctor and psychoanalyst, Professor of Psychology at UNICATT and Rome and a member of the Italian Psychoanalytical Society. He was one of the founding members and later Honorary Chairman of the A.I.E.M.P.R. mentioned before (International Association for Medical-Psychological and Religious Studies).

This Association started around 1950 with the primary objective of promoting reflection born from the encounter between psychiatry, psychology and psychoanalysis with theological reflection. That reflection started from a basic premise: the new contributions from psychiatry and psychoanalysis, on many occasions with a critical questioning character, did not necessarily mean disqualifying the religious experience or its reduction to infantilising or psychopathic dimensions. The attempt was more necessary as conservative sectors of the Catholic Church were urging the condemnation of the new psychological theories, particularly psychoanalysis. Prominent figures in the psychiatric, psychological and psychoanalytic fields, such as G. Zilboorg, A. Godin, A. Gemelli, J. Font, López Ibor, L. Ancona, H. Ey, L. Beirnaert, M. Oraison, A. Plé, Ch. Durand, etc., joined efforts to prevent the advancement of such tendencies. After starting as a Catholic organisation (ACIEMP: Association Catholique Internationale d'Etudes

Médico-Psychologiques), it soon acquired an ecumenical status, integrating Protestant, Catholic and Orthodox members. Since 1957, International Congresses have taken place every three years. The first, with J. J. López Ibor, as chair, was held in Madrid in 1957 under the *Religious Behaviour and Mental Health* theme, and the most recent in Rome in 2022 with de theme *The sacred in the age of crisis.*

Also significant was the Symposium on Psychoanalysis and Religion organised by the Chilean Psychoanalytic Association jointly with the Pontifical Catholic University of Chile in 1995. As Ana-Maria Rizzuto, to whom we are so much in debt also on these problems, pointed out, it was the first Symposium that the International Psychoanalytical Association organised on the theme of religion since its foundation by S. Freud. We had there the opportunity to evaluate the complex relations between psychoanalysis and the religious experience.

Perhaps the most significant conclusion after those days of joint reflection was that psychoanalysis has not yet faced the challenge of giving an ear and listening to the religious experience. One of the participants in the Symposium referred to the analytical experience she was going through at the time. She confessed she found it harder to deal with the theme of his religious experience than with that of her sexual life. She felt that her analyst had more difficulty listening to the first than the second theme. Thus, she was signalling a critical problem, which still affects a good part of contemporary psychoanalysis at the counter-transference level. Therefore, the road still ahead for both parties, psychoanalysis and religion, presents resistances concerning both poles in the relationship. Psychoanalysis should question itself in the same way that psychiatry has done (Neeleman & Persaud, 1995).

From the theological field

"My desire to make pastoral-care analysis the common property of all pastors failed almost entirely. The theologians prefer to busy themselves with the baggage of dogma and questions of church law rather than with the living souls of human beings! It is a pity, how dreadfully things are bungled in pastoral care. Oh well, it is God's concern. I do not believe that my life work was only a vain attempt". With these words of disappointment but of religious hope, Oskar Pfister addressed his friend H. W. Kienast ten years after Freud's death and seven years before his own death (Kienast, 1973, 1974). They reveal the profound resistances suffered in theological reflection in front of what psychoanalysis could mean.

We cannot count Theology among the more sensible disciplines for the anthropological issues derived from psychoanalytic research. Not that there were no reasons for it, perhaps more than others. Among them is that religion was one of the focal points on which psychoanalysis centred its attention and applied its more radical criticism.

The bibliography of theological works offering reflections after the anthropological revolution of psychoanalysis is short (Vande Kemp, 1984), especially if we compare it with the extensive production available on the psychoanalysis of religion (Meissner, 1961). The latter works, otherwise, come mainly from authors who, being believers and working essentially in the field of psychoanalysis, have necessarily questioned themselves on what belief means after facing the psychoanalytic challenge. But the theologians seem to have yet to consider that psychoanalysis could offer relevant data for their research from their own reflection and theological work. "We are afraid of it. It causes anxiety in us", joked a theologian faced with the question. Probably he expressed a good part of the truth in that widespread evasion from matters of the unconscious.

From an institutional point of view, the Catholic hierarchy has always shown misgivings and distrust towards psychoanalysis, without making any official condemnation of it. Mistrust, however, was permanent (Ancona, 1983; Homans, 1970; Plé, 1974). Pope Pius XII made more than one statement in somewhat derogatory terms about the new discipline; one of the occasions was the first International Congress on the Histopathology of the Nervous System. Another was the International Congress on Psychotherapy and Clinical Psychology. Pope Paul VI spoke in similar terms. In these papal interventions, the threat of pansexualism was always the dominant topic. This choice is significant since what Freud stressed in his critical psychoanalytic view were the dogmatic problems more than the moral ones.

The *Monitum* of the Holy Office dated 15 July had a particular echo on the international press: It dealt with the psychological education given to priests and religious order members and followed the contested intervention with a psychoanalytic experience in the Mexican Benedictine monastery of Cuernavaca. The intervention was initiated by G. Lemercier, prior of the monastery, who introduced a group therapy with two analysts (man and woman) for the sixty monks in the community. Lemercier himself and forty other monks abandoned religious life; Pope Paul VI shut down the monastery, and from that moment, he took a somewhat hostile attitude towards psychoanalysis. The assertion by Cardinal Felici (Felici, 1954) that it would be hard to excuse from mortal sin any person that would submit out of their own free will to psychoanalysis also resonated in the worldwide press. The same happened when the Holy Office, under Pope Pius XII, included in the *Index* the book by Marc Oraison (Oraison, 1952).
when the latter was in Rome with the Jesuit L. Beirnaert and the Dominican A. Plé in a congress organised by Maryse Choisy on psychoanalysis and religion matters. Marc Oraison was forced to correct his errors in a self-criticism incorporated into the second edition of his *Vie chrétienne et problèmes de la sexualité* (Oraison, 1972).

The words of Mgr. Méndez Arceo stand out as a call in the desert against this background of mistrust and suspicion towards psychoanalysis. In the days of Vatican II, at the Counciliary Hall, he said: "I can not explain the silence of Schema XIII on psychoanalysis… we cannot ignore the psychoanalytic revolution, not less than the technical one. The psychoanalytical discourse is part of human culture, entails a renewal of the concept of man and raises problems on which nothing was known". The Mexican bishop even recalled that the same mistake made with Galileo could be made again with psychoanalysis. Still more surprising, and away from the usual practice in Catholic circles, the bishop warned on taking a concordist position by assimilating the new discipline to a previous doctrine on man. (As happened with V.E. Frank, I. Caruso, P. R. Hofstäter, and W. Daim, members of Vienna Working Circle for Depth Psychology, who tried for a synthesis between psychoanalysis and Catholicism). He said: "There is no shortage of Catholics who harbour the illusion of Christian or Catholic psychoanalysis, when true science is neither Christian nor un-Christian" (Acta Synodalia, 1978) [translated for this edition].

Also, in the Protestant field, there were attitudes of rejection. Most of the churches did not assume Freudian options. An example, told by Marta Robert (Robert, 1964), was the pastor of the Presbyterian Church of Sidney, who tried to form a group open to that sensibility and gave lectures on psychoanalysis in diverse societies. Less lucky than Oskar Pfister, he soon resigned as pastor.

Naturally, many social and cultural factors have weighed in this lack of resonance of psychoanalysis in the panorama of Christian thought. In Spain, in particular, we cannot forget that during Franco's dictatorship, the country's culture was deprived of psychoanalytic contributions on a general level and in psychological and psychiatric research. We already mentioned Ángel Garma (Garma, 2013), the most relevant figure of the rising Spanish psychoanalysis, who was forced into exile in 1936 to Argentina, where he became a key person in the important psychoanalytic movement developed in that country (Moulines, 1972). At that time, Spain lost so the possibility of seeing the start of a psychoanalytic school similar to those rising in the rest of Europe.

During the dictatorship, other currents, some phobically anti-psychoanalytic, were encouraged at the expense of Freudian theory. Sexuality, converted into a taboo like in any type of tyranny (whether political or otherwise), played an essential role in the proscription of the whole Freudian psychology. Consequently, Spanish theology did not feel questioned by the changed view of man that the new discipline set in.

The political situation of dictatorship, which impinged on such basic human dimensions as justice and liberty, took up (mainly after the 1960s) almost the whole field of concern for the best Spanish theology. The social, economic, and political issues took preference over others, more anthropologic, in which psychoanalysis would have found a place to be heard. Also, the impact of Latin-American theology, marked by social and political urgencies, still strengthened the described situation. On the other hand, Marxism offers a vision of the present time as pregnant with the future, while psychoanalysis' view is pregnant with the past, which helps Marxism find a stronger echo in the realm of theology. As we have noted elsewhere, only those directly concerned with more anthropological matters paid attention to the proposal of psychoanalysis in the Spanish scene: A. Tornos,

E. Freijo, J. Rof Carballo (Rof Carballo, 1969), P. F. Villamarzo, and A. Vázquez were among them.

Psicoanálisis y Dios (Tornos, 1968), stands out in this picture. In effect, this work deeply resonated in the psychoanalysis-faith debate in Spain. It was the first time that, in this context, the psychoanalytic questioning of faith was approached beyond the usual purely defensive positions taken until that moment. Unlike previously, *Psicoanálisis y Dios* was more interested in Freud's hits than in his mistakes, with a clear view that the errors concerned Freud while the hits affected us all. Beyond the shock and the defence, Tornos knew how to face psychoanalysis' questioning of faith in a new manner in Spain's intellectual context, avoiding the temptation of previously taming the challenge which needed an answer.

Another distinguished Spanish name is Enrique Freijo Balsebre (Freijo Balsebre 1966a), a priest, medical doctor, philosopher, and theologian. He founded the School of Psychology at the Salamanca Pontifical University. He was a Freud scholar who was decisive in introducing the psychoanalytic view in the study of religion. Also, in Spain, it is necessary to mention Antonio Vázquez (Vázquez, 1982, 2014), the driving force and Dean of the same School of Psychology in Salamanca. He raised attention on the psychology of religion in Spain and Latin America. He was an expert and disseminator of Erik Erikson, William James, Antoine Vergote, Freud, and Jung.

However, the voice of these men was not strong enough to be heard in the fields of theological work, besieged by other voices and concerns. The exceptions can be counted on one's fingers (Estrada, 1997; Torres Queiruga, 1986).

It is nonetheless surprising, even if paradigmatic of the situation, that in a work such as *Las nuevas antropologías. Un reto a la teología*, by the theologian J. L. Ruiz de la Peña, there is no mention of psychoanalysis. This author, who showed rigour and depth on other occasions, reviews the anthropological views derived from existentialism, structuralism, Marxism, anthropologic biology, etc. He does this without considering Freud's work or what psychoanalysis globally represents worthy of having a place among the new visions of man that defy theological thought, even if no one of the visions reviewed has paid so full, preferential attention or so radical a criticism to theology as the one psychoanalysis represents. Still more surprising if we consider that in the chapter dedicated to structuralism, the review covers the anthropological ideas of M. De Foucault, Levi-Strauss or L. Althusser, without mentioning that great figure of structuralism, J. Lacan, who precisely represents the psychoanalytic version of that current of thought.

Also, in other countries, the production about religious faith is incomparably more abundant in the psychoanalytic field than in the theological one. There was a particular sensitivity to taking in psychoanalysis in philosophy and theology in France. Besides the psychoanalytic authors we have already mentioned, we should address those that worked in theology and spirituality. Keeping just the more eminent figures, we should point to Paul Ricoeur (Ricoeur, 1970), Jacques Pohier

(Pohier, 1972), Albert Plé (Plé, 1968), Maurice Bellet (Bellet, 1973), J. B. Lecuit (Lecuit, 2007), or L. Lemoine (Lemoine, 2002) if we wish to summarise the theological production concerned with psychoanalysis.

We know the dramatic path of the Dominican theologian J. Pohier (Pohier 1972) through his approach, interrogation and reflection on psychoanalysis and theology. With his conviction on the close interrelation between dogma and ethics, he found in psychoanalysis the light for understanding some of the paradoxes, contradictions and dark areas in many traditional theological formulations. In his excellent *Au nom du Père* (Pohier 1972), he showed, among other things, the close links between specific versions of Christian soteriology and the Catholic considerations on sexual morality. In his next book, *Quand je dis Dieu* (Pohier 1977), in an original, creative, certainly free (for many, disconcerting), way, he deals with questions about God, the creation, and the death and resurrection of Jesus. The book was condemned by the Vatican on 13 April 1979. Disciplinary sanctions of extreme severity followed the public condemnation: he was forbidden to preach, preside the Eucharist, and preach theology, depriving him, as a member of the Order of Preachers, presbyter, and theologian, of the three functions that served as the basic frame of his vocation and his life. The condemnation and tough sanctions caused this honest and passionate man to suffer a crisis which, in living flesh, he presented (indecently for some) in his more disturbing and provoking book: *God in Fragments* (Pohier, 1986). There, he renders a personal and self-critical confession of his entire route, with reflections, always live and thought-provoking, about God, death, sexuality, guilt, etc.

Beyond the evaluation and discussion needed on this polemic case (Pohier, 1978) beyond the objections that from psychoanalysis and theology could be made against certain positions of J. Pohier, this theologian, who stands out because of the loneliness of his commitment, appears in a certain sense as a martyrdom case which attests the difficulty inherent to the theology-psychoanalysis confrontation. In *God in Fragments*, he recognises that his highly doubtful position, based on psychoanalytic data, on the theme of resurrection, is revisable.

In an area close to theology but with a philosophical preference, the writings of P. Ricoeur are an inspiring example of a profound approach to the Freudian critique of religion. His already mentioned book, *Freud and Philosophy: An Essay on Interpretation* (Ricoeur, 1970), still is one of the most honest and rigorous studies ever undertaken from philosophical reflection to examine what the problem of the false conscience, as formulated by psychoanalysis, can mean in any intellectual elaboration.

Although not so comprehensively and systematically as Ricoeur, other theologians have approached the psychoanalytic challenge in specific work moments. Among them, Christian Duquoc, mentioned above, has shown excellent sensitivity to capturing crucial questions that the unconscious poses to dogma, above all in his *Dieu different* (Duquoc, 1977). Also, A. Plé (Plé, 1968), from the field of ethics, has worked closely with Freud's texts to extract elements for a wise interrogation of moral proposals. The ample work of the psychiatrist M. Oraison (Oraison, 1952), is also marked by psychoanalytic issues, even though it would belong to the area of the psychology of religion rather than among the theologians interested in psychoanalysis for their theological elaboration. He must be credited with opening, not without difficulties, the French theological field to the issues of psychiatry and psychoanalysis. Also worth mentioning is Maurice Bellet in his theological work. Working more from the psychoanalytic experience than from Freud's texts as space for theological thought on the theme, Bellet has interrogated the experience of faith in its latent meanings and fundamental risks.

Surrounded by hard-to-define knowledge delimitations, it is necessary to refer to the French Jesuit Michel de Certeau (Certeau, 1986). A historian in his first intellectual journey, he then travelled the spaces of philosophy, anthropology, theology and psychoanalysis. An innovative critic (causing him institutional questioning), always original and creative, de Certeau searched from the history of mysticism and religious currents in the XVI and XVII centuries until the hermeneutics of May 1968 in France. From 1970 onwards, he began to look into the epistemological nature of historiography, particularly from a psychoanalytic perspective. Along with Jacques Lacan, he was one of the founders of l'École Freudienne de Paris, though he never practised as a psychoanalyst. De Certeau examined the Freudian legacy, discussed the history of madness with Michel de Foucault and glossed critically over Géza Roheim's anthropologic tradition. His work remains a source of inspiration in broad areas of Europe and America after teaching in Paris, Geneva and San Diego, CA.

In the Netherlands stands J. A. Belzen (Belzen, 1997a), who, with a solid education in social and religious sciences, history and philosophy, took the professorship of Psychology of Religion at Amsterdam University and the chair at the (European initially) International Association for the Psychology of Religion. In this field, he has done intense research with psychoanalytic hermeneutical tools.

Still in the Netherlands, Herman Westerink (Westerink, 2009b) is relevant as well. A researcher and professor of psychology of religion at the Titus Brandsma Institute, Radboud University in Nijmegen, he has worked on spirituality at length, and on mystical experience in particular, with a special contribution to the study of Freud's position on guilt feelings and its reception by theological circles. He also stands in his studies of Lacan's work and reformist thought.

In Italy, the psychology of religion, including psychoanalysis, also had substantial contributions. A must is a reference to Agostino Gemelli (Gemelli, 1955). Before becoming a Franciscan friar, he received a degree in medicine in Pavia and a doctorate in philosophy in Louvain and then concentrated on psychology. He was the founder and first Rector of the Università Cattolica del Sacro Cuore of Milan and the leading Institute of Psychology. Under Pope Pius XI, he became the first Chairman of the Pontificia Accademia Delle Scienze. Despite his efforts to serve well science and faith, some of his positions caused heated debates, especially those related to his activities during World War I (Colombo, 2003).

The case of E. Drewermann is more complex and would require a more detailed analysis than what these pages allow. E. Drewermann, in his prolific work, conducts a full orchestra consisting of theology, philosophy, Freud's psychoanalysis, Jung's analytical psychology, Biblical exegesis, history of religions and even literature and cinema. But, sometimes, we have the impression that the final result of this complex orchestration lacks the required harmony, that psychoanalysis is used with too little rigour, and that the reader can notice a tendency to manipulate psychoanalytic theory in favour of previously established postulates. We critically reviewed this utilisation of psychoanalysis in a joint work (González Faus et al., 1996, pp. 61–128) in which we critically analysed his book *Kleriker. Psychogramm eines Ideals* (Drewermann, 1989).

In Drewermann's writings, there is an undue theologisation of psychology and an undue psychologisation of theology. These bring forth a peculiar concordism, this time (what is, indeed, less usual) in favour of critical theology. But the work loses force and rigour. It is deplorable because the thought possesses a highly stimulating and healthy character for theologians and the church community. Otherwise, its methodological deficiencies should not be an alibi to try to invalidate forthwith many conclusions, which certainly could have been more solidly and more rigorously. Drewermann confronts the problems gallantly, lucidly questions certain church positions on significant moral issues (abortion, conscientious objection, divorce) and, in particular, denounces the psychological and institutional locks preventing theologians, pastors, and moralists from listening attentively to human problems.

Philosophers and theologians in Brazil reflected on the impact of psychoanalysis on religious belief. We already mentioned Ricardo Torri (Torri de Araújo, 2015), a Jesuit theologian and psychoanalyst. In addition, Karin Wondracek (Wondracek, 2003a) is a psychoanalyst and theologian. On his part, Fabiano Veliq (Veliq, 2016), from the philosophy field, also worked on the influence of psychoanalysis in philosophy and theology.

We have already noticed the powerful bibliographic production in the United States concerning the relations between psychoanalysis and religion. But clearly, the interest of psychoanalysis and other human sciences in the research on religion has been far more significant than the theologian's interest in studying the challenges that psychoanalysis would bring for them. Most of the theological reflections have come from theologians who, at the same time, worked in the psychoanalytic area, as illustrated by the example of William W. Meissner.

Also from theological work comes Donald E. Capps (Capps, 1997), ordained minister of the Evangelic Lutheran Church in America, Professor de Pastoral Theology at the Princeton Theological Seminary and Doctor Honoris Causa by the University of Uppsala (Sweden) for his significant contribution to the psychology of religion.

Peter Homans, a theologian and Professor of Psychology and Religious Studies at the University of Chicago, made engaging contributions such as *Theology after*

Freud: An Interpretive Inquiry (Homans, 1970) and *The Ability to Mourn: Disillusionment and the Social Origins of Psychoanalysis* (Homans, 1989), in which he showed a particular erudition and, above all, great sensitivity towards the socio-cultural dimensions of our time and the light that psychoanalysis throws upon them. Also worth noting is the work of Ryan LaMothe (LaMothe, 1998b), president of the Society for Pastoral Theology and professor of pastoral care and counselling at the Saint Meinrad Seminary and School of Theology in Indiana. He is the author of many publications about psychoanalysis' relation to the psychology of religion and pastoral theology.

Two figures come forward from Jewish thought and theology: Richard Lowell Rubenstein and Mortimer Ostow. The first, a Massachusetts-ordained rabbi, outstands for his psychoanalytic interpretations of biblical themes, his studies on the cabala, Judeo-Christian relationships, and his contribution to a theology of the holocaust. His *The Religious Imagination* (Rubenstein, 1967a) constitutes a suggestive psychoanalytic approach to Jewish theology. On his part, Mortimer Ostow, professor of pastoral psychiatry at the Jewish Theological Seminary in Manhattan, is also competent in neuroscience, getting thus a multidisciplinary view of undoubtful interest. He researched the psychological sources of anti-Semitism and other religious and racial fanaticism expressions. He also carried out substantial work integrating mental health training into Jewish clergy education. In his last book, *Spirit, Mind, & Brain: A Psychoanalytic Examination of Spirituality and Religion* (Ostow, 2007), he applied neurophysiological knowledge to what he called the "religious instinct" in man.

The road covered by the theological side has been long, as it was the psychoanalytic one. There is a long stretch between the positions on religion of Freud and Françoise Dolto, the one between Oskar Pfister and figures like E. B. Barrett, W. Meissner, D. Capps, L. Beirnaert, D. Vasse, R. Sublon, J. Font, ministers, and psychoanalysts as he was. The difficulties were great, and progress was often hampered by endangering setbacks. Oskar Pfister, who so often felt disappointed by the scant echo that his inquiries found in the theological field, would not be elated with enthusiasm today but would undoubtedly have kept firm in his hope. And would have also recognised that the relationship between psychoanalysis and religion moves now in more adequate parameters than those he and Freud established at the beginning of their long unfinished dialogue.

Opening up to permanent questioning

The intriguing ambiguity of illusion

After Freud and Pfister, one of the main methods followed by psychoanalysis for higher clarification of the object of their debate was precisely the one the Swiss pastor signalled in his criticism of Freud's concept of illusion. Pfister insisted in The Illusion of a Future that realistic thinking and desire live together and are forced to do so in many of life's dimensions, science included. We already pointed out how this was one of the elements that ensuing psychoanalysis would, in time, develop once liberated from the narrow epistemological frame in which Freud had enclosed it.

Illusion, which Freud presented as opposed to reality, came to be understood as a necessary and powerful force for human development and food for mental health. From being considered as a mere resistance of the pleasure principle against that of reality, Winnicott saw it as a possible source of creativity. Man always plays with reality, illusorily anticipates it, and even distorts what he dislikes. And this, to one degree or another, is needed to sustain oneself, becoming a necessary process and, in a way, unavoidable. Illusion, therefore, can be conceived as a means of transit to reality and not as a mere obstacle to reaching it (Winnicott, 1971, 1988; Wulff, 1991). It is a significant aspect of the human capacity to get involved in the world of experience, which finds more and more its best expression in the person's creativity and ability to give sense to his reality. In this context, the concept of the *transactional object* arises, describing a third area of intermediate experience between pure subjectivity and the experience of the relation with the other. Something present in the external and internal childhood world that, from an element of transition and encounter with reality, will stay and play a role in adult life. Faith, the experience of God, the use of symbols and the experience of prayer can be understood as transactional experiences, very pertinently stressed by W. Meissner and Ana-Maria Rizzuto (Meissner, 1984; Rizzuto, 1979).

From other psychoanalytic perspectives, Freud's concept of illusion was also questioned. For instance, Julia Kristeva, belonging to the J. Lacan school, affirms that the analyst's function is to awaken the imaginary and make the world of illusions possible. The analyst's position, differing from that of Freud, would consist of restoring its total therapeutic and epistemological value to illusion, even though, for this author, this does not mean an invitation to religious faith or atheism. "Repression can be atheist; atheism is repressive, whereas the experience of psychoanalysis can lead to renunciation of faith with clear understanding" (Kristeva, 1987, p. 26).

But illusion and belief are there as fundamental structures of human dynamism. Only the dead do not believe ("il n'y a que les morts pour ne croire à rien."), affirms J. B. Pontalis (Pontalis, 1971, pp. 3–11; Pontalis, 1978, p. 7). Trying to live without belief, religious or otherwise, would be a grotesque confusion of the scientific spirit requirements with the cult of militant and lethal rationality – a dire consequence, otherwise, of the dichotomy between knowledge and belief that marks our culture. To believe is equivalent to not wanting to die. That is why, like Pontalis rightly affirms, the "I believe" is not said. It is ante-predicative. And perhaps for that reason, the belief that nothing is believed can become one of the firmest beliefs.

Belief, illusion, wish-fulfilment are involved in most of the options and decisions of the persons' lives. Also (we should not forget) that of adhering to psychoanalysis. Not only pure logic reasons move in that direction. They are also taken (and not in the last place) because psychoanalysis is likeable; it is a seductive and intelligent theory, inspires prejudices in favour of one's truth, satisfies unconscious desires, and Freud imposes and satisfies the longing for a father. None of these speaks against the value and truth of psychoanalysis. The only problem would be if the adhesion were exclusively due to these motives (Costecalde et al., 1999; Görres, 1974, p. 72).

And belief always nests illusion. What is more, an illusion that should be understood and protected. "I believe that any religious faith's essence consists of that faith forming illusions about reality", affirms Scharfenberg. "In other words: faith does not make do with the reality it finds, such as it is; it is not satisfied with that and goes a bit out of reality. I don't see this as childish chimerical thought that we can disqualify. Far from it, I have the impression that we need, even urgently need, that attitude for the future and mastery of the future (Scharfenberg, 1974, p. 313) [translated for this edition]. Of course, it is not an invitation to chimerical fantasy but – like Pfister told us – to harmonically articulate desire and reality in a dynamic process in which, dialectically, desire inspires reality, and the latter organises and limits desire. "One can aim at the gratification of wishes in a way very much in keeping with reality", Pfister wrote in *The Illusion of a Future* (Pfister, 1993, p. 564).

In this way, illusion appears with that significant equivocal character that the term holds in Spanish, unlike in other European languages. Illusion can be a misleading mirage but also an imaginary aspiration, the fantasised expectation. In effect, we find illusion in the María Moliner Dictionary defined as an "image, formed in the mind, of something non-existent", but also as "joy, happiness felt from the possession, contemplation or hope of something" (Moliner, 1998, s.v. Ilusión) [translated for this edition]. Illusion, then, can be a mental creation, an exclusive product of desire, or, by contrast, arise from the encounter between desire and reality, supported by the two poles.

The psychoanalysts of Spanish language should undertake a reflection (scarce enough also from other disciplines or fields) on this bipolarity that the term illusion holds for us in Spanish. Starting from its Latin etymology related to play (*illusio*, from *illudere*, whose simple form is *ludere*, to play), it progressively acquired the meaning of deception. We can already see this in Sebastián de Covarrubias ("something that appears different from what it is") (Covarrubias, 1611, p. 75) [translated for this edition] and then gains force in the baroque literature of the Golden Age, especially in the language of the ascetics and mystics. The devil is a master at creating illusions and cunning ploys for unwary souls. But, as María Moliner explains, illusion in Spanish also has a different, positive, and valuable meaning: "tener ilusión" (having illusion) is, in effect, something quite different from "hacerse ilusiones" (make oneself illusions). And "no ser un iluso" (not being a dreamer, a dupe) is not the same as "desilusionado" (disillusioned).

With precise words, Julián Marías, in his brief treaty on illusion, gives his account of the strange and original semantic change in the use of the Spanish language from the arrival of romanticism, a move that the dictionaries picked up late. Marías writes: "Is it not extraordinary that the word *illusio*, deception, mockery, derision or mistake, a wary, cautious, sceptical, word, has come to bear the innocent, active, trustful, loving, meaning towards reality, above all, personal reality?" (Marías, 1984) [translated for this edition].

The subject's attitude towards the world depends on the "illusioned" or "disillusioned" mode of interpreting reality. Reality, let us not forget, is always interpreted one way or another. Illusion, then, can correspond to a look and an approach in which the future appears as a possibility for fulfilling still unfulfilled expectations. That is what Pfister, for instance, reminded Freud about when he was referring to that yearning for achievement which characterises human beings and is shown in the aspiration "to climb higher, over the dead and the images of our parents, while the ape, in so far as he is not urged forward by the not completely conservative nature of his phylogenesis, is content to go on hanging to his father's tail" (Meng & Freud, 1961, p. 136). Illusion, therefore, is an anticipatory force. It tries to make present in fantasy what still is not present. It obviously tries from incertitude (showing its distance to delirium) and with all the risk to fall and pervert itself into the illusory.

Illusions are inseparable from desire, "Leaves fallen from the worn tree of the heart" as beautifully expressed by Espronceda in his poem, and translated by Fernando Pessoa into English (Espronceda, 1840; Pessoa/Barbosa López, 2018).

Espronceda	*Pessoa*	*Pessoa (variant)*
Hojas del árbol caídas	Leaves that from the tree have fallen	Leaves that from the tree have fallen
juguetes del viento son	Are playthings of the wind's art	Are the playthings of the wind
Las ilusiones perdidas	Are dreams that lives hath stolen	Are illusions lost and stolen
¡ay! son hojas desprendidas	Oh, they are leaves that have fallen	Oh, they are leaves that have fallen
del árbol del corazón.	From the worn tree of the heart.	From the worn tree of the heart.

However, against the proposals from Freud and the Enlightenment, there is no reason to reduce illusion to desire necessarily. Like Julián Marías says, desire is a necessary but not sufficient condition. Illusion adds something, an argument, which is not in the desire itself and brings a dramatic character that desire, by itself, does not possess. It is something *happening to someone* and concerns the projective configuration of his life. It is not possible to narrate a desire but only to describe or analyse it; it is possible to tell an illusion (Marías, 1984, pp. 57–62).

Like Pfister remarked in his criticism of Freudian interpretation, realistic thought and desire are forced to live together in many essential dimensions of life. Because illusion, in the positive meaning highlighted by the Spanish language, belongs to the very essence of life and therefore, like also Pfister said, we cannot live without illusions.

But furthermore, as remarked by Remedios Ávila in her lucid analysis of philosophy as an exercise in disillusion, illusion owns a semantic scope almost coinciding with that of value. Illusion, on its positive side, tells us about the vital and motivating force of the subject. Under the mask of Zarathushtra, Remedios Ávila says, Nietzsche himself is also a creator of symbols, of values; an enchanter, a telling wizard, a creator of illusions ("Eternal recurrence, superman and will to power are the names of those symbols that fulfil the same function of those other value-illusions projected by art, metaphysics and ethics" (Ávila, 1999, p. 158) [translated for this edition]). So, we understand "to live disillusioned" – from the semantic nearness between illusion and value – as equivalent to living demoralised, discouraged, and deprived of enough vital energy. The relationship between illusion and the super-ego, particularly in its Ego-Ideal dimension, is thus brought forward.

We know that Freud did not appear fully convinced by his own theory on illusion. He seemed somehow conscious that the relation and contact with reality did not necessarily take place under the form of *Ananke*-like stoic submission or infantilising illusion. He even doubted that his own proposal of radical eviction of all illusion would not, itself, be illusory. So, the relations of illusion with cultural values and, from there, with sublimation, reveal a whole field of problems against which Freud struggled without finding a response. Pfister presented those problems to him from his different vital options, generating all the ambivalence we have analysed here.

In respect of all this, there is a text by Freud extremely revealing about the ambiguity in his approach to the relationship with reality. It is a short work, *Humour* (Freud, 1927d), written quite close in time to *The Future of an Illusion*. We find: "The ego refuses to be distressed by the provocations of reality, to let itself be compelled to suffer. It insists that it cannot be affected by the traumas of the external world; it shows, in fact, that such traumas are no more than occasions for it to gain pleasure. (…) Humour is not resigned; it is rebellious" (Freud, 1927d, pp. 162–163). In this refusal to submit to the conditions of reality, humour (in the same way as illusion) would seem, from a psychopathological perspective, to show a regressive and reactionary strand. How does humour escape from this, refuse to suffer, assert the Ego over and against the real world, and victoriously maintain the pleasure principle? To answer this enigma, Freud curiously appeals to the ego structure, specifically the Super-Ego, telling us: "in other connections we knew the super-ego as a severe master. It will be said that it accords ill with such a character that the super-ego should condescend to enabling the ego to obtain a small yield of pleasure. It is true that humorous pleasure never reaches the intensity of the pleasure in the comic or in jokes, that it never finds vent in hearty laughter. It is also true that, in bringing about the humorous attitude, the super-ego is actually repudiating reality and serving an illusion. But (without rightly knowing why) we regard this less intense pleasure as having a character of very high value; we feel it to be especially liberating and elevating" (Freud, 1927d, p. 166). The Super-Ego, then, comes to play a comforting and protective role for the Ego when it feels overwhelmed by the weight of reality. A protective role that Freud considers also linked to the paternal instance in the origin of the Super-Ego. Freud's conclusion of it all is clear: "If it is really the super-ego which, in humour, speaks such kindly words of comfort to the intimidated ego, this will teach us that we have still a great deal to learn about the nature of the super-ego" (Freud, 1927d, p. 166).

Therefore, humour appears as a non-pathological means of rejecting reality "serving an illusion". It is not a repressive denial of reality (through disregard or hallucination) but an attempt to look at it from another perspective, not from that of the Ego, but of the Super-Ego, which, as a paternal instance, appears caring and protective. The result is a healthy and "elevating" liberation.

All of this leads us to think that, for Freud himself, contact with reality is not fatally condemned to occur under the stoical submission that only science can drive or in the illusory mode of infantile denial of life's acceptance. An interpretation of reality favoured by desire is possible, without pathological connotation, and even more, through the intervention of the Super-Ego, the instance which, in Freudian analysis, accounts for cultural values and plays a determinant role both in sublimation and in the religious formulation. Illusion, Super-Ego, sublimation and belief show their intimate connections and the possibility of a reading of reality that breaks free from the fatal alternative of either deception or resignation.

The suggestive ambiguity of the term illusion in Spanish has captured something essential in the life of desire. A careful analysis of the term runs necessarily into that problem that, time and again, Pfister claimed before Freud in his theoretical and technical analysis: sublimation. In effect, in that impregnation of a subject's life project, illusion refers directly to the world of (aesthetic, moral, or religious) values and the intervention of desire in its cultural projection through sublimation. Pfister succeeded in opening a field of analysis barely understood by the ensemble of Freudian metapsychology.

Letting experience speak

Of course, all these questions have undeniable consequences in the psychoanalytic treatment of religious belief. Because now it would not be so much a matter of whether belief, as an illusion, is compatible or not with the analysed person but rather one of determining the sense of that illusion rightly: if that of the mirage arising from the unresolved infantile needs or wishes, or that which springs from a healthy contact with reality and can experience the expectation of something beyond that reality (although hinted there) in which one knows how to live and accommodate his own desire. Widlöcher puts it this way: "Perhaps the question, always latent in Freud's dialogue with Oskar Pfister, of whether the analysed subject can believe in God or not, should be abandoned, and turn instead on the modalities along which the person recognises what, Verb or Destiny, Logos or Ananke, defines his own contingency" (Widlöcher, 1966, p. 42) [translated for this edition].

It is there that psychoanalysis poses its most decisive requirement. It is not anymore a matter of believing or not in God but of trying to understand the motivations underlying that belief or unbelief. An issue that is not solved by a theoretical debate or through the input of proofs or arguments but in the new epistemic field opened by psychoanalysis. The analytic experience is thus the only place to approach the problems concerning psychoanalysis and faith. One place which, as we saw, took a decidedly secondary position in the debate initiated by Freud and Oskar Pfister.

We find thus an approach that escapes from the mere opposition between unbelief and faith, following the Enlightenment model response, which we also saw in the Pfister and Freud debate. Neither are we in the concordist attempt, so dear to the Swiss pastor, willing to see in psychoanalysis just an instrument for faith's purification. This attempt, outlasting Pfister, is based on a contestable assumption: psychoanalysis rediscovers Christianity. From this basis, the concordist has read psychoanalysis in a way that denies any opposition. The violence made to the fundamental concepts of metapsychology becomes then the rule. It is the only way to "baptise" those elements and take away from them everything which could question the faith one defends. Once this basic denaturing of the most essentially psychoanalytic is done, everything seems fit to go on. Through Freud towards God would be then the message. The attempt can still be seen in some religious sectors.

Otherwise, that bid to "purify" faith through psychoanalysis contains a good dose of illusion in its most Freudian sense; because it is indeed an illusion to think of an experience of faith free from any unconscious component, any connection with the infantile world and any magic or superstitious element. As illusory as a human relation equally liberated from the whole personal history weight, including its wounds.

The religious experience has no other anchoring place than those personal dynamics, always the result of individual biography and singular vicissitudes in its development and maturity; therefore, the space of a subject determined in his discourse by unconscious connections which will inevitably appear in his thoughts, in his feelings and his religious activity. And all that is happening not because of pathology but because of nature. It is not possible then, as attempted on other occasions, to sideline the psychoanalytic questioning on religion out to the neurotic behaviour field, to psychopathology, trying to save the so-called "normal" subject this way. The subject who speaks, precisely because he does, is determined by other words spoken inside him but unknown to him.

Any cultural discourse, the religious one included, is a human discourse; whether neurotic or sublime, academic or vulgar, highly formal or banal, is a discourse that, being human, is subject to the laws that psychoanalysis has brought to the fore discovering the unconscious. In other words, submitted to the intervention of an area excluded, but determinant, of all saying. In this way, any discourse admits at least a double listening. Psychoanalysis takes care of one of them. It does not – it should not – try to rule on what is true or false, good or bad. It only listens to detect the other discourse, which, independently of the truth or falsehood in what is said, can amount to a lie in that said, since, from this perspective, it is possible to tell truths in a false way.

So, the problem is to determine where faith speaks from. Furthermore, we face a fundamental fact that we cannot forget: religious language, in general, and Christian faith, in particular, use an ensemble of expressions intimately linked to the most potent determinants of the emotional world. Christian faith, for instance, tells us about one God who manifests Himself as *Father*; a Son who, with the same nature, comes to offer salvation; a *virgin-mother*, Mary, through whom the Word came and who appears as privileged maternal representation, and our *brothers* with whom we form a single human *family*. That is to say, faith expresses itself by embracing the fundamental instances of our affective structures: "father", "son", "mother", "brothers", and "family", to sink its roots in the deepest levels of our personal dynamics. The problem, then, is that these representations can be lived in very different registers of our experience. They can respond to very childish, paralysing dynamics if at the level of the "imaginary"; that is, of the pure infantile desire that, ignoring intersubjectivity, pretends to be free from any limiting structuring mode. Or can be lived at the level of the "symbolic", that is, in the context of an affective world already matured in the interhuman relations and the acceptance of its limits, making those representations work as ideal, not illusory, references. That is the fundamental question only the analytical experience and not mere speculation or discourse (psychoanalytic or theological) confrontation can elucidate.

That analytic experience can deliver very diverse and always particular courses. It would not support a global discourse to answer what psychoanalysis allows or forbids faith. Building any thesis for or against religion from that epistemic space is impossible. We shall not find any proof of the neurotic or healthy character that religious faith in itself may entail. It is only possible to raise questions on what that faith may mean in the single case of each speaking subject. As well as what an atheist position, an atheist belief, may be hiding under its manifest saying. In sum, it is a matter of understanding that we are on a ground where it is no longer a question of finding "theoretical responses" to the respective discrepancies between psychoanalysis and theology but rather, as A. Tornos asserts in a prescient way, of the theologians and psychoanalysts upholding the question on where their dialogue comes from (Tornos, 1971).

Starting from these particular experiences, it will be possible to bring out general interrogations about what specific religious beliefs can activate in the individual or groups. It will not be possible, however, to establish any general thesis. For example, it could be asked how Christian, Jewish, Islamic, or any other dogmatic or moral doctrines may establish connections with specific vicissitudes of child development and to what extent they could provoke fixations or regressions that could prevent a healthy dynamic evolution of the subjects. In this respect, Freud's intuitions, as expressed in *Totem and Taboo* or *Moses and Monotheism*, or perhaps even more, those shown in his clinical analyses (such as the Schreber or Wolf-Man cases), will keep providing critical clues on the modalities in which theology or popular religiousness formulate their beliefs in a God the Father who saves from sin and death and communicates His divine life. Or on the significations latent in certain manners of presenting theological anthropology, Mariology, or sacramental doctrine and practice. The suspicion on what infantile omnipotence feelings can involve in religion and their diversions in ambivalence and guilt conflicts will always be a key of particular interest for the analysis and understanding of the theological discussion. However, we shall always make do with what is the interpretation of a specific field of human discourse. Nothing else corresponds to psychoanalysis.

References

Acta Synodalia Sacrosancti Concilii Oecumenici Vaticani II: Periodus quarta, pars VI (1978), 626–627.

Aletti, M. (1992a). *Psicologia, psicoanalisi e religione. Studi e Richerche*, Bologna: Dehoniani.

Aletti, M. See further References in the Bibliography at the end of the book.

Alexander, F. (1935). Buddhistic training as an artificial catatonia. *The Psychoanalytic Review*, *18*: 129–145.

Ancona, L. (1983). Psicoanalisi e mondo catolico. *Medicina e Morale*, *3*: 241–253.

Ancona, L. (2006). *Il debito della Chiesa alla psicoanalisi*, Milano: Franco Angelli.

Ancona, L. See further References in the Bibliography at the end of the book.

Anzieu, D. (1980). Du code et du corp mystique et leurs paradoxes. *Nouvelle Revue De Psychanalyse*, *22*: 159–177.

Anzieu, D., Chauvin, R. G., Cordonnier, G. & Desoille, R. (1976). *Les pouvoirs inconnus de l'homme: Les Extra-sensoriels*, Paris: Tchou.

Arènes, J. (1999). *Accueillir la faiblesse*, Paris: Desclée De Brouwer, 1999.

Arènes, J. See further References in the Bibliography at the end of the book.

Ávila, R. (1999). *Identidad y tragedia. Nietzsche y la fragmentación del sujeto*, Barcelona: Crítica.

Balmary, M. (1979). *L'homme aux statues. Freud et la faute cachée du Père*, Paris: Grasset.

Balmary, M. (2005). *Le moine et la psychanalyse*, Paris: Albin Michel.

Balmary, M. (2010). *Freud jusqu'à Dieu*, Arles: Actes Sud.

Balmary, M. See further References in the Bibliography at the end of the book.

Barrett, E. B. (1924). *Psychoanalysis and Christian Morality*, London: Catholic Truth Society.

Barrett, E. B. See further References in the Bibliography at the end of the book.

Barrutia, A. (1989), Introduction to P. Gay, *Freud. Una vida de nuestro tiempo*, Barcelona, Paidós.

Beirnaert, L. See further References in the Bibliography at the end of the book.

Beirnaert, L. (1987). *Aux frontières de l'acte analytique. La Bible, Saint Ignace, Freud et Lacan*, Paris: Seuil.

Beit-Hallahmi, B. (1992). *Between Religious Psychology and the Psychology of Religion*, Westport, CT: Praeger Publishers/Greenwood Publishing Group, Inc.

Beit-Hallahmi, B. See further References in the Bibliography at the end of the book.
Beit-Hallahmi, B. (1996). *Psychoanalytic Studies of Religion: A Critical Assessment and Annotated Bibliography*, Westport, CT: Greenwood Press.
Bellet, M. (1973). *Foi et psychanalyse*, Paris: Desclée de Brouwer.
Bellet, M. See further References in the Bibliography at the end of the book.
Belzen, J. A. (Ed.) (1997a). *Hermeneutical Approaches in Psychology of Religion*, Amsterdam: Rodopi.
Belzen, J. A. See further References in the Bibliography at the end of the book.
Birman, J. (1994). *Psicanálise, ciência e cultura*, Rio de Janeiro: Zahar.
Birman, J. See further References in the Bibliography at the end of the book.
Black, D. M. (2011). *Why Things Matter: The Place of Values in Science, Psychoanalysis and Religion*, London/New York, NY: Routledge.
Black, D. M. See further References in the Bibliography at the end of the book.
Blass, R. B. (2003). The puzzle of Freud's puzzle analogy: Reviving a struggle with doubt and conviction in Freud's *Moses and monotheism. International Journal of Psychoanalysis, 84*: 669–682.
Blass, R. B. See further References in the Bibliography at the end of the book.
Boehlich, W. (Ed.) (1990). *Sigmund Freud, the Letters of Sigmund Freud to Eduard Silberstein, 1871–1881*, Cambridge, MA: Harvard University Press.
Bourdin, D. (1999). Filiation et humanisation. *Lumen Vitae, 241*: 7–23.
Bourdin, D. & Souletie, J. L. (1999). *Dieu le Père (Tout simplement)*, Paris: Les Éditions de l'Atelier.
Brabant, E., Falzeder, E. & Giampieri-Deutsch, P. (Eds.) (1993). *The Correspondence of Sigmund Freud and Sándor Ferenczi, Volume I, 1908–1914*, Cambridge, MA: Harvard University Press.
Capps, D. (1997). *Men, Religion, and Melancholia: James, Otto, Jung and Erikson*, New Haven, CT: Yale University Press.
Capps, D. See further References in the Bibliography at the end of the book.
Caruso, I. (1946). *Religion und Psychotherapie*, Innsbruck: Buckdruckerei Tyrolia.
Carveth, D. L. (2013). *The Still Small Voice: Psychoanalytic Reflections on Guilt and Conscience*, London: Karnac.
Carveth, D. L. See further References in the Bibliography at the end of the book.
Castilho Pereira, W. C. (2004). *A formação religiosa em questão*, Petropolis: Vozes.
Castilho Pereira, W. C. See further References in the Bibliography at the end of the book.
Causse, J. D. (1999). *La Haine et l'amour de Dieu*, Genève: Labor et Fides.
Causse, J. D. See further References in the Bibliography at the end of the book.
Certeau, M. de (1986). *Heterologies. Discourse on the Other*, Minneapolis, MN: University of Minnesota Press.
Certeau, M. de, See further References in the Bibliography at the end of the book.
Choisy, M. (1950). *Psychanalyse et Catholicisme*, Paris: l'Arche.
Choisy, M. (1955). *Le chrétien devant la psychanalyse*, Paris: Téqui.
Clément, C. & Kakar, S. (1999). *La folle et le saint*, Paris: Seuil.
Colombo, D. (2003). Psychoanalysis and the Catholic Church in Italy: the role of Father Agostino Gemelli, 1925–1953. *Journal of the History of the Behavioral Sciences, 39 (4)*: 333–348.
Cooper, P. C. (1999a). Sense and Non-sense: Phenomenology, Buddhist and psychoanalytic. *Journal of Religion and Health, 35 (4)*: 351–370.
Cooper, P. C. See further References in the Bibliography at the end of the book.

Corveleyn, J. (1996). The psychological explanation of religion as a wish-fulfilment. A test-case: the belief in immortality. In H. Grzymala-Moszczynska & B. Beit-Hallahmi (Ed.), *Religion, Psychopathology, and Coping*. Atlanta, GA: Rodopi Press.
Corveleyn, J. See further References in the Bibliography at the end of the book.
Costecalde, A., Gárate-Martínez, I., Lachaud, D. & Trono, C. (1999). *Hacerse psicoanalista*, Madrid: Alianza.
Covarrubias, S. (1611). *Tesoro de la lengua castellana o española*, Madrid: Biblioteca Nacional de España.
Dadoun, R. (1972). *Géza Róheim et l'essor de l'anthropologie psychanalytique*, Paris: Payot.
Dadoun, R. (1980). Un vol d'Upanishads au-dessus de Sigmund Freud. *Nouvelle Revue De Psychanalyse, 22*: 143–154.
Dobbs, T. (2008). Transformation in psychoanalysis and religion as "persons in relationship": The influence of John Macmurray. *Psychoanalytic Inquiry, 28*: 590–598.
Dobbs, T. (2009). *Faith, Theology, and Psychoanalysis: The Life and Thought of Harry S. Guntrip*, London: James Clarke.
Dolto, F. See further References in the Bibliography at the end of the book.
Dolto, F. & Séverin, G. (1978). *L'Evangile au risque de la psychanalyse*, Paris: Seuil.
Domínguez-Morano, C. (2020a). *Mística y psicoanálisis. El lugar del Otro en los místicos de Occidente*, Madrid: Trotta.
Domínguez-Morano, C. (2020b). *The Myth of Desire. Sexuality, Love, and the Self*, Lanham, MD: Lexington.
Domínguez-Morano, C. See further References in the Bibliography at the end of the book.
Domínguez-Morano, C. (1991). *El psicoanálisis freudiano de la religión*, Madrid: Paulinas.
Drewermann, E. (1989). *Kleriker: Psychogramm eines Ideals*, Olten: Walter Verlag.
Duquoc, C. (1977). *Dieu différent: Essai sur la symbolique trinitaire*, Paris: Cerf.
Eigen, M. (1998). *The Psychoanalytic Mystic*, London/New York, NY: Free Association Books.
Eigen, M. See further References in the Bibliography at the end of the book.
Espronceda, J. (1840). *El estudiante de Salamanca*, Madrid: Yenes (see Pessoa).
Estrada, J. A. (1997). *La imposible Teodicea*, Madrid: Trotta, 155–158.
Felici, P. (1954). Psicoanalisi. In: P. Palazzini & F. Roberti (Eds.) *Dizionario di teologia morale, 2*, pp. 1163–1166, Roma: Studium.
Font i Rodon, J. (1983). *Psicopatología de la experiencia religiosa*, Barcelona: Fundació Vidal i Barraquer.
Font i Rodon, J. See further References in the Bibliography at the end of the book.
Frankl, V. (1967). *Psychotherapy and Existentialism: Selected Papers on Logotherapy*, New York, NY: Simon & Schuster.
Frankl, V. (1975). *The Unconscious God*, New York, NY: Simon and Schuster.
Frankl, V. (2000). *Man's search for ultimate meaning*, Cambridge, MA: Perseus Pub.
Freijo Balsebre, E. (1966a). *El problema religioso en la historia de la psicología médica contemporánea. psicología y religión en la obra de Sigmund Freud*, Vitoria: Ed. Eset.
Freijo Balsebre, E. See further References at the end of the book.
Freud, S. (1921c). *Group Psychology and the Analysis of the Ego*, S.E., 18: 69–133, London: Hogarth.
Freud, S. (1927d). *'Humour'*, S.E., 21: 159, London: Hogarth.
Frick, E. (1993). *Wer ist schuld? Das Problem der Kausalität in Psychiatrie und Psychoanalyse. eine Untersuchung zu Martin Heideggers Zollikoner Seminaren*, Hildesheim: Olms.

Frick, E. See further References at the end of the book.
Fromm, E. (Ed.) (1947). *Man for Himself. An Inquiry into the Psychology of Ethics*, New York, NY: Holt, Rinehart and Winston Inc.
Fromm, E. (1950b). *Psychoanalysis and Religion*, New Haven, CT: Yale University Press.
Fromm, E. See further References at the end of the book.
García Cabero, M. (1976). *Freud o la irreligiosidad imposible*, Estella: Verbo Divino.
Gargiulo, G. (2004). *Psyche, Self and Soul: Rethinking Psychoanalysis, the Self and Spirituality*, London: Whurr.
Gargiulo, G. See further References at the end of the book.
Garma, A. (1966). Psicoanálisis y Religión. (La correspondencia entre Freud y Pfister). *Revista De Psicoanálisis, 23*: 318–333.
Garma, A. (2013). Repetición de traumas ancestrales e identificaciones destructivas en la religión y en el antijudaísmo. *Revista de la Asociación Española de Neuropsiquitría, 33*: 173–191.
Gay, P. (1987). *A Godless Jew, Freud, Atheism, and the Making of Psychoanalysis*, New Haven, CT: Yale University Press.
Gay, P. (1988). *Freud: A Life for Our Time*, New York, NY: W.W. Norton.
Gay, P. (1995). *The Enlightenment: The Rise of Modern Paganism*, New York, NY: Peter Smith Pub.
Gay, P. (1996). *The Enlightenment: An Interpretation: The Science of Freedom*, New York, NY: Peter Smith Pub.
Gay, P. (1999). *Enlightenment, Passion, Modernity: Historical Essays in European Thought and Culture*, New York, NY: Norton&Co.
Gemelli, A. (1955). *Psychoanalysis Today*, New York, NY: P. J. Kenedy.
Godin, A. (1986). *Psychologie des expériences religieuses*, Paris: Le Centurion.
Godin, A. See further References at the end of the book.
González Faus, J. I., Domínguez Morano, C. & Torres Queiruga, A. (1996). Psicoanálisis clerical, in: *Clérigos en debate*, Madrid: PPC.
Görres, A. (1974). *Jesús de Nazaret y Sigmund Freud*, Estella: Ed. Verbo Divino.
Görres, A. (1983). *Kennt die Religion den Menschen? Erfahrungen zwischen Psychologie und Glauben*, München: Serie Piper.
Görres, A. See further References at the end of the book.
Görres, A. & Rahner, K. (1982). *Das Böse. Wege zu seiner Bewältigung in Psychotherapie und Christentum*, Freiburg: Herder.
Grotstein, J. (1997). "The sins of the fathers …": human sacrifice and the inter- and trans-generational neurosis/psychosis. *International Journal of Psychotherapy, 2*: 11–26.
Grotstein, J. (2001). *Who Is the Dreamer Who Dreams the Dream? A Study of Psychic Presences*, Hillsdale, NJ: The Analytic Press.
Grotstein, J. See further References at the end of the book.
Guntrip, H. (1956a). *Psychotherapy and Religion*, New York, NY: Harper and Brothers.
Guntrip, H. See further References at the end of the book.
Hernández Ramírez, V. (2020). Psicoanálisis y teología reformada. Diálogo y desafío. *Revista de información y análisis teológico. CMIRP, 11*: 45–52.
Hernández Ramírez, V. See further References at the end of the book.
Homans, P. (1970). *Theology after Freud: An Interpretive Inquiry*, New York, NY: Bobbs-Merrill Co.
Homans, P. (1989). *The Ability to Mourn: Disillusionment and the Social Origins of Psychoanalysis*, Chicago, IL: University of Chicago Press.

Homans, P. See further References at the end of the book.
Hood, R. W. Jr. (2001). *Dimensions of Mystical Experiences: Empirical Studies and Psychological Links*, Amsterdam: Rodopi.
Hood, R. W. Jr. See further References at the end of the book.
Infante, J. A. (1996). Dios y la religión en el psicoanálisis. *Teología y Vida, 37*: 47–56.
Irwin, J. (1968). *Ethical and Pastoral Aspects of Oskar Pfister's Correlation of Psychoanalysis and Religion*, STM-These, New York, NY: General Theological Seminary.
Irwin, J. (1973a). Pfister and Freud: the rediscovery of a dialogue. *Journal of Religion and Health, 12 (4)*: 315–327.
Irwin, J. See further References at the end of the book.
Jeammet, N. (1993a). *Les destins de la culpabilité. Une lecture de l'histoire de Moïse aux frontières de la psychanalyse et de la théologie*, Paris: PUF.
Jeammet, N. See further References at the end of the book.
Jones, E. (1923). *Essays in Applied Psycho-Analysis*, London: International Psycho-Analytical Press.
Jones, E. (1951) *Essays in Applied Psycho-Analysis II.* London: Hogarth.
Jones, E. (1974), *Psycho-myth, Psycho-history: Essays in Applied Psycho-Analysis II*, New York, NY: Hillstone.
Jones, E. See further References at the end of the book.
Jones, E. (1953–1957). *The Life and Work of Sigmund Freud, Volumes I to III*, New York, NY: Basic Books.
Jones, J. W. (1991a). *Contemporary Psychoanalysis and Religion: Transference and Transcendence*, New Haven, CT: Yale University Press.
Jones, J. W. See further References at the end of the book.
Jonte-Pace, D. (2001a). *Speaking the Unspeakable: Religion, Misogyny, and the Uncanny Mother in Freud's Cultural Texts*, Berkeley, CA. University of California Press.
Jonte-Pace, D. See further References at the end of the book.
Julien, Ph. (2008). *La psychanalyse et le religieux: Freud, Jung, Lacan*, Paris: Cerf.
Julien, Ph. See further References at the end of the book.
Kakar, S. (1981). *The Inner World; A Psychoanalytic Study of Childhood and Society in India*, Oxford: Oxford University Press.
Kakar, S. (2007). *The Analyst and the Mystic*, Gurugram: Penguin Books.
Kakar, S. See further References at the end of the book.
Kienast, H. W. (1973). Oskar Pfister's centennial. *The Proceedings of the Institute of Medicine of Chicago, 29 (10)*: 353.
Kienast, H. W. (1974). The significance of Oskar Pfister's in-depth pastoral care. *In Journal of Religion and Health, 13*: 94.
Kirkpatrick, L. A. (2004). *Attachment, Evolution, and the Psychology of Religion*, New York, NY: Guilford Press.
Kirkpatrick, L. A. See further References at the end of the book.
Kristeva, J. (1987). *In the Beginning Was Love: Psychoanalysis and Faith*, New York, NY: Columbia University Press.
Kristeva, J. See further References at the end of the book.
La Barre, W. (1962). *They Shall Take Up Serpents: Psychology of the Southern Snake-Handling Cult*, Minneapolis, MN: University of Minnesota Press.
La Barre, W. (1968) *Géza Róheim. El psicoanálisis y la antropología* en *Historia del psicoanálisis*, IV, Buenos Aires: Paidos, 64–78.
La Barre, W. See further References at the end of the book.

LaMothe, R. (1998b). Sacred objects as vital objects: transitional objects reconsidered. *Journal of Psychology and Theology, 26*: 159–167.
LaMothe, R. See further References at the end of the book.
Leavy, S. A. (1980). *The Psychoanalytic Dialogue*, New Haven, CT: Yale University Press.
Leavy, S. A. See further References at the end of the book.
Lecuit, J. B. (2007). *L'anthropologie théologique à la lumière de la psychanalyse. la contribution majeure d'Antoine Vergote*, Paris: Cerf.
Lecuit, J. B. See further References at the end of the book.
Lemoine, L. (2002). Le dialogue foi chrétienne/Psychanalyse dans le discernement des vocations entre 1950 et 1975. *Le Supplément, 222*: 69–101.
Lemoine, L. See further References at the end of the book.
Mannoni, O. (1972). Freud y la religión. *Cuadernos Sigmund Freud, 2–3*: 57–72.
Mannoni, O. (1976). L'athéisme de Freud. *Ornicar? 6*: 21–32.
Marías, J. (1984). *Breve tratado de la ilusión*, Madrid: Alianza.
Matte-Blanco, I. (1975a). *The Unconscious as Infinite Sets*, London: Karnac.
Matte-Blanco, I. See further References at the end of the book.
McDargh, J. (1983). *Psychoanalytic Object Relations Theory and the Study of Religion: On Faith and the Imaging of God*, Lanham, MD: University Press of America.
McDargh, J. (1992). Commentary on returning words to flesh and contemporary psychoanalysis and religion. *Pastoral Psychology, 40*: 391–399.
McDargh, J. See further References at the end of the book.
McGuire, W. (1974). *The Correspondence between Sigmund Freud and C.G. Jung*, Princeton: Princeton University Press.
Meissner, W. W. (1961). *Annotated Bibliography in Religion and Psychology*, New York, NY: The Academy of Religion and Mental Health.
Meissner, W. W. (1984). *Psychoanalysis and Religious Experience*, New Haven, CT: Yale University Press.
Meissner, W. W. (1987). *Life and Faith: Psychological Perspectives on Religious Experience*, Washington, DC: Georgetown University Press.
Meissner, W. W. (1992a). *Ignatius of Loyola: The Psychology of a Saint*, New Haven, CT: Yale University Press.
Meissner, W. W. (1999). *To the Greater Glory: a Psychological Study of Ignatian Spirituality*, Milwaukee, WI: Marquette University Press.
Meissner, W. W. See further References in the Bibliography at the end of the book.
Meng, H. & Freud, E. L. (Eds.) (1961). *Psychoanalysis and Faith: The Letters of S. Freud & O. Pfister*, London: Hogarth [reprinted New York, NY: Basic Books, 1963].
Merkur, D. (1988a). The prophecies of Jeremiah. *American Imago, 42*: 1–37.
Merkur, D. (1999). *Mystical Moments and Unitive Thinking*, New York, NY: State University of New York Press.
Merkur, D. (2010). *Explorations of the Psychoanalytic Mystic*, Amsterdam, New York, NY: Rodopi.
Merkur, D. See further References in the Bibliography at the end of the book.
Moliner, M. (1998). *Diccionario de uso de español* (*2 vols.*) (2nd ed.), Madrid: Gredos.
Moulines, U. (1972). El psicoanálisis en España y latinoamérica, in Dierkens, J., *Freud. Antología sistemática*. Barcelona: Oikos-Tau.
Neeleman, J. & Persaud, R. (1995). Why do psychiatrists neglect religion?. *British Journal of Medical Psychology, 68*: 169–178.
Noth, I. (2008). Albert Schweitzer und die Psychoanalyse. *Luzifer-Amor. Zeitschrift zur Geschichte der Psychoanalyse, 43*: 133–143.

Noth, I. See further References in the Bibliography at the end of the book.
Noth, I. & Morgenthaler, C. (2014b). The friendship between Sigmund Freud and Oskar Pfister as seen in the correspondence between the Jewish atheist founder of psychoanalysis and the Swiss Pastor who pioneered Pastoral Psychology. *Pastoral Psychology, 63*: 81–90.
Oraison, M. (1952). *Vie chrétienne et problèmes de la sexualité*, Paris: Lethielleux.
Oraison, M. (1957). Le médecin psychanalyste et le confesseur. *Recherches et Débats du Centre Catholique des Intellectuels Français, 21*: 153–172.
Oraison, M. (1972). *Vie chrétienne et problèmes de la sexualité* (2nd ed.), Paris: Lethielleux-Fayard.
Ostow, M. (2007). *Spirit, Mind, & Brain: A Psychoanalytic Examination of Spirituality and Religion*, New York, NY: Columbia University Press.
Ostow, M. See further References in the Bibliography at the end of the book.
Padrón Estarriol, C. (1997). La croyance. *Revue Française de Psychanalyse, 56*: 787–810.
Pargament, K. (2007). *Spiritually Integrated Psychotherapy: Understanding and Addressing the Sacred*, New York, NY: Guilford Press.
Pargament, K. See further References in the Bibliography at the end of the book.
Parsons, W. B. (2013). *Freud and Augustine in Dialogue: Psychoanalysis, Mysticism, and the Culture of Modern Spirituality*, Charlottesville, VA: University of Virginia Press.
Parsons, W. B. (2021). *Freud and Religion: Advancing the Dialogue*, New York, NY: Cambridge University Press.
Parsons, W. B. See further References in the Bibliography at the end of the book.
Paul, R. A. (1996). *Moses and Civilization: The Meaning Behind Freud's Myth*, New Haven, CT: Yale University Press.
Paul, R. A. See further References in the Bibliography at the end of the book.
Pessoa, F. (2018). "The Student of Salamanca": an English Translation, in N. Barbosa López, *Pessoa Plural: Journal of Fernando Pessoa Studies*, 318–551.
Pfister, O. (1948). *Christianity and Fear: a Study in History and in the Psychology and Hygiene of Religion*, London: Allen & Unwin.
Pfister, O. (1993) [1927]. The Illusion of a Future: A Friendly Disagreement with Prof. Sigmund Freud. *The International Journal of Psychoanalysis, 74*: 557–599.
Plé, A. (1968). *Freud et la religion*, Paris: Cerf.
Plé, A. (1974). Les variations de l'Église à l'égard de la psychanalyse. *Concilium, 99*: 119–124.
Plé, A. See further References in the Bibliography at the end of the book.
Pohier, J. (1972). *Au nom du Père. Recherches théologiques et psychanalytiques*, Paris: Cerf.
Pohier, J. (1977). *Quand je dis Dieu*, Paris: Seuil.
Pohier, J. (1978). *Pohier: Quand je dis Dieu. Debat*: Le Supplément 126.
Pohier, J. (1986). *God in Fragments*, London: SCM Press.
Pohier, J. See further References in the Bibliography at the end of the book.
Pontalis, J. B. (1971). L'illusion maintenue. *Nouvelle Revue de Psychanalyse, 4*: 3–11.
Pontalis, J. B. (1978). Se fier à… sans croire en…. *Nouvelle Revue de Pyschanalyse, 18*: 5–14.
Pruyser, P. W. (1973). Sigmund Freud and His Legacy: Psychoanalytic Psychology of Religion. In: C. Glock & P. Hammond (Eds.) *Beyond the Classics? Essays in the Scientific Study of Religion*, pp. 243–290, New York, NY: Harper & Row.
Pruyser, P. W. See further References in the Bibliography at the end of the book.
Putnam, J. J. (1915). *Human Motives*, Boston, MA: Little Brown and Co.
Raguse, H. (1992). Der Ödipus-Komplex und die depressive Position. Psychoanalytische Reflexionen zur Wirkungsgeschichte des 12. Kapitels der Apokalypse des Johannes. *Zeitschrift für Psychoanalytische Theorie und Praxis/Journal for Psychoanalytical Theory and Practice, 7*: 126–144.

Raguse, H. See further References in the Bibliography at the end of the book.
Reik, T. (1931). *Ritual: Psychoanalytic Studies*, London: Hogarth Press.
Reik, T. (1940). *From Thirty Years with Freud*, New York, NY: Farrar & Rinehart.
Reik, T. (1946). *The Psychological Problems of Religion*, New York, NY: Farrar, Straus & Co.
Reik, T. See further References in the Bibliography at the end of the book.
Reineke, M. J. & Goodman, D. M. (Eds.) (2017). *Ana-María Rizzuto and the Psychoanalysis of Religion. The Road to de Living God*, Lanham, MD: Lexington.
Ricoeur, P. (1970). *Freud and Philosophy: An Essay on Interpretation*, New Haven, CT: Yale University Press.
Ricoeur, P. See further References in the Bibliography at the end of the book.
Rieff, P. (1961). *Freud: The Mind of the Moralist*, New York, NY: Anchor Books.
Rieff, P. See further References in the Bibliography at the end of the book.
Rizzuto, A. M. (1974). Object relations and the formation of the image of God. *The British Journal of Medical Psychology, 47 (1)*: 83–99.
Rizzuto, A. M. (1979). *The Birth of the Living God: A Psychoanalytic Study*, Chicago, IL: University of Chicago Press.
Rizzuto, A. M. (1998a). *Why Did Freud Reject God? A Psychodynamic Interpretation*, New Haven, CT: Yale University Press.
Rizzuto, A.-M., See further References in the Bibliography at the end of the book.
Robert, M. (1964). *La révolution psychanalytique. La vie et oeuvre de Freud*, Volume 2, Paris: Payot.
Rodrigué, E. (1996). *Sigmund Freud. El siglo del psicoanálisis*, Volume 2, Buenos Aires: Ed. Sudamericana.
Rodríguez Amenabar, S. M. (1979). *Metapsicología y hecho religioso*, Buenos Aires: Eudeba.
Rodríguez Amenabar, S. M. (1995). *Psicoanálisis, cristianismo y religiosidad*, Buenos Aires: Paulinas.
Rof Carballo, J. (1969). Psicoanálisis y religión. Estudio Introductorio. In: A. Plé (Ed.) *Freud y la religion*, pp. 3–93, Madrid: BAC.
Róheim, G. (1921). Das Selbst. *Imago*, 7: 1–39.
Róheim, G. (1925). *Australian Totemism: a Psychoanalytic Study in Anthropology*, London: Allen and Unwin.
Róheim, G. (1971). *The Origin and Function of Culture*, Garden City, NY: Doubleday.
Róheim, G. See further References at the end of the book.
Roland, A. (1972). Imagery and symbolic expression in dreams and art. *International Journal of Psychoanalysis, 53*: 531–539.
Roland, A. (1988). *In Search of Self in India and Japan: Toward a Cross-Cultural Psychology*, Princeton, NJ: Princeton University Press.
Roland, A. See further References at the end of the book.
Rosolato, G. (1987). *Le sacrifice*, Paris 1987, P.U.F.
Rosolato, G. See further References in the Bibliography at the end of the book.
Roudinesco, E. & Plon, M. (1997). *Dictionnaire de la psychanalyse*, Paris: Fayard.
Rubenstein, R. L. (1967a). *The Religious Imagination*, New York, NY: Bobbs-Merrill.
Rubenstein, R. L. See further References in the Bibliography at the end of the book.
Rubin, J. B. (1992). *Psychoanalytic Treatment with a Buddhist Meditator*, Westport, CT: Praeger Publishers/Greenwood Publishing Group, Inc.
Rubin, J. B. See further References in the Bibliography at the end of the book.
Saussure, T. (2009). *L'inconscient, nos croyances et la foi chrétienne. Études psychanalytiques et bibliques*, Paris: Cerf.

Saussure, T. See further References in the Bibliography at the end of the book.
Scharfenberg, J. (1974), Encuentro entre el psicoanálisis y la teología. Balance provisional, in *Jesús de Nazaret y Sigmund Freud*, Estella, Verbo Divino.
Scharfenberg, J. (1988). *Sigmund Freud and His Critique of Religion*, Philadelphia, PA: Fortress Press.
Scharfenberg, J. See further References at the end of the book.
Shafranske, E. P. (1992). God-representation as a transformational object. In: M. Finn & J. Gartner (Eds.) *Objects Relations Theory and Religion, Clinical Applications*, pp. 52–72, Westport, CT/London: Praeger.
Shafranske, E. P. See further References at the end of the book.
Sibony, D. (2001). *Psychanalyse et judaïsme*, Paris: Flammarion.
Sibony, D. See further References at the end of the book.
Simmonds, J. G. (2006b). The oceanic feeling and a sea change: historical challenges to reductionist attitudes to religion and spirit from within psychoanalysis. *Psychoanalytic Psychology, 23*: 128–142.
Simmonds, J. G. See further References at the end of the book.
Sorenson, A. L. (1990). Psychoanalytic perspectives on religion: The illusion has a future. *Journal of Psychology and Theology, 18*: 209–217.
Sorenson, A. L. See further References at the end of the book.
Spero, M. H. (1985). The reality of the image of God in psychotherapy. *American Journal of Psychology, 39*: 75–85.
Spero, M. H. See further References at the end of the book.
Spero, M. H. (1992). *Religious Objects as Psychological Structures: A Critical Integration of Object Relations Theory, Psychotherapy, and Judaism*, Chicago, IL: The University of Chicago Press.
Sublon, R. (1975). *Le temps de la mort. savoir, parole, désir*, Strasbourg: Cerdic Pub.
Sublon, R. See further References at the end of the book.
Symington, N. (1994a). *Emotion and Spirit: Questioning the Claims of Psychoanalysis and Religion*, London: Cassels.
Symington, N. See further References at the end of the book.
Tornos, A. (1968). *Psicoanálisis y Dios*, Bilbao: Mensajero.
Tornos, A. (1971). *Sociedad y teología*, Bilbao: Desclée de Brouwer.
Tornos, A. See further References at the end of the book.
Torres Queiruga, A. (1986) *Creo en Dios Padre*, Sal Terrae, Santander.
Torri de Araújo, R. (2015). *Experiência mística e psicanalise*, São Paulo: Ed. Loyola.
Torri de Araújo, R. See further References at the end of the book.
Vande Kemp, H. (1984). *Psychology and Theology in Western Thought 1672–1965*, New York, NY: Kraus Int. Publ.
Vandermeersch, P. (1991b). *Unresolved Questions in the Freud/Jung Debate. On Psychosis, Sexual Identity and Religion*, Leuven: Leuven University Press.
Vandermeersch, P. See further References at the end of the book.
Vasse, D. (1991). *L'autre du désir et le Dieu de la foi: Lire aujourd'hui Thérèse d'Avila*, Paris: Seuil.
Vasse, D. See further References at the end of the book.
Vázquez, A. (1982). *Notas para una lectura de las "Moradas" de Santa Teresa desde la psicología profunda*, Salamanca: Universidad Pontificia.
Vázquez, A. (2014). Teresa de Lisieux (1873–1897). In: AA. VV, *Maestros y Testigos*, pp. 83–110, Valencia: Tirant.

Veliq, F. (2016). Religião e projeção em Freud: elementos para o debate entre psicanálise e religião. *Synesis, 8* (*2*): 49–65.
Veliq, F. See further References at the end of the book.
Vergote, A. (1988). *Guilt and Desire: Religious Attitudes and Their Pathological Derivatives*, New Haven, CT: Yale University Press.
Vergote, A. (1997a). *La psychanalyse à l'épreuve de la sublimation*, Paris: Cerf.
Vergote, A. See further References at the end of the book.
Villamarzo, P. F. (1979). *Psicoanálisis de la experiencia ético-religiosa*, Madrid: Marova.
Vitz, P. C. (1977). *Psychology as Religion*, Grand Rapids, MI: Eerdmans.
Vitz, P. C. (1988). *Sigmund Freud's Christian Unconscious*, New York, NY: Guilford Press.
Vitz, P. C. See further References at the end of the book.
Westerink, H. (2009b). *A Dark Trace. Sigmund Freud on the Sense of Guilt*, Leuven: Leuven University Press.
Westerink, H. See further References at the end of the book.
Whitebook, J. (2017c). *Freud: An Intellectual Biography*, New York, NY: Cambridge University Press.
Whitebook, J. See further References at the end of the book.
Widlöcher, D. (1966). quoted by him in *Préface à l'edition française de la Correspondence avec le pasteur Pfister 1909–1939.* Editor: Heinrich Meng, Paris: Gallimard.
Winnicott, D. W. See further References at the end of the book.
Winnicott, D. W. (1971). *Playing and Reality*, London: Tavistock.
Winnicott, D. W. (1988). *Human Nature*, London: Free Association Books.
Wondracek, K. H. K. (2003a). *O futuro e a ilusão. Um embate com Freud sobre Psicanálise e Religião*, Petrópolis, RJ: Vozes.
Wondracek, K. H. K. See further References at the end of the book.
Wulff, D. M. (1991). *Psychology of Religion. Classic and Contemporary Views*, New York, NY: John Wiley & Sons.
Wulff, D. M. (1999). Psychologists define religion. Patterns and prospects of a century quest. In: G. Platvoet & A. L. Molendijk (Eds.) *The Pragmatics of Defining Religion. Contexts, Concepts and Contents*, pp. 207–224, Leiden-Boston-Köln: Brill.
Wyss, D. (1968), *Las escuelas de Psicología Profunda*, Madrid: Gredos.
Yerushalmi, Y. H. (1989). Freud on the Historical Novel: From the manuscript draft (1934) of Moses and Monotheism. *International Journal of Psychoanalysis, 70*: 375–395.
Yerushalmi, Y. H. (1991). *Freud's Moses: Judaism Terminable and Interminable*, New Haven, CT: Yale University Press.
Yerushalmi, Y. H. See further References at the end of the book.
Zilboorg, G. (1962). *Psychoanalysis and Religion*, New York, NY: Farrar, Straus, & Cudahy.

CONCLUSION

The dialogue between psychoanalysis and faith, initiated with the encounter of Sigmund Freud with Oskar Pfister, has covered a long road. On one side, it was necessary to shed off the epistemology in which the personal options of the founder of psychoanalysis interfered with the more specific one of the discipline he founded. Another need was to move the dialogue away from the theoretical level in which both figures remained and restart from the more limited but more profound and specifically psychoanalytic ground of clinical experience. It was equally required to strip it from the concordist intentions of the pastor in his attempt to turn psychoanalysis into a mere instrument for faith purification. Multiple resistances had to be defeated, conceptual ambiguities clarified, and well-rooted prejudices overcome to finally reach what Freud expressed in his far-sighted and precise words (inevitably blurred in so many other moments) before getting to know Dr. Pfister personally: "In itself, psychoanalysis is neither religious nor non-religious, but an impartial tool which both priest and layman (*der Geistliche wie der Laie*) can use in the service of the sufferer". Or in the service of whoever tries to know the truth about himself, we would add today.

It is an impartial tool which does not have – should not have, on the risk of self-perversion – messages nor intentions, and which does not try, therefore, either to support or reduce faith, but only to listen to it to restore the veiled elements, forgotten in the text, and also elucidate the motives to carry out such deletions and veiling. Nothing more and nothing less. Because an omnipotent attempt is given up: to know what happens with religion as if it could be enclosed as a part of the discourse. And at the same time, it stays at the level of suspicion and questioning, which will necessarily raise non-negligible defences and resistances since we are called this way to a difficult ascesis of self-dispossession.

DOI: 10.4324/9781003389804-8

Neither religion – Oskar Pfister often forgot it – can pretend to know beforehand what psychoanalysis is and can contribute. Religion also faces a renouncement: that of trying to include in its own discourse a knowledge that escapes it and that, from a place other than its own, poses the problem of its truth. Not truth as adequacy to any external reality but as adequacy to itself.

Faith will not be reduced to the condition of a defendant anxious to give an account of himself before a court. It is a matter of faith paying account just before itself, becoming able to understand itself better and make itself understood by others. As it pretends by its own dynamism, on its part, it will also have to show its interrogation and suspicion towards psychoanalysis, as gallantly done by Pfister before his admired Freud. Thus, it will reduce the pretension which, in so many ways and occasions, psychoanalysis displayed as the holder of one truth, taken simply as "the" truth.

Otherwise, religion stays there, a huge challenge to psychoanalysis and to the knowledge that psychoanalysis always has pretended to have over faith. Especially a challenge to a problem, that of sublimation, which remains a significant unknown in need of clarification. Pfister pointed to it repeatedly, and Freud seemed paralysed in front of the interpellation, probably because this Freudian concept involves a series of essential aporias in understanding culture in general and religion in particular.

Perhaps psychoanalysis also ignores much about the modalities in which the religious experience can be lived. It has not shown interest in approaching them to know them in some depth; this is serious as ignorance and lack of attention often seem to result from the shameful defences and resistances appearing in front of religion.

In this respect, it is undoubtedly significant and exemplary that a convinced atheist like Jacques Lacan showed great interest and fascination in religious phenomena such as mysticism or the baroque era of Roman Catholicism. Or that he wished to learn the history of religions (incidentally, something that Freud always considered advisable in the training of analysts) and even tried to obtain, through his brother, Benedictine monk François Lacan, an audience with the Pope. Furthermore, he had in his ranks several Jesuits, such as Louis Beirnaert or Michel de Certeau, the great historian of mysticism. Perhaps Lacan was revealing a deep intuition in all this. If psychoanalysis considers that the strategies of desire are a vital area of research, religion can teach a lot about it. To this end, psychoanalysis would have to master the eventual unconscious resistances that religion frequently seems to rise.

We referred above to that woman that during psychoanalysis was having more difficulties with her psychoanalyst addressing the issues related to her religious experience than those related to her sexual life. She was convinced that, in this case, the resistance to the analytic process came from the other side. The datum merits, at least, interrogation. Because it probably indicates the negative countertransferential reaction that psychoanalysis has shown so many times towards religion.

We saw many times that countertransferential reaction appear in Freud on his relationship with Oskar Pfister, as we also saw at the same time how he valiantly tried to combat it – sometimes, controlling it enough to be able to listen to that word of faith which caused him so much perplexity and amazement. In other moments, letting himself fold up by the negativity of his countertransference and liberate the animosity that the other part mobilised in him. But the start of dialogue took place, and our pastor and analyst also had to open up, as much as he could, to the questioning from Freud and all psychoanalysis. He let himself be questioned and stood up for himself with greater or lesser skill and rationality. He found a way to initiate the dialogue, which is still open in our time.

That initial dialogue was an unfinished one from many points of view. However, it was also a starting point for a whole road to travel. At our current stage, only mutual interrogation, which reduces resistances, brings in sidelined questions, and opens to listening to the other, will be the way to go further. And perhaps we will have to recognise that if an unfinished dialogue is still maintained today, it is because, not by accident but by essence, it is called to be endless.

BIBLIOGRAPHY

1. Abbasi, A. (2008). 'Whose side are you on?': Muslim psychoanalysts treating non-Muslim patients. In: S. Akhtar (Ed.) *The Crescent and the Couch: Cross-currents Between Islam and Psychoanalysis* (pp. 335–350). New York, NY: Aronson.
2. Abasi, A. (2012). The Analyst at Work. 'A very dangerous conversation': The patient's internal conflicts elaborated through the use of ethnic and religious differences between analyst and patient. *International Journal of Psychoanalysis, 93*: 515–534.
3. Abitbol, S. (2020). The Jew, the woman, and the psychoanalyst: A model of non-segregative social bond. *Ágora. Estudos em Teoria Psicanalítica, 23*: 11–19.
4. Abraham, K. (1912). Amenhotep IV: A psychoanalytic contribution to the understanding of his personality and the monotheistic cult of Aton. *Psychoanalytic Quarterly, 4*: 538–569.
5. Ackerman, N. W. & Jahoda, M. (1948a). The dynamic basis of anti-Semitic attitudes. *Psychoanalytic Quarterly, 17*: 240–260.
6. Ackerman, N. W. & Jahoda, M. (1950). *Anti-Semitism and Emotional Disorder; a Psychoanalytic Interpretation*, New York, NY: Harpers & Brothers.
7. Ackerman, S. (2017). Exploring Freud's resistance to The Oceanic Feeling. *American Journal of Psychoanalysis, 65* (*1*): 9–31.
8. Ackermann, N. W. & Jahoda, M. (1948b). Toward a dynamic interpretation of anti-Semitic attitudes. *American Journal of Orthopsychiatry, 18*: 163–173.
9. Adam, M. (2010). Ouverture: Lacan, un athéisme du Pas-tout. *Champ Lacanien, 8*: 13–21.
10. Aist, C. S. (2012). The recovery of religious and spiritual significance in American Psychiatry. *Journal of Religion and Health, 51* (*3*): 615–629.
11. Akhtar, S. & Parens, H. (Eds.) (2001). *Does God Help? Development and Clinical Aspects of Religious Belief*, Northvale, NJ/London: Jason Aronson.
12. Akhtar, S. (2005). *Freud Along the Ganges: Psychoanalytic Reflections on the People and Culture of India*, New York, NY: Other Press.
13. Akhtar, S. (2008). *The Crescent and the Couch: Cross-Currents Between Islam and Psychoanalysis*, New York, NY: Jason Aronson.
14. Akhatar, S. (2015). Where is India in my psychoanalytic work? *Psychoanalytic Review, 102*: 873–911.

15. Albuquerque, B. (2017). *Sigmund Freud e Oskar Pfister: Um diálogo sobre psicanálise e religião*, Rio de Janeiro: Universidad do estado do Rio de Janeiro.
16. Alburquerque, B. (2018a). Mística e psicanálise: Uma introdução, de Freud a Lacan. *Psicanálise & Barroco em Revista, 16 (1)*: 196–202.
17. Albuquerque, B. (2018b). Blue like jazz: singularidades de uma experiência religiosa e musical. *Psicanálise & Barroco em Revista, 16 (2)*: 61–87.
18. Aletti, M. & De Nardi, F. (Eds.) (2002). *Psicoanalisi e Religione. Nuove Prospettive Clinico-Ermeneutiche*, Torino: Centro Scientifico Editore.
19. Aletti, M. & Fagnani, D. (1998). La metáfora religiosa e i fenomeni transizionali. Una prospettiva per la psicología della religione. *Orientamenti Pedagogici, 45*: 623–632.
20. Aletti, M. & Rossi, G. (1999). *Ricerca di sé e trascendenza. Approcci psicologici alla identità religiosa in una società pluralista*, Torino: Centro Scientifico Editore.
21. Aletti, M. & Rossi, G. (Eds.) (2001). *L'Illusione religiosa: Rive e Derive*, Torino: Centro Scientifico Editore.
22. Aletti, M. (1992a). *Psicologia, psicoanalisi e religione. Studi e Richerche*, Bologna: Dehoniani.
23. Aletti, M. (1992b). The psychology of religion in Italy. *The International Journal for the Psychology of Religion, 2*: 171–189.
24. Aletti, M. (Ed.) (1994). *Religione o psicoterapia? Nuovi fenomeni e movimenti religiosi slla luce della psicología*, Roma: LAS.
25. Aletti, M. (1998). La religione como vissuto psichico. In: A. Fabris & M. Gronchi (Eds.) *Il pluralismo religioso. Una prospettiva interdisciplinare* (pp. 74–99). Cinisello Balsamo: San Paolo.
26. Aletti, M. (2000). La representazioni di Dio come oggetto transizionale illusorio. *Rivista Di Psicologia Analitica, 9*: 109–134.
27. Aletti, M. (2005). Religion as an illusion: Prospects for and problems with psychoanalytical model. *Archive for the Psychology of Religion, 27*: 1–18.
28. Aletti, M. (2009). Psicoanalisi e teoría dell'attaccamento: Due approci a religión e spiritualità. In: M. aletti & G. Rossi (Ed.) *Psicologia della religione e teoría dellàttacamento* (pp. 105–126). Roma: Aracne.
29. Aletti, M. (2010). *Percorsi di psicologia della religione alla luce della psicoanalisi*, Torino: Aracne, Torino.
30. Aletti, M. (2012). My concern with psychology of religion: Defending psychology, respecting religion. In: J. A. Belzen (Ed.) *Psychology of Religion: Autobiographical Account* (pp. 19–41). New York, NY: Springer.
31. Aletti, M. (2014). Religion, illusion, and their future in the light of psychoanalysis. *Psicologia Della Religione. e-journal/Psychology of Religion e-Journal, 1 (1)*: 1–17.
32. Aletti, M. (2015). L'eredità di Lou Andreas Salomé e Donald Winnicott come contributo psicoanalitico allá ricerca teologica. Alcune considerazioni. *Psicologia Della Religione e-Journal, 2*: 41–46.
33. Aletti, M. (2017). Becoming a believer, becoming an unbeliever. In: M. J. Reineke & D. M. Goodman (Eds.) *Ana-María Rizzuto and the Psychoanalysis of Religion. The Road to de Living God* (pp. 47–64). Lanham, MD: Lexington.
34. Alexander, F. (1935). Buddhistic training as an artificial catatonia. *The Psychoanalytic Review, 18*: 129–145.
35. Haghi, A. (2017). God and man in Freudian psychoanalysis: A critical examination of Freud's The Future of an Illusion. *Religious Inquiries, 6*: 41–55.
36. Al-Jadidi, S. (2021). Islamic religion and psychoanalysis: An overview. *Middle East Journal of Family Medicine, 19*: 148–150.
37. Alonso del Campo, U. (1976). Psicoanálisis y religión. *Proyección, 23*: 131–150.
38. Amado Lévy-Valensi, E. (1984). *Le Moïse de Freud ou la référence occulté*, Mónaco: Rocher.
39. Amati Mehler, J. (1985). Oggeti transizionale e area transizionale. *Rivista di psicoanalisi, 31*: 375–390.

40. Anatrella, T. (1999). *Psychanalyse et christianisme*, Paris: Flamarion.
41. Ancona, L. (1983). Psicoanalisi e mondo catolico. *Medicina e Morale, 3*: 241–253.
42. Ancona, L. (1991). *Psicoanalisi, bisessualità e sacro*, Castrovillari: Teda.
43. Ancona, L. (2003). C'è un genere in Dio? Paternità-maternità di Dios. In: C. Domínguez-Morano & R. Briones (Eds.) *Másculino-femenino y hecho religioso* (pp. 15–28). Granada: Universidad de Granada.
44. Ancona, L. (2006). *Il debito della Chiesa alla psicoanalisi*, Milano: Franco Angelli.
45. Anderson, J. W. (2007). Harmful versus beneficial religion: A psychoanalytic perspective. *The Annual of Psychoanalysis, 35*: 121–136.
46. Andreae, S. (1974). *Pastoraltheologische Aspekte der Lehre Sigmund Freuds von der Sublimierung der Sexualität*, Kevelaer: Butzon & Bercker.
47. Andreas-Salomé, L. (1913). Von frühem Gottesdienst. *Imago, 2*: 457–467.
48. Andreas- Salomé, L. (2016). *Sex and Religion: Two Texts of Early Feminist Psychoanalysis*, Piscataway, NJ: Transaction Publishers.
49. Andresen, J. J. (1984). The motif of sacrifice and the sacrifice complex. *Contemporary Psychoanalysis, 20*: 526–559.
50. Anzieu, D. (1980). Du code et du corp mystique et leurs paradoxes. *Nouvelle Revue de Psychanalyse, 22*: 159–177.
51. Anzieu, D., Chauvin, R., Cordonnier, G. & Desoille, G. (1976). *Les pouvoirs inconnus de l'homme: Les Extra-sensoriels*, Paris: Tchou.
52. Aparicio, S. (2010). L'athéisme, pointe de la psychanalyse? *Champ Lacanien, 8*: 33–39.
53. Apolito, A. (1970). Psychoanalysis and religion. *American Journal of Psychoanalysis, 30*: 115–23.
54. Appelbaum, J. (2012). Father and son: Freud revisits his Oedipus complex in Moses and monotheism. *American Journal of Psychoanalysis, 72 (2)*: 166–184.
55. Aragno, A. (2014). The roots of evil: A psychoanalytic inquiry. *Psychoanalytic Review, 101 (2)*: 249–288.
56. Arènes, J. (1999). *Accueillir la faiblesse*, Paris: Desclée De Brouwer.
57. Arènes, J. (2004). Vie psychique et vie spirituelle. *La Vie Spirituelle, 752*: 251–264.
58. Arènes, J. (2006). Marie de la Trinité ou l'épreuve du nihilisme. In: E. T. Clermont-Tonnerre (Ed.) *Marie de la Trinité. Lecture d'une expérience et d'une oeuvre* (pp. 105–124). Paris: Cerf.
59. Arènes, J. (2011). *La quête spirituelle hier et aujourd'hui. Un point de vue psychanalytique*, Paris: Cerf.
60. Arènes, J. (2012a). *Croire au temps du Dieu fragile. Psychanalyse du deuil de Dieu*, Paris: Cerf.
61. Arènes, J. (2012b). Marie de la Trinité et la question du Père: aperçus psychanalytiques. *Laval théologique et philosophique, 68*: 553–565.
62. Argent, M. (2021). Spiritual direction and Bion's idea of O. In: R. Manning (Ed.) *Mutual Enrichment Between Psychology and Theology* (pp. 176–189). London/New York, NY: Routledge.
63. Argyle, M. & Beit-Hallahmi, B. (1975). *The Social Psychology of Religion*, London/New York, NY: Routledge and Kegan Paul.
64. Arlow, J. A. (1964). The Madonna's conception through the eyes. *Psychoanalytic Study of Society, 3*: 13–25.
65. Armengol, R. (1999). El fanatismo, una perversión del narcisismo. *Temas de Psicoanálisis, IV*: 131–166.
66. Armstrong, S. (2008). Freud's Hannibal: New light on Freud's Moses. *Psychoanalytic Review, 95 (2)*: 231–257.
67. Aron, L. (2004). God's influence on my psychoanalytic vision and values. *Psychoanalytic Psychology, 21*: 442–451.
68. Aron, L. & Henik, L. (Eds.) (2010). *Answering a Question with a Question: Contemporary Psychoanalysis and Jewish Thought*, Brighton, MA: Academic Studies Press.

69. Aron, W. (1956). Notes on Sigmund Freud's ancestry and Jewish contacts. *Yivo Annual of Jewish Social Science, 11*: 286–295.
70. Ashbach, C., Fraley, K., Koehler, P. & Poulton, J. (2020). *Suffering and Sacrifice in the Clinical Encounter*, Quezon: Phoenix.
71. Assmann, J. (1997). *Moses the Egyptian: The Memory of Egypt in Western Monotheism*, Cambridge, MA: Harvard University Press.
72. Assoun, P. L. (1980). Freud et la mystique. *Nouvelle Revue de Psychanalyse, 22*: 29–67.
73. Assoun, P. L. (2009). Le démon à l'épreuve de la psychanalyse. *Lumière et Vie, 282*: 81–89.
74. Ater, M. (1979). A new look at 'Moses and monotheism'. *The Israel Journal of Psychiatry and Related Sciences, 20*: 179–191.
75. Ater, M. (1992). *The Man Freud and Monotheism*, Jerusalem: The Magnes Press.
76. Atura, A. (2017). Unpleasant business: Rat, Jew, payment, and covenant in Freud's rat Man. *Journal of the American Psychoanalytic Association, 65 (2)*: 173–193.
77. Auque, H. (2003). Dieu: un Père? In: C. Domínguez-Morano & R. Briones (Eds.) *Másculino-femenino y hecho religioso* (pp. 29–37). Granada: Universidad de Granada.
78. Ausping Birch, J. (2001). *Psicoanálisis, religión y espiritualidad*, México: Universidad Iberoamericana.
79. Avedaño Amador, C. R., González Montoya, S. & Herrera Obregón, I. (Eds.) (1999). *Psicología y religión. Tensiones y tentaciones*, Buenos Aires: Kairós.
80. Avis, P. (1995). A hermeneutic of suspicion: Sigmund Freud. In: P. Avis (Ed.) *Faith in the Fires of Criticism. Christianity in Modern Thought* (pp. 63–79). London: Longman and Todd.
81. Ayaquica Martínez, J. (2006). Dos miradas a la religión: Freud y Trías. *Interscicios, 11*: 149–158.
82. Azevedo, G. (2018). Psicologia da religião e sistema de crenças. *Numen: Revista de Estudos e Pesquisa da Religião, 21 (2)*: 59–65.
83. Babonneau, M. (2003). Un futur sans illusion? *Revue Française de Psychanalyse, 57*: 617–645.
84. Bakan, D. (1958). *Sigmund Freud and the Jewish Mystical Tradition*, New York, NY: Van Nostrand.
85. Bakan, D. (1965). Some thoughts on reading Augustine's Confessions. *Journal for the Scientific Study of Religion, 5*: 149–152.
86. Bakan, D. (1966). *The Duality of Human Existence. An Essay on Psychology and Religión*, Chicago, IL: Rand Mc Nally.
87. Bakan, D. (1968). *Disease, Pain, and Sacrifice: A Psychology of Suffering*, Boston, MA: Beacon Press.
88. Bakan, D. (1971). *Slaughter of the Innocents*, San Francisco, CA: Jossey-Bass.
89. Baker, M. W. (1999a). The psychodynamic treatment of resistance with a religious patient from the perspective of intersubjectivity theory. *Journal of Psychology and Theology, 27*: 291–299.
90. Baker, M. W. (1999b). Jesus as object: Christian conversion as interpreted through the perspective of intersubjectivity theory. *Journal of Psychology and Theology, 27*: 300–308.
91. Balmary, M. (1986). *Le sacrifice interdit: Freud et la Bible*, Paris: Desclée.
92. Balmary, M. & Marguerat, D. (2016). *Nous irons tous au Paradis, le Jugement dernier en question*, Paris: Albin Michel.
93. Balmary, M. (1993). *La divine origine. dieu n'a pas créé l'Homme*, Paris: Grasset.
94. Balmary, M. (1997). *L'homme aux statues. Freud et la faute cachée du Père*, Paris: Grasset.
95. Balmary, M. (1999). *Abel oú la traversée de l'Eden*, Paris: Grasset.
96. Balmary, M. (2005). *Le moine et la psychanalyse*, Paris: Albin Michel.
97. Balmary, M. (2010). *Freud jusqu'à Dieu*, Arles: Actes Sud.
98. Balmary, M. et al. (2009). *Le Sacré, cet obscur objet du désir?* Paris: Albin Michel.
99. Balmès, F. (2006). Athéisme et noms divins dans la psychanalyse. *Cliniques méditerranéennes, 1 (73)*: 39–60.

100. Bancaud-Besoin, S. (2012). *L'athéisme des psychanalystes: les acceptions du terme athéisme dans la théorie psychanalytique*, Toulouse: Université Toulouse le Mirail.
101. Bar Nes, A. (2021). *Psychoanalysis, Mysticism, and the Problem of Epistemology: Defining the Indefinable*, London/New York, NY: Routledge.
102. Barillot, P. (2010). L'athéisme à l'épreuve. *Champ lacanien, 8*: 109–116.
103. Baron, M. (1999). *Oskar Pfister, "pasteur à Zürich" (1873-1956): Psychanalyse et protestantisme*, Puteaux: Éditions du Monde.
104. Baron, S. W. (1939). Review of Freud's Moses and Monotheism. *American Journal of Sociology, 45*: 471–477.
105. Barrett, E. B. (1924). *Psychoanalysis and Christian Morality*, London: Catholic Truth Society.
106. Barrett, E. B. (1925). *Man: His Making and Unmaking*, New York, NY: T. Seltzer.
107. Barrett, E. B. (1929). The psychoanalysis of ascetism. In: V. F. Calverton & S. Schamalhausen (Eds.) *Sex in Civilization* (pp. 490–503). New York, NY: Macauly.
108. Barrett, E. B. (1930). *The Magnificent Illusion*, New York, NY: I. Washburn.
109. Barrios, J. (1991). *Freud ante el fenómeno de la religión*, Buenos Aires: Distal.
110. Barruel de Lagenest, J. P. (2004). *Psicologia Analítica Freudiana e Vivência Da Fé*, Sao Paulo: Loyola.
111. Bartemeier, L. H. (1965). Psychoanalysis and religion. *Bulletin of the Menninger Clinic, 29*: 237–244.
112. Bartoli, E. (2003). Psychoanalytic practice and the religious patient: A current perspective. *Bulletin of the Menninger Clinic, 67*: 347–366.
113. Bartoli, E. (2007). Off the beaten path? Psychoanalysts' religious and spiritual perspectives: Implications for training. *Annual of Psychoanalysis, 35*: 9–23.
114. Bartolomei, M. C. (1992). *Psicoanalisi e teologia. Ermeneutiche a confronto*, Milano: Cuem.
115. Baruk, H. (1965). La signification de la psychanalyse et le Judaïsme. *Revue d'Histoire de la Médecine Hébraïque, 19*: 15–28, 53–65.
116. Bassler, M. (2000). *Psychoanalyse und Religion. Versuch einer Vermittlung*, Stuttgart/Berlin: Kohlhammer.
117. Baumann, K. (2007). Zwangsstörung und Religion aus heutiger Sicht. *Fortschritte Der Neurologie-Psychiatrie, 75 (10)*: 597–592.
118. Bauzá, J. (2017). *lacan y la mística*, Barcelona: Fundació Vidal i Barraquer.
119. Beck, S. J. (1963). Abraham's ordeal. *Psychoanalytic Review, 50*: 175–185.
120. Beck, s. J. (1971). Cosmic optimism in some Genesis myth. *American Journal of Orthopsychiatry, 41*: 380–389.
121. Bedford-Strohm, D. (2020). Ruth's creations in the sand: Deconstructing & reconstructing parental and divine imagos. *Journal of Sandplain Therapy, 29*: 105–119.
122. Beers, W. (1992). *Women and Sacrifice: Male Narcissism and the Psychology of Religion*, Detroit, MI: Wayne State University Press.
123. Beier, M. (2004). *A Violent God-Image: An Introduction to the Work of Eugen Drewermann*, New York, NY/London: Continuum.
124. Beier, M. (2006). On the psychology of violent Christian fundamentalism: Fighting to matter ultimately. *Psychoanalytic Review, 93*: 301–27.
125. Beier, M. (2020). Countering antisemitism and religious violence. *Psychoanalytic Review, 107 (1)*: 1–34.
126. Beirnaert, L. (1965). La psychanalyse et le concile. *Études, 323*: 578–580.
127. Beirnaert, L. (1952a). L'Église et la psychanalyse. *Étude, 275*: 229–237.
128. Beirnaert, L. (1973). Psychanalyse et vie de foi. Essai sur le problématiques. In: Vergote, A., Ortigues, E., Trotignon, P. et al. *Problèmes de psychanalyse* (pp. 103–204). Paris: Desclée de Brouwer.
129. Beirnaert, L. (1949). Sens chrétien du péché et fausse culpabilité. *Études Carmélitaines, 2*: 31–41.

130. Beirnaert, L. (1952b). La signification du symbolisme conjugal dans la vie mystique. *Études Carmélitaines, 1*: 380–389.
131. Beirnaert, L. (1957). Freud, la religion et la civilization. *Recherches et débats du centre catholique des intellectuels français, 21*: 173–183.
132. Beirnaert, L. (1964a). *Expérience chrétienne et psychologie*, Paris: EPI.
133. Beirnaert, L. (1964b). The mythic dimension in Christian sacramentalism. In: W. Birmingham & J. E. Cunnen (Eds.) *Cross Currents of Psychiatry and Catholic Morality* (pp. 7–30). New York, NY: Pantheon.
134. Beirnaert, L. (1964c). De l'incertitude à la totales assurance chez saint Ignace. *Christus, 42*: 195–208.
135. Beirnaert, L. (1968a). Introduction à la psychanalyse freudienne de la religion. *Études, 328*: 200–210.
136. Beirnaert, L. (1968b). L'Inconscient dans la religion. *Études, 329*: 278–286.
137. Beirnaert, L. (1987). *Aux frontières de l'acte analytique. La Bible, Saint Ignace, Freud et Lacan*, Paris: Seuil.
138. Beirnaert, L. (Ed.) (1989). *L'expérience du désir et la naissance du sujet (Psychanalyse, éthique et mystique)*, Paris: Médiasèvres.
139. Beirnaert, L., (1950). *Note sur les attaches psychologiques du symbolisme du coeur chez Sainte Marguerite-Marie: Études Carmélitaine, Le Cœur,*Paris, Desclée de Brouwer, 228–233.
140. Beit-Hallahmi, B. (1992). *Between Religious Psychology and the Psychology of Religion*, Westport, CT: Praeger Publishers/Greenwood Publishing Group, Inc.
141. Beit-Hallahmi, B. (1977). Curiosity, doubt, and devotion: The beliefs of psychologists and the psychology of religion. In: H. N. Malony (Ed.) *Current Perspectives in the Psychology of Religion* (pp. 381–391). Grand Rapids, MI: W. B. Eerdmans.
142. Beit-Hallahmi, B. (1985). Religiously based differences in approach to the psychology of religion: Freud, Fromm, Allport and Zilboorg. In: Brown L. B. (Ed.) *Advances in the Psychology of Religion. International Series in Experimental Social Psychology* (Vol. 11, pp. 18–33). Oxford: Pergamon Press, Inc.
143. Beit-Hallahmi, B. (1987). *Prolegomena to the Psychological Study of Religion*, Lewisburg, PA: Bucknell University Press.
144. Beit-Hallahmi, B. (1989). *Prolegomena to the Psychological Study of Religion*, Lewisburg, PA: Bucknell University Press.
145. Beit-Hallahmi, B. (1992c). Between psychology and religion. In: M. Finn & J. Gartner (Eds.) *Object Relations Theory and Religion* (pp. 119–128). Westport, CT: Praeger.
146. Beit-Hallahmi, B. (1994). The foundations of Judaism: Psychoanalytic interpretations. *The Israel Journal of Psychiatry and Related Sciences, 31 (3)*: 200–210.
147. Beit-Hallahmi, B. (1995). *Object Relations Theory and Religious Experience*, Birmingham, AL: Religious Education Press, Inc.
148. Beit-Hallahmi, B. (1996). *Psychoanalytic Studies of Religion: A Critical Assessment and Annotated Bibliography*, Westport, CT: Greenwood Press.
149. Beit-Hallahmi, B. & Argyle, M. (1975). God as father projection: The theory and evidence. *British Journal of Medical Psychology, 48*: 71–75.
150. Beit-Hallahmi, B. & Argyle, M. (1997). *The Psychology of Religious Behaviour, Belief and Experience*, London/New York, NY: Routledge.
151. Beit-Hallahmi, B. (2006). Freud. object-relation theory. Psychoanalytic approaches. In: E. M. Dowling & W. G. Scarlett (Eds.) *Encyclopedia of Religious and Spiritual Development* (pp. 172–174, 326–327, 356–358). Thousand Oaks, CA/London: Sage.
152. Beit-Hallahmi (2007). Triggering metamorphosis: Freud and Sidhartha. *The Annual of Psychoanalysis, 35*: 151–63.
153. Beit-Hallahmi, B. (2009a). Freud, Sigmund. In: D. A. Leeming, K. Madden & S. Marlan (Eds.) *Encyclopedia of Psychology and Religion* (pp. 336–339). New York, NY: Springer.

154. Beit-Hallahmi, B. (2009b). Women and religion. In: D. A. Leeming, K. Madden & S. Marlan (Eds.) *Encyclopedia of Psychology and Religion* (pp. 978–981, 336–379). New York, NY: Springer.
155. Beit-Hallahmi, B. (2021). Challenges to an evolutionary perspective on religion. In: J. R. Liddle & T. K. Shackelford (Eds.) *The Oxford Handbook of Evolutionary Psychology and Religion* (pp. 356–373). New York, NY: Oxford University Press.
156. Beit-Hallahmi, B. & Argyle, M. (1997). *The Psychology of Religious Behaviour. Belief and Experience*, London/New York, NY: Routledge.
157. Beivers, A. & Frick, E. (2019). Spiritual care im Gesundheits- und Krankenhausmarkt: Wichtiges Change-Element und Rückbesinnung auf den Ursprung der Versorgung. In: A. Büssing, M. Warode & H. Bolsinger (Eds.) *Spiritualität in der Managementpraxis* (pp. 189–205). Freiburg: Herder.
158. Bellet, M. (1969). Psychologie et spiritualité. *Christus, 64*: 495–509.
159. Bellet, M. (1973). *Foi et psychanalyse*, Paris: Desclée de Brouwer.
160. Bellet, M. (1974). Incidences de la crise analytique sur le vécu de la foi. *Concilium, 99*: 43–52.
161. Bellet, M. (1987). *Le Dieu pervers*, Paris: Cerf.
162. Bellet, M. (1989). *L'écoute*, Paris: Desclée de Brouwer.
163. Belzen, J. A. & Van der Lans, J. M. (Eds.) (1986). *Current Issues in the Psychology of Religion. Proceedings of the Third Symposium on the Psychology of Religion in Europe*, Amsterdam: Rodopi.
164. Belzen, J. A. (Ed.) (2012). *Psychology of Religion: Autobiographical Account*, New York, NY: Springer.
165. Belzen, J. A. & Geels, A. (Eds.) (2008). *Mysticism. A Variety of Psychological Perspectives*, New Delhi: Overseas Press.
166. Belzen, J. A. & Wikström, O. (Eds.) (1988). *Taking a Step Back. Assessments of the Psychology of Religion*, Amsterdam: Rodopi.
167. Belzen, J. A. (1997b). How to assess the identity of the psychology of religion. In: J. A. Belzen & O. Wikström (Eds.) *Taking a Step Back: Assessments of the Psychology of Religion* (pp. 17–35). Uppsala: Uppsala University Library.
168. Belzen, J. A. (1997c). Reflections on the passing away of a trailblazer: Joachim Scharfenberg 1927–1996. *The International Journal for Psychology of Religion*, 7: 53–55.
169. Belzen, J. A. (1999). Paradoxes. An essay on the object of the psychology of religion. In: J. G. Platvet & A. L. Molendijk (Eds.) *The Pragmatics of Defining Religion. Contexts, Concepts, and Contests* (pp. 93–122). Leiden-Boston-Köln: Brill.
170. Belzen, J. A. (2004). *Religie, melancholie en zelf. een historische en psychologische studie over een psychiatrisch ego-document uit de negentiende eeuw*, Kampen: Kok.
171. Belzen, J. A. (2005). In defense of the object: On trends and directions in the psychology of religion. *The International Journal for the Psychology of Religion, 15*: 1–16.
172. Belzen, J. A. (Ed.) (1997a). *Hermeneutical Approaches in Psychology of Religion*, Amsterdam: Rodopi.
173. Belzen, J. A. (Ed.) (2009). *Changing and Scientific Study of Religion: Beyond Freud? Theoretical, Empirical and Clinical Studies from Psychoanalytic Perspectives*, New York, NY: Springer.
174. Benedetti, G. (1992). *Psycotherapie als existentielle Herausforderung*, Göttingen: Vandenhoeck and Ruprecht.
175. Benkö, A. (1981). *Psicologia da religião*, São Paulo: Loyola.
176. Benson, P. & Spilka, B. (1973). God image as a function of self-esteem and locus of control. *Journal for the Scientific Study of Religion, 12*: 297–310.
177. Benyamini, I. (2012). *Narcissist Universalism – A Psychoanalytic Reading of Paul's Epistles*, New York, NY: T&T Clark International.
178. Bergeret, J. (1997). Prélude à une étude psychanalytique de la croyance. *Revue française de psychanalyse, 61 (3)*: 877–896.

179. Bergin, A. E. (1983). Religiosity and mental health: A critical evaluation and meta-analysis. *Professional Psychology: Research & Practice, 14*: 170–184.
180. Bergmann, M. S. (1976). Moses and the evolution of Freud's Jewish identity. *The Israel Annals of Psychiatry and Related Disciplines, 14 (1)*: 3–26.
181. Bergmann, M. S. (1992). *In the Shadow of Moloch: The Sacrifice of Children and Its Impact on Western Religions*, New York, NY: Columbia University Press.
182. Bergmann, M. S. (2006). The taming of God's aggression and the need for a loving God. *The Annual of Psychoanalysis, 35*: 111–119.
183. Berguer, G. (1920). *Some Aspects of the Life of Jesus from the Psychological and Psycho-Analytic Point of View*, New York, NY: Harcourt.
184. Berke, J. H. (1996). Psychoanalysis and Kabbalah. *Psychoanalytic Review, 83 (6)*: 849–863.
185. Berkower, L. R. (1968). Sigmund Freud's Jewish background and his influence on him. *Sinai Hospital Detroit Bulletin, 4*: 141–144.
186. Bernstein, R. (1998). *Freud and the Legacy of Moses*, Cambridge: Cambridge University Press.
187. Bertola, A. & Casadei, A. (2018). *Psicoanalisi e spiritualità. Trauma, crisi e motivi di speranza*, Milano: Franco Angeli.
188. Bertolus, M., Ledoux, A., Lemaire, E., Pohier, J. & Beirnaert, L. et al. (1968). *La Relation Pastorale*. Paris: Cerf.
189. Bertrand, M. (2011). Le maternel dans le religieux. *Revue Française de Psychanalyse, 75*: 1703–1710.
190. Beth Fletcher, B. & Keith, E. (1994). The relationship of God image to level of object relations development. *Journal of Psychology and Theology, 22 (4)*: 352–371.
191. Bettelheim, B. (1982). *Freud and Man's Soul*, New York, NY: Alfred A Knof.
192. Beuchot, M., Blanco, R. & Sierra, a. L. (2011). *Hermenéutica y analogía en psicoanálisis-Una aproximación psicológica*. México: Universidad Nacional Autónoma de México.
193. Biale, D. (2013). Freud's Moses: The enlightenment Bible of a Godless Jew. In: C. Nadom (Ed.) *Enlightenment and Secularism: Essays on the Mobilization of Reason* (pp. 365–376). Lanham, MD: Lexington.
194. Bianco, A. C. & Vidal, N. (2014). Novas expressões da religiosidade: o que elas dizem sobre o sujeito em sociedade hoje. *Ágora. Estudos em Teoria Psicanalítica, 17*: 177–186.
195. Bidaud, É (1988). *Anorexia mental, ascese, mística: Uma abordagem psicanalítica*, Rio de Janeiro: Companhia de Freud.
196. Bier, W. C. (1957). *Freud and Catholics*, New York, NY: American Press.
197. Bilbao, F. & Giannakopoulos, P. (2005). Influence de la culture religieuse sur la symptomatologie du trouble obsessionnel compulsif. *Revue Medicale Suisse, 43*: 2818–2821.
198. Bingaman, K. A. (2003). *Freud and Faith: Living in the Tension*, Albany, NY: State University of New York Press.
199. Binkowski, G., Rosa, M. D. & Baubet (2020). A discursividade evangélica e alguns de seus efeitos: Laço social, psicopatologia e impasses teóricos e transferenciais. *Rev. latinoam. psicopatol. fundam,23 (2)*. https://doi.org/10.1590/1415-4714.2020v23n2p245.6
200. Binkowski, G., Abumanssur, E. & Silva, E. (Eds.) (2022). *Religião e psicanálise: para além do futuro de uma ilusão*, São Paulo: Recriar.
201. Bion, R. W. (1970). *Attention and Interpretation. A Scientific Approach to Insight in Psychoanalysis and Groups*, London: Tavistock.
202. Birky, I. T. & Ball, S. (1988). Parental trait influence on God as an object representation. *Journal of Psychology, 122*: 133–137.
203. Birman, J. (1988). Desejo e promessa, encontro impossível: O discurso freudiano sobre a Religião. In. J. c. Moura (Ed.) *Hélio Pellegrino. A-Deus. Psicanalise e religião* (pp. 116–143). Petrópolis: Vozes.
204. Birman, J. (1984). Sobre a correspondência de Freud com o pastor Pfister. *Religião e Sociedade, 11 (2)*: 30–53.

205. Birman, J. (1987). Psicanalise e judaísmo. *Tempo psicoanalítico, 10 (3)*: 79–85.
206. Birman, J. (1994). *Psicanálise, ciência e cultura*, Rio de Janeiro: Zahar.
207. Birman, J. (2013). Discurso freudiano e tradição judaica. *Ágora. Estudos em Teoria Psicanalítica, 16*: 11–23.
208. Bishop, L. C. (1992). C. S. Lewis on psychoanalysis: Through darkest Zeitgeistheim. *Journal of Psychology and Christianity, 1*: 44–56.
209. Bitter, W. (1954). *Vorträge über Das Vaterproblem in Psychotherapie Religion Und Gesellschaft*, Stuttgart: Hippokrates.
210. Bitter, W. (1958). *Meditation in Religion und Psychotherapie*, Stuttgart: Ernst Klett Verlag.
211. Bitter, W. (1962). *Krisis und Zukunft der Frau. Psychotherapie, Religion, Gesellschaft*, Stuttgart: Klett Verlag.
212. Bitter, W. (1965). *Psychotherapie und religiöse Erfharung*, Stuttgart: E. Klett Verlag.
213. Bitter, W. (1973). *Der Verlust der Seele: Ein Psychotherapeut analysiert die moderne Gesellschaft*, Freiburg: Herder.
214. Black, D. M. (1998). Which earth given and human hands have made: Differentiating psychoanalysis and the religions. *British Psycho-analytic Society Bulletin, 34*: 11–19.
215. Black, D. M. (1993). What sort of a thing is a religion? A view from object-relations theory. *International Journal of Psychoanalysis, 74*: 613–625.
216. Black, D. M. (2011). *Why Things Matter: The Place of Values in Science, Psychoanalysis and Religion*, London/New York, NY: Routledge.
217. Black, D. M. (2015). Religion as the affirmation of values. *British Journal of Psychotherapy, 31*: 510–523.
218. Black, D. M. (2016). Who founded Buddhism? Notes on the psychological effectiveness of religious objects. *The International Journal of Psychoanalysis, 98*: 435–455.
219. Black, D. M. (2020). The working of values in ethics and religion. *International Journal of Psychoanalysis, 101*: 992–1013.
220. Black, D. M. (Ed.) (2006). *Psychoanalysis and Religion in the 21st Century: Competitors or Collaborators*, London/New York, NY: Routledge.
221. Blanco, R. (2009). Freud y Pfister: un conflicto irresoluble, una amistad incuestionable. *Litoral, 42*: 57–72.
222. Blanco, R. (2001). Tiempo bíblico y tiempo psicoanalítico. ed., *Anales del Congreso*, México, UNAM: XV Congreso Asociación Filosófica de México.
223. Blanco, R. (2002). Antropología judeocristiana, psicoanálisis y miedo. In: I. Jaidar (Ed.) *Los dominios del miedo* (pp. 41–52). México, U.A.M: Xochimilco.
224. Bland, E. D. & Strawn, B. D. (Eds.) (2014). *Christianity & Psychoanalysis. A New Conversation*, Downers Grove, IL: IVP Press.
225. Blass, R. B. (2003). The puzzle of Freud's puzzle analogy: Reviving a struggle with doubt and conviction in Freud's *Moses and monotheism. International Journal of Psychoanalysis, 84*: 669–682.
226. Blass, R. B. (2004). Beyond illusion: Psychoanalysis and the question of religious truth. *The International Journal of Psychoanalysis, 85*: 615–634.
227. Blass, R. B. (2019). Psychoanalytic thinking on religious truth and conviction. In: R. Gipp & M. Lacewing (Eds.) *The Oxford Handbook of Philosophy and Psychoanalysis* (pp. 553–570). New York, NY: Oxford University Press.
228. Blatt, D. S. (1988). The development of the hero: Sigmund Freud and the reformation of the Jewish tradition. *Psychoanalysis and Contemporary Thought, 11*: 639–703.
229. Blazer, D. (2002). *Freud versus Deus: Como a psiquiatría perdeu a alma e o cristianismo perdeu a cabeça*, Viçosa: Ultimato.
230. Blevins, J. (2008). Different subjects: Postmodern selves in psychology and religion. *Pastoral Psychology, 57*: 25–44.
231. Blum, E. (1956). Über Sigmund Freud: Der Mann Moses und die monoteische Religion. *Psyche, 10*: 367–390.

232. Blum, F. (1995). Psychoanalysis and religion; a historical view of Freud. *International Record of Medicine and General Practice Clinics, 168 (12)*: 754–759.
233. Blumenberg, Y. (2012). *Der auszug aus Ägypten bleibt unser ausgangspunkt« die verborgene Tradition in Sigmund Freuds "Der Mann Moses und die monotheistische Religion"*, Frankfurt/M: Brandes & Apsel.
234. Boccanegra, L. (2001). Funzione paterna e senso del destino. In: Ferrarotti (Ed.) *Le figure del padre* (pp. 197–220). Roma: Armando.
235. Bocock, R. (2002). Freud's social theory. In: R. Bocock (Ed.) *Sigmund Freud* (pp. 49–91). London/New York, NY: Routledge.
236. Boer, R. (2007). The search for redemption: Julia Kristeva and Slavoj Žižek on Marx, Psychoanalysis, and Religion. *Filozofija i Društvo, 18*: 153–176.
237. Bomford, R. (1990). The attributes of God and the characteristics of the unconscious. *International Review of Psychoanalysis, 17*: 485–492.
238. Bomford, R. (1999). *The Symmetry of God*, London/New York, NY: Free Association Book.
239. Bomford, R. (2006). God and the unconscious. *British Journal of Psychotherapy, 18*: 339–348.
240. Bonaparte, M. (1947). Saint Christopher patron of the motor car drivers. *American Imago, 4*: 49–77.
241. Bonaparte, M. (1958). Psychoanalysis in relation to social, religious, and natural forces. *International Journal of Psychoanalysis, 39*: 513–515.
242. Boné, I. (2013). Mística o locura ¿Es posible distinguirlas? In: M. I. Rodríguez (Ed.) *La experiencia mística* (pp. 193–213). Burgos: Monte Carmelo.
243. Bonomi, C. (2010). Castration, circoncision et origines de la psychanalyse. *Le Coq-Héron, 203*: 16–44.
244. Bori, P. C. (1976). Una pagina inedita di Freud: La premessa al romanzo storico su Mosè. *Rivista di storia contemporanea, 7*: 1–16.
245. Bori, P. C. (1989). *L'stasi del profeta ed altri saggi tra ebraismo e cristianismo dalle origini sino al "Mosès" di Freud*, Bolonia: Il Mulino.
246. Bori, P. C. (1990). Oskar Pfister, "Pfarrer in Zurich" e analista laico. *Psicoterapia e Scienze Unmane, 2*: 33–57.
247. Bori, P. C. (1994). Moses the Great Stranger. In: P. C. Dori (Ed.) *From Hermeneutic to Ethical Consensus Among Cultures* (pp. 155–164). Atlanta, GA: Scholars Press.
248. Bornhausen, K. (1909). Amerikanische Religionspsychologie in Deutschland. Die Christliche Welt. *Evangelisches Gemeindeblatt für Gebildete aller Stände, 42*: 992–995.
249. Bortoloni, M. (2020). The return of the repressed. On Robert N. Bellah, Norman O. Brown, and religion in human evolution. *Journal of the History of the Behavioral Sciences, 56 (1)*: 20–35.
250. Bourdin, D. (1999). Filiation et humanisation. *Lumen Vitae, 241*: 7–23.
251. Bourdin, D. & Souletie, J. L. (1999). *Dieu Le Père (Tout simplement)*, Paris: Les Éditions de l'Atelier.
252. Bousseyroux, M. (2010). Quitte de Dieu, pas de sa jouissance. *Champ lacanien, 8*: 41–47.
253. Boyarin, J. (1997). Another Abraham: Jewishness and the Law of the Father. *Yale Journal of Law & the Humanities, 9*: 345–394.
254. Braunias, P. (2010). *Oskar Pfister: Ein vergessener Pionier der psychoanalytischen Pädagogik? Überblick über sein pädagogisches Werk*, Wien: Universität Wien.
255. Braunstein, N. (2006). The God of psychoanalysts. *Journal of European Psychoanalysis, 22*: 63–75.
256. Brenner, A. B. (1950). The Great Mother Goddess: Puberty initiation rites and the covenant of Abraham. *Psychoanalytic Review, 37*: 320–340.
257. Brenner, A. B. (1952). The covenant with Abraham. *Psychoanalytic Review, 39*: 34–52.
258. Breuner, N. F. (1992). The cult of the Virgin Mary in Southern Italy and Spain. *Ethos, 20*: 66–95.

259. Brickman, C. (2002). Primitivity, race, and religion in psychoanalysis. *Journal of Religion, 82*: 53–74.
260. Bridgman, L. P. & Carter, J. D. (1989). Christianity and psychoanalysis: Original sin-Oedipal or Preoedipal? *Journal of Psychology and Theology, 17*: 3–8.
261. Britton, R. (1995). Psychic reality and unconscious belief. *International Journal of Psychoanalysis, 76*: 19–23.
262. Britton, R. (2005). The use of theological concepts in psychoanalytic understanding. In: N. Field (Ed.) *Ten Lectures on Psychotherapy and Spirituality* (pp. 91–106). London: Karnac.
263. Brokaw, B. F. & Edwards, K. J. (1994). The relationship of God image to level of object relations development. *Journal of Psychology and Theology, 22*: 352–371.
264. Bronheim, H. E. (1994). Psychoanalysis and faith. *The Journal of American Academic for Psychoanalysis and Dynamic Psychiatry, 22 (4)*: 681–697.
265. Brown, L. B., (Ed.) (1985). *Advances in the Psychology of Religion*, Oxford: Pergamon Press.
266. Brown, N. O. (1958). *Life Against Death: The Psychoanalytic Meaning of History*, Middletown, CT: Wesleyan University Press.
267. Brown, S. (1981). A look at Oskar Pfister and his relationship to Sigmund Freud. *Journal of Pastoral Care, 35 (4)*: 220–233.
268. Browning, D. S. (1987). *Religious Thought and the Modern Psychologies: A Critical Conversation in the Theology of Culture*, Philadelphia, PA: Fortress Press.
269. Browning, D. S. (1973). *Generative Man: Psychoanalytic Perspectives*, Philadelphia, PA: Westminster Press.
270. Browning, D. S. & Cooper, T. D. (2004). *Religious Thought and the Modern Psychologies* (2nd ed.). Minneapolis, MN: Fortress Press.
271. Brunner, J. (1991). The (ir)relevance of Freud's Jewish identity to the origins of psychoanalysis. *Psychoanalysis and Contemporary Thought, 14*: 655–684.
272. Bucchini-Giamarchi, M. (1997). De la croyance religieuse à l'athéisme. *Revue française de psychanalyse, 61*: 981–988.
273. Buckley, P. (1981). Mystical experience and schizophrenia. *Schizophrenia Bulletin, 7*: 516–521.
274. Budden, A. (2008). Pathologizing possession: An essay on mind, self, and experience in dissociation. *Anthropology of Consciousness, 14*: 27–59.
275. Buri, J. R. & Mueller, R. A. (1993). Psychoanalytic theory and loving God concepts: Parent referencing versus self-referencing. *The Journal of Psychology: Interdisciplinary and Applied, 127 (1)*: 17–27.
276. Burnham, J. C. (1985). The encounter of Christian theology with deterministic psychology and psychoanalysis. *Bulletin of the Menninger Clinic, 49 (4)*: 321–352.
277. Bustamante, C. (2006). María Magdalena: Literatura, psicoanálisis y teología. *Teología y Vida, 17*: 304–418.
278. Caballero Arencibia, A. (1994). *Psicoanálisis y Biblia. El psicoanálisis aplicado a la investigación de textos bíblicos*, Salamanca: Universidad Pontificia.
279. Cabezas de Herrera, R. (1989). *Freud, el teólogo negativo*, Salamanca: Universidad Pontificia.
280. Cabral, A. C. (2007). A abordagem Freudiana da ilusão e da crença: A posição religiosa e a posição do analista. *Revista de Psicanálise da Sociedade Psicanalítica de Porto Alegre, 14*: 541–555.
281. Caldwell, R. (1989). *The Origin of the Gods*, New York, NY: Oxford University Press.
282. Camus-Donnet (2011). Havvah, la vie. Quelle origine? *Revue Française de Psychanalyse, 75*: 1711–1717.
283. Cantor, J. (2008). Vision and virtue in psychoanalysis and Buddhism: Anatta and its implications for social responsibilities. *Psychoanalytic Inquiry, 28*: 532–540.
284. Cantz, P. (2012). Towards a biblical psychoanalysis: a second look at the first book: Mental health. *Religion & Culture, 15*: 779–797.

285. Cantz, P. & Castle, M. (2013). A psycho-biblical response to death anxiety: Separation and individuation dynamics in the Babel narrative. *Journal of Psychology and Theology, 41 (4)*: 327–339.
286. Capps, D. (1985). Agustine as narcissist. *Journal of the American Academy of Religion, 53*: 115–127.
287. Capps, D. (1997). *Men, Religion, and Melancholia: James, Otto, Jung and Erikson*, New Haven, CT: Yale University Press.
288. Capps, D. (2000). *Jesus: A Psychological Biography*.St, Louis, MO: Chalice.
289. Caaps, D. (2000b). *Social Phobia: Alleviating Anxiety in an Age of Self-Promotion*, St. Louis, MO: Chalice; Wipf & Stoc.
290. Capps, D. (Ed.) (2001). *Freud and Freudians on Religion: A Reader*, New Haven, CT: Yale University Press.
291. Capps, D. (2002). *Men and their Religion: Honor, Hope, and Humor*, Harrisburg, PA: Trinity Press International.
292. Capps, D. (2004). Leonardo's Mona Lisa: Iconic center of male melancholic religion. *Pastoral Psychology, 53*: 107–137.
293. Capps, D. (2005). *Young Clergy: A Biographical-Developmental Study*, New York, NY: Haworth.
294. Capps, D. (2006). The 'Reversal of Generations' phenomenon as illustrated by the lives of John Henry Newman and Abraham Lincoln. *Pastoral Psychology, 55*: 3–25.
295. Capps, D. (2007a). The making of a reliably religious boy. *Pastoral Psychology, 55*: 253–270.
296. Capps, D. (2007b). Augustine's Confessions: Self-reproach and the melancholy self. *Pastoral Psychology, 55*: 571–592.
297. Capps, D. (2012). The path of least resistance. In: J. A. Belzen (Ed.) *Psychology of Religion: Autobiographical Accounts* (pp. 43–52). New York, NY: Springer Science.
298. Capps, D. (2013). *At Home in the World: A Study in Psychoanalysis, Religion, and Art*, Eugene, OR: Lutterworth Press.
299. Capps, D. & Carlin, N. (2007c). Mental illness publications in major pastoral care journals from 1950 to 2003. *Pastoral Psychology, 55*: 593–600.
300. Capps, D., Capps, W. H. & Bradford, M. G. (Eds.) (1977). *Encounter With Erikson: Historical Interpretation and Religious Biography*, Santa Barbara, CA: Scholar Press.
301. Cardoso Bertoldo, F. (2017). *Sigmund Freud e Jürgen Moltmann – Da ilusão à maturidade cristã: Um estudo interdisciplinar entre teologia e psicanálise*, Porto Alegre: PUCRS.
302. Carr, W. (2000). Some reflections on spirituality and mental health. *Mental Health, Religion & Culture, 3 (1)*: 1–12.
303. Carroll, M. P. (1986). *The Cult of the Virgin Mary: Psychological Origins*, Princeton, NJ: Princeton University Press.
304. Carroll, M. P. (1987). "Moses and Monotheism" revisited Freud's "Personal Myth". *American Imago, 44*: 15–35.
305. Carroll, M. P. (1987). Praying the Rosary: The anal-erotic origin of a popular Catholic devotion. *Journal for the Scientific Study of Religion, 26*: 486–498.
306. Carroll, M. P. (1989). *Catholic Cults and Devotions: A Psychological Inquiry*, Montreal: McGill-Queens Press.
307. Carroll, M. P. (1991). Ernest Jones on Holy Communion: Refurbishing an early psychoanalytic insight. *Journal of Psychohistory, 18*: 307–315.
308. Carroll, M. P. (1999). *Irish Pilgrimage, Holy Wells and Popular Catholic Devotion*, Baltimore, MD: The Johns Hopkins University Press.
309. Carroll, M. P. (2010). Love the mother, hate the father: Understanding sociology's of Freud on religion. Invehement rejection. In: G. Kaplan & W. Parson (Eds.) *Disciplining Freud on Religion: Perspectives from the Humanities and Sciences* (pp. 87–105). Lanham, MD: Lexington Books.
310. Carter, J. D. & Narramore, B. (1976). *The Integration of Psychology and Theology: An Introduction*, Grand Rapids, MI: Zondervan.

311. Carulli, R. G. (2012). Psicoterapia e religione. Difficoltà d'indagine e indicazioni tecniche. *Psichiatria e Psicoterapia, 31*: 192–204.
312. Caruso, I. (1946). *Religion und Psychotherapie*, Insbruck: Buckdruckerei Tyrolia.
313. Caruso, I. & Tango Duque, R. (1960). Valores espirituales y psicoanálisis. *Revista de Espiritualidad, 19*: 51–55.
314. Carveth, D. L. (1994). Dark Epiphany: The encounter with finitude or the discovery of the object in the body. *Psychoanalysis and Contemporary Thought, 17*: 215–250.
315. Carveth, D. L. (1998). Freud's flawed philosophy of religion: A reply to Rempel. *Canadian Journal of Psychoanalysis, 6*: 141–147.
316. Carveth, D. L. (1999a). Is there a future in disillusion? Constructionist and deconstructionist approaches in psychoanalysis. *Journal of the American Academy of Psychoanalysis, 27*: 325–358.
317. Carveth, D. L. (1999b). Christianity: A Kleinian perspective. *Canadian Journal of Psychoanalysis, 7*: 187–121.
318. Carveth, D. L. (2013). *The Still Small Voice: Psychoanalytic Reflections on Guilt and Conscience*, London: Karnac.
319. Carveth, D. L. (2020). Psychoanalysis is spirituality. *Vestigia, 2*: 19–61.
320. Carveth, D. L. (1996). Psychoanalytic conceptions of the Passions. In: J. O'Neil (Ed.) *Freud and the Passions* (pp. 25–51). University Park, PA: The Pennsylvania State University.
321. Casement, P. (2020). *Religion and Psychoanalysis*, London: Aeon Books Ltd.
322. Casey, R. P. (1942). Oedipus motivation in religious thought and fantasy. *Psychiatry, 5*: 219–228.
323. Casey, R. P. (1938). The psychoanalytic study of religion. *Journal of Anormal and Social Psychology, 33*: 437–452.
324. Castilho Pereira, W. C. (2004). *A formação religiosa em questão*, Petropolis: Vozes.
325. Castilho Pereira, W. C. (2012). *Sofrimento psíquico dos presbíteros. Dor institucional*, Petropolis: Vozes.
326. Castilho Pereira, W. (2021). *Os Sete pecados capitais à luz da psicanálise*, Petropolis: Vozes.
327. Castillo Ramírez, J. D. (2007). Réplica. In: C. Domínguez Morano (Ed.) *Reflexiones sobre religión y psicoanálisis* (pp. 185–229). Puebla: Universidad Iberoamericana.
328. Castillo Ramírez, J. D. (2008). Gradiva, Moisés, Rain Man y el ocurrente Lacan. reflexión crítica sobre el psicoanálisis aplicado. México: ITESO.
329. Castro Álvarez, E. (2016). Una mística en análisis con Lacan. *Revista de la Escuela lacaniana de Psicoanálisis,28*. http://elpsicoanalisis.elp.org.es/
330. Catalan, J. F. (1986). Psychisme et vie spirituelle. In: *Dictionnaire de Spiritualité, XII*, (pp. 2569–2605). Paris: Beauchesne.
331. Catalan, J. F. (1991). *Expérience spirituelle et psychologie*, Paris: Desclée de Brouwer.
332. Catalan, J. F. (1993). *L'homme et sa religion. Approche psychologique*, Paris: Desclée de Brouwer.
333. Catalan, J. F. (2003). Illusion? La part du rêve. *Christus, 197*: 55–61.
334. Cataldo, L. M. (2007). Religious experience and the transformation of narcissism: Kohutian theory and the life of St. Francis of Assisi. *Journal of Religion & Health, 46*: 527–540.
335. Cataldo, L. M. (2019a). Where God is between us: Religious experience, surrender, and the third in clinical perspective. *Psychoanalytic Perspectives, 16*: 113–133.
336. Causse, J. D. (1999). *La Haine et l'amour de Dieu*, Genève: Labor et Fides.
337. Causse, J. D. (2007). Métaphore paternelle: judaïsme et christianisme. Une lecture de Jacques Lacan. *Études théologiques et religieuses, 82*: 249–266.
338. Causse, J. D. (2012). Lacan avec saint Paul. Loi, désir et grâce. *Laval théologique et philosophique, 68*: 541–551.
339. Causse, J. D. (2014). Le corps et l'expérience mystique. Analyse à la lumière de Jacques Lacan et de Michel de Certeau. *Cahiers d'études du religieux. Recherches Interdisciplinaires, 13*: 1–11.

340. Causse, J. D. (2018). *Lacan et le christianisme*, Paris: Campagne Première.
341. Causse, J.-D. & Cuvillier, É (2015). *Viaje a través del cristianismo: exégesis, antropología, psicoanálisis*, Santander: Sal Terrae.
342. Cavell, M. (2007) Comment on "The Return of the Repressed: Narcissism, Religion, and the Ferment in Psychoanalysis" by James W. Jones. *The Annual of Psychoanalysis 35*:61–65.
343. Cavell, M. (2016). Freud and the Buddha: the couch and the cushion. *The Psychoanalytic Quarterly, 85 (3)*: 793–800.
344. Cazacu, O. (2013). *Orthodoxy and Psychoanalysis. Dirge or Polychronion to the Centuries-Old Tradition?* Frankfurt am Main: Internationaler Verlag der Wissenschaften.
345. Ceccarelli, P. R. (2014). Religião ou Ilusão?: O embate Freud x Pfister. *Reverso, 36*: 75–83.
346. Cecero, J. J., Marmon, T. S., Beitel, M., Hutz, A. & Jones, C. (2004). Images of mother, self, and God as predictors of dysphoria in non-clinical samples. *Personality and the Individual Differences, 36*: 1669–1680.
347. Cenacchi, G. (1985). Ermeneutica del raportto tra religione e psicoanalisi nel pensiero di Sigmund Freud. *Sapienza, 38*: 155–175.
348. Certeau, M. de (1975). Ce que Freud fait de l'histoire. A propos de "Une névrose démoniaque au XVII siècle". In. M. de Certeau, *L'écriture de l'histoire* (pp. 291–314). Paris: Gallimard.
349. Certeau, M. (1977). Le corps folié. Mystique et folie aux XVI et XVII siècles. In: A. Verdiglione (Ed.) *La folie dans la psychanalyse* (pp. 189–203). Paris: Payot.
350. Certeau, M. (1986). *Heterologies. Discourse on the Other*, Minneapolis, MN: University of Minnesota Press.
351. Certeau, M. (1988). *The Writing of History*, New York, NY: Columbia University Press.
352. Certeau, M. (1992). Mysticism. *Diacritics, 22*: 11–25.
353. Certeau, M. (2000). *The Possession at Loudun*, Chicago, IL: *University of Chicago Press.*
354. Chamoun, M. (2005). Islam et Psychanalyse dans la culture arabo-musulmane. *Pratiques Psychologiques, 11*: 3–13.
355. Chandler, T. (1962). Ikhnaton and Moses. *American Imago, 19*: 127–139.
356. Chapman, C. (1977). Freud's critique of religion: Neglect of the anxiety theory. *Psychoanalysis and Contemporary Thought, 20 (1)*: 147–160.
357. Charles, M. (2003). On Faith, hope, and possibility. *The Journal of the American Academy of Psychoanalysis and Dynamic Psychiatry, 31*: 687–704.
358. Charles, M. (2009). Working with a patient claiming a direct relationship with God: Encountering otherness. *Journal of the American Academy of Psychoanalysis & Dynamic Psychiatry, 37*: 21–34.
359. Charme, S. L. (1983). Religion and the theory of masochism. *Journal of Religion and Health, 22*: 221–233.
360. Charron, J. M. (1992). *De narcisse à Jésus. La quête de l'identité chez François d'Assise*, Paris: Cerf.
361. Chartier, M. & Goehner, L. (1976). A study in the relationship of parent-adolescent communication, Self-esteem, and God image. *Journal of Psychology and Theology, 4*: 227–232.
362. Chasseguet-Smirgel, J. (1988). Some thoughts on Freud's attitude during the Nazi period. *Psychoanalysis and Contemporary Thought, 11*: 249–265.
363. Chessick, R. D. (1988). Prolegomena to the study of Paul Ricoeur's Freud and philosophy. *Psychoanalytic Review, 75 (2)*: 299–318.
364. Chaves, W. C. & Nani Gonçalves, R. H. (2008). Considerações a respeito da concepção de religião nos textos freudianos 'O futuro de uma ilusão' e 'O mal-estar na cultura'. *Revista Mal-estar e Subjetividade, 8*: 453–473.
365. Chemouni, J. (1991). *Freud, la psychanalyse et le judaisme. Un messianisme sécularisé*, Paris: Editions Universitaires.

366. Choisy, M. (1950). *Psychanalyse et Catholicisme*, Paris: l'Arche.
367. Choisy, M. (1955). *Le chrétien devant la psychanalyse*, Paris: Téqui.
368. Chemouni, J. (1988). *Freud et le Sionisme: terre psychanalytique, terre promise*, Paris: Solin.
369. Chorne, D. & Goldenberg, M. (Eds.) (2006). *La creencia y el psicoanálisis*, Buenos Aires: Fondo de Cultura Económica.
370. Christensen, C. W. (1963). Religious conversion. *Archives of General Psychiatry, 9*: 207–216.
371. Christensen, L. W. (1999). Suffering and the dialectical Self in Buddhism and relational psychoanalysis. *American Journal of Psychoanalysis, 59*: 37–57.
372. Cimino, C. (2010). The ecstatic mind. *The International Journal of Psychoanalysis, 91*: 585–595.
373. Clack, B. (2007). After Freud: Phantasy and imagination in the philosophy of religion. *Philosophy Compass, 3*: 203–221.
374. Clemens, N. A. (2013). Psyche-the meeting of mind and soul: current psychoanalytic views on the mental representation of God. *Journal of Psychiatric Practice, 19 (6)*: 495–497.
375. Clément, C. & Kakar, S. (1999). *La folle et le saint*, Paris: Seuil.
376. Clemente, M. (2020). *Eros Crucified: Death, Desire, and the Divine in Psychoanalysis and Philosophy of Religion*, London/New York, NY: Routledge.
377. Coelho, D. M. (2002). O texto freudiano como analisador da cultura: Uma resposta aos discursos totalizantes da ciência e da religião. *Revista Mal estar e Subjetividade, 2*: 123–144.
378. Cohen, M. & Gereboff, J. (2004). Orthodox Judaism and psychoanalysis: Toward dialogue and reconciliation. *The Journal of American Academic for Psychoanalysis and Dynamic Psychiatry, 32 (2)*: 267–286.
379. Cohen, M. (2002). Convergence: maturation and integration in the course of a religious conversion. *The Journal of American Academic for Psychoanalysis and Dynamic Psychiatry, 30 (3)*: 383–400.
380. Cohen, M. (2003). The affirmation of a religious (not merely spiritual!) orientation in clinical treatment. *Journal of the American Academy of Psychoanalysis and Dynamic Psychiatry, 31*: 269–273.
381. Cohen, M. (2005). The bibliography to Spero's comments should stand on its own as a review of the pertinent literature on psychoanalysis and religion. *The Journal of American Academic for Psychoanalysis and Dynamic Psychiatry, 33*: 561–565.
382. Cohen, M. (2006). Opening psychoanalytic space to the spiritual. *Psychoanalytic Review, 93 (3)*: 505–509.
383. Cohen, M. (2009). An old God awakens, briefly. *The Journal of American Academic for Psychoanalysis and Dynamic Psychiatry, 37*: 35–43.
384. Cohen, M. (2019). Working with religion: Often neglected aspects of transference and countertransference. *The American Journal of Psychoanalysis, 79*: 103–113.
385. Col, J. J. (1996). *Psicoanálisis de Freud y religión. Estado actual de ambigüedades por resolver*, Bahía Blanca: Instituto Juan XXIII.
386. Cole, W. G. (2017). *Sex, Christianity, and Psychoanalysis*, London/New York, NY: Routledge.
387. Collins, B. (2020). *The Other Rāma: Matricide and Genocide in the Mythology of Paraśurāma*, Albany, NY: N.Y. State University of New York Press.
388. Colombo, D. (2003). Psychoanalysis and the Catholic Church in Italy: The role of Father Agostino Gemelli, 1925–1953. *Journal of the History of the Behavioral Sciences, 39 (4)*: 333–348.
389. Coltart, N. (1994). The practice of psychoanalysis and Buddhism. In: J. Didion (Ed.) *Slouching Towards Bethlehem* (pp. 164–175). New York, NY: The Guilford Press.
390. Combres, L. (2013). Function(s) of religion in the contemporary world: psychoanalytic perspectives: About new types of religious conversions. *Journal of Religion and Health, 52 (4)*: 1396–1381.

391. Conde Díaz, A. (2006). *La religión en el diván*, Madrid: Biblioteca Nueva.
392. Contardi, R. (2012). II giovane Freud studente di religione: I'apprendistato filosofico via di accesso al continente psichico. *Rivista di Psicoanalisi, 58*: 821–842.
393. Cooper, P. C. (1998). The disavowal of the spirit: Integration and wholeness in Buddhism and psychoanalysis. In: A. Molino (Ed.) *The Couch and the Tree: Dialogues in Psychoanalysis and Buddhism* (pp. 231–246). New York, NY: North Point Press.
394. Cooper, P. C. (1999a). Sense and non-sense: Phenomenology, Buddhist and psychoanalytic. *Journal of Religion and Health, 35* (*4*): 351–370.
395. Cooper, P. C. (1999b). Buddhist meditation and countertransference: A case study. *American Journal of Psychoanalysis, 59*: 71–86.
396. Cooper, P. C. (2000). Unconscious process: Zen and Psychoanalytic Versions. *Journal of Religion and Health, 51*: 57–69.
397. Cooper, P. C. (2001a). Clouds into rain. *Journal of Religion and Mental Health, 40*: 167–184.
398. Cooper, P. C. (2001b). The gap between: Being and knowing in Zen Buddhism and psychoanalysis. *American Journal of Psychoanalysis, 61*: 341–362.
399. Cooper, P. C. (2002). Between wonder and doubt: Psychoanalysis in the goal-free zone. *American Journal of Psychoanalysis, 62*: 95–118.
400. Cooper, P. C. (2004). The abyss becoming well: psychoanalysis and reversals in perspective. *Psychoanalytic Review, 91*: 157–177.
401. Cooper, P. C. (2014). Zen meditation, reverie, and psychoanalytic listening. *Psychoanalytic Review, 101* (*6*): 795–813, 147–161.
402. Cooper, P. C. (2016). Zen Musings on Bion's "O" and "K". *Psychoanalytic Review, 103* (*4*): 515–538.
403. Cooper, P. C. (2020). Realizational perspectives: Bion's psychoanalysis and Dogen's Zen. *American Journal of Psychoanalysis, 80*: 37–52.
404. Cooper-White, P. (2014). Why didn't Freud reject Pfister? A response to Isabelle Noth and Christoph Morgenthaler. *Pastoral Psychology, 63*: 91–95.
405. Cooper-White, P. (2018). *Old and Dirty Gods: Religion, Antisemitism, and the Origins of Psychoanalysis*, London/New York, NY: Routledge.
406. Cordero Pando, J. (1976). *Psicoanálisis de la culpabilidad*, Estella: Verbo divino.
407. Cordero Pando, J. (1986). Una interpretación psicoanalítica del fenómeno religioso. *Cuaderno de realidades sociales, 27–27*: 77–88.
408. Córdova, C. (1992). De los salmos a las sutras: El itinerario espiritual de Fromm. *Salud Mental, 15*: 1–9.
409. Cortés, Á (1999). Antecedents to the conflict between psychology and religion in America. *Journal of Psychology and Theology, 27* (*1*): 20–32.
410. Corveleyn, J. (1996). The psychological explanation of religion as a wish-fulfilment. A test-case: the belief in immortality. In H. Grzymala–Moszczynska & B. Beit-Hallahmi (Eds.) *Religion, Psychopathology, and Coping* (pp. 57–70). Atlanta, GA: Rodopi Press.
411. Corveleyn, J. (1997). The obsessional episode in the conversion experience of Ignatius of Loyola: A psychobiographical contribution. In: J. A. Belzen (Ed.) *Hermeneutical Approaches in Psychology of Religion* (pp. 155–172). Atlanta, GA: Rodopi Press.
412. Corveleyn, J., Luyten, P. & Dezutter, J., (2013) Psychodynamic psychology and religion. In: Paloutzian, R. & Park, C. (Eds.) *Handbook of the Psychology of Religion and Spirituality* (2nd ed.) (pp. 94–117). New York, NY: The Guilford Press.
413. Corveleyn, J. & Hutsebaut, D. (Eds.) (1994). *Belief and Unbelief: Psychological Perspectives*, Amsterdam: Rodopi.
414. Cotti, P. (2014). 'I am reading the history of religion': A contribution to the knowledge of Freud's building of a theory. *History of Psychiatry, 25* (*2*): 187–202.
415. Cottingham, J. (2012). Freud's critique of religion: How damaging is his account? In: M. A. Holowchak (Ed.) *Radical Claims in Freudian Psychoanalysis: Point/Counterpoint* (pp. 113–128). Lanham, MD: Jason Aronson.

416. Cottingham, J. (2019). Psychoanalysis and religion. In: R. Gipps (Ed.) *The Oxford Handbook of Philosophy and Psychoanalysis* (pp. 537–552). New York, NY: Oxford University Press.
417. Crespy, G. (1968). Exégèse et psychanalyse. Considérations aventureuses sur Romains 7, 7–25. In: Bouttier, M. et al. *L'Evangile hier et aujourd'hui* (pp. 169–180). Genève: Labor et Fides.
418. Crockett, C. (2000). On Sublimation: The significance of psychoanalysis for the study of religion. *Journal of the American Academy of Religion, 68* (*4*): 837–855.
419. Crownfield, D. R. (Ed.) (1992). *Body/Text in Julia Kristeva: Religion, Women and Psychoanalysis*, New York, NY: State University of New York Press.
420. Cushman, P. (2007). A burning world, an absent God: Midrash, hermeneutics, and relational psychoanalysis. *Contemporary Psychoanalysis, 43*: 47–88.
421. Cusin, A., Fattori, L., Stanzione Modàfferi, M., & Vandi (2019). *Oltre Il senso di infinito a partire dal "sentimento oceanico"*, Roma: Alpes.
422. Cuvillier, E. (2007). Bible et psychanalyse: quelques éléments de réflexion. *Études théologiques et religieuses, 82*: 159–177.
423. Da Cunha, G. P. (2012). Qual é o futuro da ilusão? A religião no pensamento lacaniano e sua contribuição para a psicanálise com base na leitura de o triunfo da religião. *Ciências da Religião: História e Sociedade, 10*: 138–162.
424. Dadoun, R. (1980). Un vol d'Upanishads au-dessus de Sigmund Freud. *Nouvelle Revue de Psychanalyse, 22*: 143–154.
425. Dalbiez, R. (1950). *L'angoisse de Luther*, Paris: Téqui.
426. Daly, C. D. (1950). The psycho-biological problems of circumcision. *International Journal of Psychoanalysis, 31*: 217–236.
427. Dansereau, M. (1971). *Freud et l'athéisme*, Paris: Desclée.
428. Dansereau, M. (2006). *Un psy sur le divan de la foi*, Montreal: Médiaspaul.
429. Daquino, G. (1980). *Religiosità e psicoanalisi*, Torino: Sei.
430. David, S. N. (2003). *Freud e a religião*, Rio de Janeiro: Jorge Zahar Ed.
431. Davids, M. F. (2009). The impact of Islamophobia. *Psychoanalysis and History, 11* (*2*): 175–191.
432. Davis, C., Pound, M. & Crockett, C. (Eds.) (2014). *Theology after Lacan: The Passion for the Real*, Cambridge: James Clarke & Co.
433. Day, F. (1944). The future of psychoanalysis and religion. *Psychoanalytic Quarterly, 13*: 84–92.
434. Dayringer, R. & Oler, R. (2005). *The Image of God and the Psychology of Religion*. London/New York, NY: Routledge.
435. De Carvalho Pereira, K. S. & Chaves, W. C. (2016). Freud e a religião: A ilusão que conta uma verdade histórica. *Tempo Psicanalítico, 48*: 112–127.
436. De Piano, F., Mukherjee, A., Kamilar, S. M., Hagen, L. M., Hartsman, E. & Olson, R. P. (2002). *Religious Theories of Personality and Psychotherapy: East Meets West*, London/New York, NY: Routledge.
437. Deconchy, J. P. (1968). God and parental images: The masculine and feminine in religious free association. In: A. Godin (Ed.) *From Cry to Word* (pp. 85–94). Brussels: Lumen Vitae.
438. Dein, S. & Pargament, K. (2012). On not praying for the return of an amputated limb: conserving a relationship with God as the primary function of prayer. *Bulletin of the Menniger Clinic, 76* (*3*): 235–259.
439. DeLay, T. (2015). *God Is Unconscious: Psychoanalysis and Theology*, Eugene: Wipf and Stock.
440. Del Col, J. J. (1996). *Psicoanálisis de Freud y religión. Estado actual de ambigüedades por resolver*, Buenos Aires: Instituto Superior Juan XXIII.
441. Delouya, D. (2000). *Entre Moisés e Freud. Tratados de origens e de desilusão do destino*, São Paulo: Via Lettera/Fapesp.

442. Dempsey, P. J. (1956). *Freud, Psychoanalysis, Catholicism*, Chicago, IL: H. Regnery.
443. Dennis, P. M. (2019). Bishop Fulton J. Sheen: America's public critic of psychoanalysis, 1947–1957. *Journal of the History of the Behavioral Sciences, 56*: 36–51.
444. Desai, P. & Collins, A. (2007). The Gita dialogue between guru and disciple: A paradigm of transformation of the Self. *The Annual of Psychoanalysis, 35*: 257–271.
445. Desmazières, A. (2009). La psychanalyse à l'Index? Sigmund Freud aux prises avec le Vatican (1921–1934). *Vingtième Siècle. Revue d'histoire, 102*: 79–91.
446. Desmazières, A. (2011). *L'Inconscient au paradis. Comment les catholiques ont reçu la psychanalyse*, Paris: Payot.
447. Deutsch, H. (1989). On satisfaction, happiness, and ecstasy. *The International Journal of Psychoanalysis, 70*: 715–723.
448. Devereux, G. (Ed.) (1974). *Psychoanalysis and the Occult*, London: Souvenir Press.
449. DeVille, A. (2019). The shrink and the spiritual director: Freud and the Jesuits, https://www.americamagazine.org/faith/2019/12/13/shrink-and-spiritual-director-freud-and-jesuits
450. Dey, D. (2019). *Freud and His Discontents. An Etiology of Psychoanalysis*, Malurthaven: Smashwords.
451. Di Censo, J. J. (1999). *The Other Freud: Religion, Culture and Psychoanalysis*, London/New York, NY: Routledge.
452. Di Censo., J. J. (1994). Symbolism and subjectivity: A Lacanian approach to religion. *Journal of Religion, 74*: 45–64.
453. Di Ciaccia, A. (1993). Théologie et psychanalyse. *Quarto, 52*: 85–92.
454. Diana, M. (2002). *Angoscia e libertà. Psicologia del profondo e religions nellópera di Eugen Drewermann*, Torino: Centro Scientifico Editore.
455. Diel, P. (1962). *La Divinité. Étude psychanalytique*, Paris: PUF.
456. Diel, P. (1986). *Symbolism in the Bible: The Universality of Symbolic Language and Its Psychological Significance*, San Francisco, CA: Harper & Row.
457. Dines, A. (2003). Duas peças de câmera. In: M. O. França. (Ed.) *Freud, a cultura judaica e a modernidades* (pp. 191–218). São Paulo: Senac São Paulo.
458. Dip, P. C. (2018). La religión bajo sospecha: Freud y Gramsci. *Praxis Filosófica*: 43–60.
459. Dobbs, T. (2009). *Faith, Theology, and Psychoanalysis: The Life and Thought of Harry S. Guntrip*, London: James Clarke.
460. Dobbs, T. (2008). Transformation in psychoanalysis and religion as "persons in relationship": The influence of John Macmurray. *Psychoanalytic Inquiry, 28*: 590–598.
461. Doehring, C. (1993). *Internal Desecration: Traumatization and Representations of God*, Lanham, ND: University Press of America.
462. Dolto, F. (1973). Psychanalyse et foi. In: Vergote, A., Ortigues, E., Trotignon, P. et al. *Problèmes de psychanalyse* (pp. 163–191). Paris: Desclée de Brouwer.
463. Dolto, F. & Séverin, G. (1978). *L'Evangile au risque de la psychanalyse*, Paris: Seuil.
464. Dolto, F. & Séverin, G. (1983). *La foi au risque de de la psychanalyse*, Paris: Seuil.
465. Domínguez- Morano, C. (2009). Teología y psicoanálisis de la experiencia religiosa. *Revista Iberoamericana de Teología, 5*: 45–67.
466. Domínguez-Morano, C. (1985). Aproximación psicoanalítica a la religiosidad tradicional andaluza. In: P. Castón (Ed.) *La religión en Andalucía* (pp. 131–175). Sevilla: Biblioteca de Cultura Andaluza.
467. Domínguez-Morano, C. (1991). *El psicoanálisis freudiano de la religión. Análisis textual y comentario crítico*, Madrid: Paulinas.
468. Domínguez-Morano, C. (1994). *Orar después de Freud*, Santander: Sal Terrae.
469. Domínguez-Morano, C. (1995a). *Teología y psicoanálisis*, Barcelona: Cristianismo y Justicia.
470. Domínguez-Morano, C. (1995b). El Dios imaginado. Psicoanálisis y figuraciones religiosas. *Razón y Fe, 231*: 29–40.

471. Domínguez-Morano, C. (1996). Psicoanálisis clerical. In: J. I. González Faus, C. Domínguez-Morano & A. Torres Queiruga (Eds.) *Clérigos en debate* (pp. 61–128). Madrid: PPC.
472. Domínguez-Morano, C. (1999a). La paternidad de Dios bajo sospecha: punto de vista psicoanalítico. In: *Dios Padre ante el reto de la injusticia y del inconsciente* (pp. 51–79). Bilbao: Universidad de Deusto.
473. Domínguez-Morano, C. (1999b). *Sigmund Freud y Oskar Pfister. Historia de una amistad y su significación teológica*, Granada: Facultad de Teología de Granada.
474. Domínguez-Morano, C. (2000). *La aventura del celibato evangélico. Sublimación o represión - Narcisismo o alteridad*, Vitoria: Frontera-Egian.
475. Domínguez-Morano, C. (2003a). *Psicodinámica de los Ejercicios Ignacianos*, Bilbao-Santander: Mensajero-Sal Terrae.
476. Domínguez-Morano, C. (2003b). Ciencia, ilusión y creencia. *Revista Portuguesa de Filosofía*, *59*: 431–453.
477. Domínguez-Morano, C. (2003c). Psicoanálisis y cristianismo. *Proyección*, *50*: 333–355.
478. Domínguez-Morano, C. (2005). Life Reform: Psychosocial Issues. *Review of Ignatian Spirituality*, *36*: 67–85.
479. Domínguez-Morano, C. (2006). *Experiencia cristiana y psicoanálisis*, Santander: Sal Terrae.
480. Domínguez-Morano, C. (2007a). Eclesiología de comunión y psicoanálisis. *Revista Iberoamericana de Teología*, *4*: 7–30.
481. Domínguez Morano, C. (2007b). *Reflexiones sobre religión y psicoanálisis*, Puebla: Universidad Iberoamericana de México.
482. Domínguez-Morano, C. (2012a). Manger et boire: salut ou condamnation: una analyse cinématographique. In: M. Vaucher, D. Bourdin, M. Durrer & O. Revaz (Eds.) *Foi de cannibale! La dévoration, entre religion et psychanalyse* (pp. 357–392). Genève: Labor et fides.
483. Domínguez-Morano, C. (2012b). Ilusos o ilusionados en la ciencia o en la creencia; reflexiones desde el psicoanálisis y la fe cristiana. In: C. Morano, J. Campos & M. M. Alcubilla (Eds.) *Ciencia, humanismo y creencia en una sociedad plural* (pp. 323–332). Oviedo: Universidad de Oviedo, Oviedo.
484. Domínguez-Morano, C. (2013). Fantasmas sexuales en torno a la feminidad y su repercusión eclesial. In: R. M. Nogués, I. Gómez Acebo, T. León & C. Domínguez-Morano (Eds.) *Mujeres en la iglesia* (pp. 211–273). Barcelona: Claret Editorial.
485. Domínguez-Morano, C. (2014). *Amores y desamores en la vida consagrada*, Vitoria: Frontera.
486. Domínguez-Morano, C. (2017). Acompanhamento espiritual e psicanalise. *Itaici*, *23*: 17–28.
487. Domínguez-Morano, C. (2018). *Belief after Freud*, London/New York, NY: Routledge.
488. Domínguez-Morano, C. (2019a). Resistance to accepting the cross: Some reflections based on psychology and ignatian anthropology. *The Way*, *58*: 67–80.
489. Domínguez-Morano, C. (2019b). El mal: dos mitos sobre el origen. Una reflexión psicoanalítica. *Proyección*, *66*: 379–39.
490. Domínguez-Morano, C. (2019c). Teología y psicoanálisis. *Ephata. Revista Portuguesa de Teología*, *1*: 169–209.
491. Domínguez-Morano, C. (2020). *Mística y psicoanálisis. El lugar del Otro en los místicos de Occidente*, Madrid: Trotta.
492. Domínguez-Morano, C. (2020). *The Myth of Desire. Sexuality, Love, and the Self*, Lanham, MD: Lexington.
493. Dominian, J. (1969). Psychanalyse et vie spirituelle. *Le Supplément*, *22*: 29–44.
494. Donard, V. (2005). Un trauma nommé demon. *Topique*, *91*: 83–91.

495. Donard, V. (2009). *Du meurtre au sacrifice*, Paris: Cerf.
496. Donard, V. (2010). Repères pour penser le martyre chrétien. *Topique, 113*: 27–41.
497. Doria Medina, R. (1991). On Freud and monotheism. *International Review of Psychoanalysis, 18*: 489–500.
498. Drawin, C. R. & Kyrillos, N. F. (2018). Psicanálise e religião: O deslocamento da problemática filosófica, de Freud a Lacan. *Tempo psicanalítico, 50*: 143–173.
499. Drawin, C., Moreira, J., Paiva, M. A. & Veliq, F. (Eds.) (2019). *Destinos da religião na contemporaneidade: Um diálogo com a psicanálise, a filosofia e as ciências da religião*, Curitiba: CRV.
500. Drewerman, E. (1989). *Kleriker: Psychogramm eines Ideals*, Olten: Walter Verlag.
501. Drewermann, E. (1982–1984). *Psychoanalyse und Moraltheologie* (3 Bd). Mainz: Grünewald.
502. Drewermann, E. (1984–1985). *Tiefenpsychologie und Exegese*, Olten: Walter Verlag.
503. Drewermann, E. (2003). *Religiös bedingte neurotische Erkrankungen*, Lengerich: Pabst Science Publisher.
504. Droguett, J. G. (2000). *O desejo de deus- Diálogo entre psicanálise e fé*, Petrópolis, RJ: Vozes.
505. Dubal, R. (1952). *La psychanalyse du diable*, Paris: Corrêa.
506. Duckham, B. (2011). Bipolar illness, God, and object relations: The treatment of M. *Smith College Studies in Social Work, 81 (2–3)*: 268–291.
507. Dundes, A. (1981). The hero pattern and the life of Jesus. *Psychoanalytic Study of Society, 9*: 49–83.
508. Earle, W. J. (1997). Illusions with futures: Jacques Lacan. In: J. L. Jacobs & D. Capps (Eds.) *Religion, Society and Psychoanalysis* (pp. 218–229). Boulder, NV: Westview Press.
509. Echavarren, G. (2003). *Freud y la antropología cristiana*, Buenos Aires: Librería Córdoba.
510. Edkins, W. (1985). Psychoanalysis and religious experience. *Journal of Psychology and Christianity, 4*: 86–90.
511. Eigen, M. (1998). *The Psychoanalytic Mystic*, London/New York, NY: Free As-sociation Books.
512. Eigen, M. & Govrin, A. (2007). *Conversations with Michael Eigen*, London: Karnac.
513. Eigen, M. (1981). The area of faith in Winnicott, Lacan & Bion. *The International Journal of Psychoanalysis, 62*: 413–433.
514. Eigen, M. (1983). Dual union or undifferentiation? A critique of Marion Milner's view of the sense of psychic creativeness. *International Review of Psychoanalysis, 10 (14)*: 415–428.
515. Eigen, M. (1985). Toward Bion's starting point: Between catastrophe and faith. *The International Journal of Psychoanalysis, 66*: 321–330.
516. Eigen, M. (1992). The fire that never goes out. *Psychoanalytic Review, 79 (4)*: 271–287.
517. Eigen, M. (1995). Stones and stream. *Psychoanalytic Review, 82 (3)*: 371–390.
518. Eigen, M. (2001). *Ecstasy*, Middletown, CT: Wesleyan University Press.
519. Eigen, M. (2002). Mysticism and psychoanalysis. *Psychoanalytic Review, 88*: 455–481.
520. Eigen, M. (2011). *Eigen in Seoul: Vol. two: Faith and Transformation*, London: Karnac.
521. Eigen, M. (2012). *Kabbalah and Psychoanalysis*, London/New York, NY: Routledge.
522. Eigen, M. (2014). *Faith*, London/New York, NY: Karnac/Routledge.
523. Elrington, A. (1933). Psychoanalysis and Catholicism. *New Blackfriars, 14*: 673–678.
524. Emmons, R. A. & Paloutzian, R. (2003). The Psychology of religion. *Annual Review of Psychology, 54*: 377–402.
525. Enckell, H. & Enckell, M. (2017). Fried and Freud on the Acropolis: on duality in the base of psychoanalytic thinking. *The Scandinavian Psychoanalytic Review, 40*: 12–18.
526. Enckell, M. (1988). Psychoanalysis and the Jewish tradition. *Scandinavian Psychoanalytic Review, 11*: 141–159.
527. Epstein, M. (1990). Beyond the oceanic feeling: Psychoanalytic study of Buddhist meditation. *International Review of Psychoanalysis, 17*: 159–166.

528. Epstein, M. (1995). Thoughts without a thinker: Buddhism and psychoanalysis. *Psychoanalytic Review, 82 (3)*: 391–406.
529. Epstein, I. (2004). Psychoanalysis and Buddism: An unfolding dialogue. *Contemporary Psychoanalysis, 40*: 299–303.
530. Erikson, E. H. (1959). *Identity and the Life Cycle*, New York, NY: International Universities Press.
531. Erikson, E. H. (1962). *Young Man Luther: A Study in Psychoanalysis and History*, New York, NY: W.W. Norton & Company.
532. Erikson, E. H. (1966). Ontogeny of ritualization in man. In: Loewenstein et al. (Ed.) *Psychoanalysis. A General Psychology: Essays in Honor of Heinz Hartmann* (pp. 337–349). New York, NY: International Universities Press.
533. Erikson, E. H. (1969). *Gandhi's Truth: On the Origin of Militant Nonviolence*, New York, NY: Norton.
534. Etezady, M. H. (2008). Faith and the couch: A psychoanalytic perspective on transformation. *Psychoanalytic Inquiry, 28*: 560–569.
535. Fabre, N. (1981). *Le signe de la baleine*, Paris: Cerf.
536. Fabre, N. (1991). *Le Dieu des enfants*, Paris: Épi-Desclée de Brouwer.
537. Fachinelli, E. (1989). *La mente estatica*, Milano:Adelphi.
538. Fagnani, D. & Rossi, M. T. (Eds.) (1998). *Simbolo, metafora, invocazione. Tra religione e psicoanalisi*, Bergamo: Moretti & Vitali.
539. Fairbairn, W. R. D. (1952) [1927]. Notes on the religious phantasies of a female patient. In: Fairbairn (Ed.) *Psychoanalytic Studies of the Personality* (pp. 183–196). London/New York, NY: Routledge.
540. Falkenström, F. (2003). A Buddhist contribution to the psychoanalytic psychology of self. *The International Journal of Psychoanalysis, 84*: 1551–1568.
541. Farrell, B. A. (1955). Psychological theory and the belief in God. *International Journal of Psychoanalysis, 36*: 187–204.
542. Fateux, K. (2008). Self-Reparation in religious experience and countertransference. *Journal of the American Academy of Psychoanalysis; Psychodynamic Psychiatry, 37*: 45–58.
543. Fattori, L. & Secchi, C. (2015). Existential crises in two religious patients: Vicissitudes of faith and the emergence of the true self. *International Journal of Psychoanalysis, 96*: 993–1011.
544. Fattori, L. & Vandi, G. (2016). *Psicoanalisi e fede. Un discorso aperto*, Roma: Franco Angelli.
545. Fauteux, K. (1994a). *The Recovery of Self: Regression and Redemption in Religious Experience*, New York, NY: Paulist Press.
546. Fauteux, K. (1994b). Regression and reparation in religious experience and therapy. *Journal of the American Academy of Psychoanalysis, 22*: 623–637.
547. Fayek, A. (2004). Islam and its effect on my practice of psychoanalysis. *Psychoanalytic Psychology, 21*: 452–457.
548. Fayek, A. (2007). The impasse between the Islamists and the West: Dreaming the same nightmare. *The Annual of Psychoanalysis, 35*: 273–286.
549. Feldman, A. A. (1944). Freud's "Moses and monotheism" and the three stages of Israelitish Religion. *Psychoanalytic Quarterly, 31*: 361–418.
550. Feldman, A. A. (1960). The Davidic dynasty ant the Davidic Messiah. *American Imago, 17*: 164–178.
551. Felici, P. (1954). Psicoanalisi. In: P. Palazzini & F. Roberti (Ed.) *Dizionario di teologia morale, 2* (pp. 1163–1166). Roma: Studium.
552. Felici, P. (1967). *Freud e il pecatto*, Roma: Ancora.
553. Fenichel, O. (1940). Psychoanalysis of antisemitism. *American Imago, 1*: 24–39.
554. Fenichel, O. (1954). "Elements of a psychoanalytic theory of antisemitism". In: H. Fenichel and D. Rapport (Eds.) *The Collected Papers of Otto Fenichel* (pp. 335–348). New York, NY: Norton.

555. Ferenczi, S. (1926). Belief, disbelief, and conviction. In: J. Rickman (Ed.) *Further Contributions to Psychoanalysis* (pp. 437–450). London: Hogath.
556. Fernandes Loureiro, L. (2013). A relação com Deus e o sinthoma: A clínica psicanalítica face ao religioso. *Revista SEPHallus, 8 (15)*: 59–68.
557. Fernández, P. (1977). *Psicoanálisis: religión y moral*, Madrid: Rivadeneyra.
558. Fernández, P. (1979). *Psicoanálisis de la experiencia ético-religiosa*, Madrid: Marova.
559. Ferreira, J. B. (1988). Caminhos da utopia e da esperança. In: J. C. Moura (Ed.) *Hélio Pellegrino A-Deus. Psicanalise e religião* (pp. 144–159). Petrópilis: Vozes.
560. Fichtner, G. (2010). Freud and the Hammerschlag family: A formative relationship. *The International Journal of Psychoanalysis, 91*: 1137–1156.
561. Figueiredo, L. C. (2008). Belief, hope, and faith. *International Journal of Psychoanalysis, 85*: 1439–1453.
562. Filho, J. (2009). *Os obstáculos ao amor e à fé*, São Paulo: Paulus.
563. Fine, A. (1989). Fluctuat nec mergitur: Les trois recommandations de Bion de l'universalisable à la part mystique et sacrée. *Revue Française de Psychanalyse, 53*: 1431–1448.
564. Finn, M. & Gartner, J. (Eds.) (1992). *Object Relations Theory and Religion: Clinical Applications*, Westport, CT: Praeger Publishers.
565. Firmino, C. E. (2018). Felicidade e religião em Freud: Uma leitura crítica. *Estudos e Pesquisas em Psicología,18 (2)*: 667–684.
566. Fizzotti, E. & Salustri, M. (2001). *Psicologia della religione. Con antologia dei testi fondamentali*, Roma: Città Nuova.
567. Florenzano, R. (2014). Tótem y tabú hoy día. *Revista Chilena de Psicoanálisis*, 31: 6–14
568. Flores Morelo, F. (1999). *Fe y psicoanálisis*. In: C. r. Avendaño Amador. *Psicología y religión: tensiones y tentaciones*. Buenos Aires: Kairós.
569. Fognini, M. (1989). Destins des émotions dans le mythe de Babel. *Revue Française de Psychanalyse, 53*: 1321–1344.
570. Fognini, M. (2009). Exploration de l'émergence du rêve dans le Livre de la Genèse. *Le Coq-héron, 126*: 28–36.
571. Font i Rodon, J. (1983). *Psicopatología de la experiencia religiosa*, Barcelona: Fundació Vidal i Barraquer.
572. Font i Rodon, J. (1989). Experiencia de Dios y psicoanálisis. In: A. Doy (Ed.) *Experiencia Religiosa* (pp. 239–254). Madrid: UPCM.
573. Font i Rodon, J. (2015). Espiritualidad y psicoanálisis. *Temas de Psicoanálisis, 10*: 1–14.
574. Font i Rodon, J. (2016). *Religión, Psicopatología y salud mental*, Barcelona: Herder.
575. Fontana, D. (2003). *Psychology, Religion, and Spirituality*, Malden, MA: Blackwell Publishing.
576. Forest, J. (2001). De quelle oreille lire l'Écriture avec Freud? *Lumen Vitae, 56*: 391–400.
577. Forster, S. & Donald, L. C. (1999). Christianity: A Kleinian perspective. *Canadian Journal of Psychoanalysis, 7*: 187–218.
578. Fortune, R. F. (1926). The symbolism of the serpent. *International Journal of Psychoanalysis, 7*: 237–243.
579. Foschi, R., Innamorati, M. & Taradel, R. (2018). "A disease of our time": The Catholic Church's condemnation and absolution of psychoanalysis (1924–1975). *Journal of the History of the Behavioral Sciences, 54*: 85–100.
580. Fowler, J. W. (1981). *Stages of Faith: The Psychology of Human Development and the Quest for Meaning*, New York, NY: HarperCollins.
581. Fowler, S. G. (2017). *Probing the Mind to Free the Soul: Toward a Psychoanalytic Protest Theology*, Eugene: Wipf and Stock.
582. Fraile, M. (1993). *Meditación budista y psicoanálisis*, Madrid: Edaf.
583. Franco, O. (1998). Religious experience and psychoanalysis: from man-as-god to man-with-god. *International Journal of Psychoanalysis, 79 (1)*: 113–131.

584. Frank Summers, F. (2006). Fundamentalism, psychoanalysis, and psychoanalytic theories. *Psychoanalytic Review, 93*: 329–352.
585. Freijo Balsebre, E. (1966a). *El problema religioso en la historia de la psicología médica contemporánea. Psicología y religión en la obra de Sigmund Freud*, Vitoria: Eset.
586. Freijo, B. (1966b). *El psicoanálisis de Freud y la psicología moral*, Madrid: Razón y Fe.
587. Freud, S. (1907). *Obsessive Actions and Religious Practices*. S. E., 9: 115–127. London: Hogarth.
588. Freud, S. (1908). *"Civilized" Sexual Morality and Modern Nervous Illness*. S. E., 9: 177–204.
589. Freud, S. (1909). *Notes upon a Case of Obsessional Neurosis*. S. E., 10: 151–249. London: Hogarth.
590. Freud, S. (1910). *Leonardo da Vinci and a Memory of his Childhood*. S. E., 11: 59–137. London: Hogarth.
591. Freud, S. (1911a). *Psycho-Analytic Notes on an Autobiographical Account of a Case of Paranoia*. S. E., 12: 9–82. London: Hogarth.
592. Freud, S. (1912–1913). *Totem and Taboo*. S. E., 13: 7–161. London: Hogarth.
593. Freud, S. (1914). *The Moses of Michelangelo*. S. E., 13: 211–238. London: Hogarth.
594. Freud, S. (1918a). *The Taboo of Virginity*. S. E., 11: 193–208. London: Hogarth.
595. Freud, S. (1918b). *From the History of an Infantile Neurosis*. S. E., 17: 7–122. London: Hogarth.
596. Freud, S. (1921). *Group Psychology and the Analysis of the Ego*. S. E., 18: 65–143. London: Hogarth.
597. Freud, S. (1923). *A Seventeenth-Century Demonological Neurosis*. S. E., 19:72–105. London: Hogarth.
598. Freud, S. (1927). *The Future of an Illusion*. S. E., 21: 1–56. London: Hogarth.
599. Freud, S. (1928a). *A Religious Experience*. S. E., 21: 169–172. London: Hogarth.
600. Freud, S. (1928b). *Dostoevsky and Parricide*. S. E., 21: 177–196. London: Hogarth.
601. Freud, S. (1930). Civilization and its *Discontents*.S. E., 21: 59–145. London: Hogarth.
602. Freud, S. (1939a). Moses and *Monotheism*. S. E., 23: 1–137. London: Hogarth.
603. Frick, E. & Fühles, M. (2009b). *Schöpferisch im Spiel vor Gott. Bibliodrama und Exerzitien*, Würzburg: Echter.
604. Frick, E. (1990). Die mystische Urkirche. Das Erleuchtungserlebnis in Manresa (1522). In: A. Falkner & P. Imhof (Eds.) *Ignatius von Loyola und die Gesellschaft Jesu* (pp. 59–64). Würzburg: Echter.
605. Frick, E. (1993). *Wer ist schuld? Das Problem der Kausalität in Psychiatrie und Psychoanalyse. eine Untersuchung zu Martin Heideggers Zollikoner Seminaren*, Hildesheim: Olms.
606. Frick, E. (1996). *Durch Verwundung heilen. Zur Psychoanalyse des Heilungsarchetyps*, Göttingen: Vandenhoeck und Ruprecht.
607. Frick, E. (2005a). *Sich heilen lassen. Eine spirituelle und psychoanalytische Reflexion*, Würzburg: Echter.
608. Frick, E. (2005b). Religiosität in der klinischen Praxis. Therapeuten berichten. In: M. Utsch (Ed.) *Religiöse Fragen in der Psychotherapie. Psychologische zugänge zu Religiosität und Spiritualität* (pp. 265–267). Stuttgart: Kohlhammer.
609. Frick, E. (2010). Macht Glaube Gesund. In: G. M. Hoff, C. Klein & M. Volkenandt (Eds.) *Zwischen Ersatzreligion und neuen Heilserwartungen. Umdeutungen von Gesundheit und Krankheit* (pp. 65–84). Freiburg/München: Alber.
610. Frick, E. (2011). *Se laisser guérir. Réflexion spirituelle et psychanalytique*, Brüssel: Lumen Vitae.
611. Frick, E. (2012). Ein psychoanalytischer Blick auf die menschlichen Motivationssysteme. In: G. Brüntrup & M. Schwartz (Eds.) *Warum wir handeln – Philosophie der Motivation* (pp. 137–152). Stuttgart: Kohlhammer.
612. Frick, E. (2017). Ist das Christentum eine Religion der Angstüberwindung? Anthropologische und psychoanalytische Überlegungen zu Eugen Bisers zentraler These.

In: G. Sans (Ed.) *Gottesbilder Eugen Biser als theologischer Grenzgänger* (pp. 131–150). Freiburg: Herder.

613. Frick, E. (2019a). Spirituelle Anamnese. In: T. Roser (Ed.) *Handbuch Der Krankenhausseelsorge* (pp. 291–300). Göttingen: Vandenhoeck & Ruprecht.
614. Frick, E. (2019b). Charting Spiritual Care – Psychiatric and psychotherapeutic aspects. In: S. Peng-Keller & D. Neuhold (Eds.) *Charting Spiritual Care – The Emerging Role of Chaplaincy Records in Global Health Care* (pp. 21–32). New York, NY: Springer.
615. Frick, E. & Hamburger, A.(Eds.) ((2014). *Freuds Religionskritik und der "Spiritual Turn". Ein Dialog zwischen Philosophie und Psychoanalyse*, Stuttgart: Kohlhammer.
616. Frick, E., Ohls, I., Stotz-Ingenlath, G. & Utsch, M. (Eds.) (2018). *Fallbuch Spiritualität in Psychotherapie und Psychiatrie*, Göttingen: Vandenhoeck & Ruprecht.
617. Frick, E. & Traugott, R.(Eds.) ((2009). *Spiritualität und Medizin. Gemeinsame Sorge für den kranken Menschen*, Sttugart: Kohlhammer.
618. Frick, H. & Huber, R. (Eds.) (1998). *Die Weise von Liebe und Tod. Psychoanalytische Betrachtungen zu Kreativität, Bindung und Abschied*, Göttingen: Vandenhoeck und Ruprecht.
619. Frie, R. (2012). Psychoanalysis, religion, philosophy, and the possibility for dialogue: Freud, Binswanger and Pfister. *International Forum of Psychoanalysis*, *21*: 106–116.
620. Friedlander, S. (1997). The confluence of psychoanalysis and religion: a personal view. In: C. Spezzano & G. J. Gargiulo (Eds.) *Soul on the Couch: Spirituality, Religion, and Morality in Contemporary Psychoanalysis* (pp. 147–161). Hillsdale, NJ: Analytic Press.
621. Fromm, E. (1950a). Freud and Jung. *Pastoral Psychology*, *1*: 11–15.
622. Fromm, E. (1950b). *Psychoanalysis and Religion*, New Haven, CT: Yale University Press.
623. Fromm, E. (1966). *You Shall Be as Gods: A Radical Interpretation of the Old Testament and Its Tradition*, New York, NY: Holt, Rinehart & Winston.
624. Fromm, E. (2004). *The Dogma of Christ: And Other Essays on Religion, Psychology and Culture*, London/New York, NY: Routledge.
625. Fuechtner, V. (2011). Wild psychoanalysis, religion, and race: Georg Groddeck talks to count Hermann von Keyserling (among others). In: V. Fuechtner (Ed.) *Berlin Psychoanalytic* (pp. 65–112). Berkeley, CA: University of California Press.
626. Fuente, A. (2016). La otra cara de Dios. *Revista de la Escuela lacaniana de psicoanálisis*, *28*. http://elpsicoanalisis.elp.org.es/
627. Fueyo Suárez, D. (1988). Dios padre y madre. Imágenes familiares y representación de Dios en la psicología contemporánea. *Revista de Estudios Filosóficos*, *37*: 235–273.
628. Fuks, B. (1999). Vocation of exile: Psychoanalysis and Judaism. *International Forum of Psychoanalysis*, *8*: 7–12.
629. Fuks, B. (2010). Violência e ethos da linguagem: Considerações sobre a teoria psicanalítica da religião. *Estudos e Pesquisas em Psicología*, *10*: 339–355.
630. Fullat, O. (2013). Sigmund Freud: la llum de la posta/Sigmund Freud: la lumière au coucher du soleil. *Temps d'Educació*, *44*: 239–258.
631. Fuller, A. R. (1994). *Psychology of Religion. Eight Points of View*, Lanham, MD: Rowman and Littlefield.
632. Fülöp-Miller, R. (1930). Jesuitismus und Psychoanalyse. *Psychoanalytische Bewegung*, *2*: 54–57.
633. Gabel, S. (2020). D.W. Winnicott and religion: The intermediate area of experiencing as a dissociative Phenomenon. *British Journal of Psychotherapy*, *36*: 4–21.
634. Gabrinetti, P. A. & Özler, S. (2014). Defenses and morality: Adam Smith, Sigmund Freud, and contemporary psychoanalysis. *Psychoanalytic Review*, *101* (*5*): 735–765.
635. Gagey, J. (1982). *Freud et le christianisme*, Paris: Desclée de Brouwer.
636. Gárate, I. (2004). Del sentimiento oceánico a la experiencia del texto. *Clínica y Análisis Grupal*, *26*: 117–129.

637. García Cabero, M. (1976). *Freud o la irreligiosidad imposible*, Estella: Verbo Divino.
638. García Callado, J. (1996). La búsqueda de lo religioso y de lo mágico en una sociedad supertecnificada. In: A. Dou Mas. *Evaluación social de la ciencia y de la técnica: análisis de tendencias* (pp. 297–302). Madrid: Universidad Pontificia de Comillas.
639. Garcia, C. A. (2007). O conceito de ilusão em psicanálise: estado ideal ou estado potencial? *Estudos de Psicologia, 12* (*2*): 169–175.
640. Gargiulo, G. (2006a). Transcending religion: Reflections on spirituality and psychoanalysis. *The Annual of Psychoanalysis, 34–35*: 97–108.
641. Gargiulo, G. (2004). *Psyche, Self and Soul: Rethinking Psychoanalysis, the Self and Spirituality*, London: Whurr.
642. Gargiulo, G. (2006). Aloneness in psychoanalysis and spirituality. *International Journal of Applied Psychoanalytic Studies, 1*: 36–46.
643. Gargiulo, G. J. (2007). Transcending religion: Reflections on spirituality and psychoanalysis. *The Annual of Psychoanalysis, 35*: 97–108.
644. Garma, A. (1966). Psicoanálisis y Religión. (La correspondencia entre Freud y Pfister). *Revista de Psicoanálisis, 23*: 318–333.
645. Garma, A. (2013). Repetición de traumas ancestrales e identificaciones destructivas en la religión y en el antijudaísmo. *Revista de la Asociación Española de Neuropsiquitría, 33*: 173–191.
646. Gauch, D. (2007). La psychanalyse au risque de la foi. *Études théologiques et religieuses, 82*: 223–233.
647. Gay, P. (1978). *Freud, Jews, and Other Germans: Masters and Victims in Modernist Culture*, New Haven, CT: Oxford University Press.
648. Gay, P. (1987). *A Godless Jew. Freud, Atheism, and the Making of Psychoanalysis*, New Haven, CT: Yale University Press.
649. Gay, P. (1988). *Freud: A Life for Our Time*, New York, NY: Norton.
650. Gay, P. (1991). *Reading Freud: Explorations and Entertainments*, New Haven, CT: Yale University Press.
651. Gay, V. P. (1975). Psychopathology and ritual: Freud's essay "obsessive actions and religious practices". *Psychoanalytic Review, 63* (*2*): 493–507.
652. Gay, V. P. (1979a). *Freud on Ritual: Reconstruction and Critique*, Missoula, MT: Scholars Press.
653. Gay, V. P. (1979b). Against wholeness: The Ego's complicity in religion. *Journal of the American Academy of Religion, 47* (*4*): 539–555.
654. Gay, V. P. (1983). *Reading Freud: Psychology, Neurosis and Religion*, Chico, CA: Scholars Press.
655. Gay, V. P. (1986). Augustine: The reader as selfobject. *Journal for the Scientific Study of Religion, 25* (*1*): 64–75.
656. Geller, J. (2006). *Atheist* jew or atheist *jew*: Freud's Jewish question and ours. *Modern Judaism, 26*: 1–14.
657. Geller, J. (2007). *On Freud's Jewish Body: Mitigating Circumcisions*, New York, NY: Fordham University Press.
658. Geller, J. (2004). The psychopathology of everyday Vienna: Psychoanalysis and Freud's familiars. *International Journal of Psychoanalysis, 85*: 1209–1223.
659. Gemelli, A. (1955). *Psychoanalysis Today*, New York, NY: P. J. Kenedy.
660. Genardière, C. D. (2009). Danser avec la femme de Loth. *Le Coq-héron, 126*: 59–67.
661. Gerber, I. (2004). O inconsciente infinito segundo Bion e Matte Blanco. *Revista Brasileira de Psicanálise*, 38: 39–58.
662. Gerber, I. (2002). *Bion, Intuition and Expansion of Psychoanalytic Theory*. London: Routledge.
663. Gerlach, A., Schlösser, A.-M. & Springer, A. (Eds.) (2004). *Psychoanalyse des Glaubens*, Gießen: Psychosozial Verlag.
664. Gibert, P. (1990). *Le récit biblique de rêve. Essai de confrontation analytique*, Lyon: Profac.

665. Lev, G., PhD. (2018). Poetics of reconcilement: Psychoanalysis and dilemmas of faith. *Psychoanalytic Psychology 35*: 38–45.
666. Gilad, S. (2015). "Freud, Religion and Messianism," Working Papers/146, Hebrew University, Jerusalem, Israel.
667. Gilet-Le Bon, S. (2010). Aime ton prochain. *Champ lacanien, 8*: 49–57.
668. Gilibert, J. (1983). L'image de Dieu. *Revue française de psychanalyse, 67*: 953–970.
669. Gillet, M. (1992). Interprétations freudiennes et analyse institutionnelle. *Lumière et Vie, 215*: 5–15.
670. Giménez Segura, M. C. (1991). *Judaísmo, psicoanálisis y sexualidad femenina*, Barcelona: Anthropos.
671. Girard, R. (1977). *Violence and the Sacred*, Baltimore, MD: Johns Hopkins University Press.
672. Glenn, J. (1960). Circumcision and antisemitism. *The Psychoanalytic Quarterly, 29*: 395–399.
673. Glover, E. (1950). *Freud or Jung*, Evanston, IL: Northwestern University Press.
674. Godin, A. (1964). *De l'expérience à l'attitude religieuse*, Bruxelles: Lumen Vitae.
675. Godin, A. (1963). *Le Dieu des parents et le Dieu des enfants*, Paris-Tournai: Casterman.
676. Godin, A. (1975). Moi perdu ou Moi retrouvé dans l'expérience charismatique: perplexité des psychologies. *Archives des Sciences Sociales des Religions, 40*: 31–52.
677. Godin, A. (1986). *Psychologie des expériences religieuses*, Paris: Le Centurion.
678. Godin, A. (1988). Du fondamentalisme comme attitude psychologique. *Lumière et Vie, 37*: 31–53.
679. Godin, A. & Hallez, M. (1964). Parental images and divine paternity. In: A. Godin (Ed.) *From Religious Experience to a Religious Attitude* (pp. 65–96). Chicago, IL: Loyola University Press.
680. Goering, J. D. (1982). Sigmund Freud, Carl Jung, and Religion. *The Mennonite Quarterly Review, 56 (1)*: 47–56.
681 Goldenberg, N. R. (1979). *Changing of the Gods: Feminism and the End of Traditional Religions*, Boston, MA: Beacon Press.
682. Goldenberg, N. R. (1993). *Resurrecting the Body: Feminism, Religion and Psychoanalysis*, New York, NY: Crossroad.
683. Goldenberg, N. R. (2010). A gentle critique of mourning religion. *Pastoral Psychology, 59*: 373–377.
684. Goldenberg, N. R. (1990). *Returning Words to Flesh: Feminism, Psychoanalysis, and the Resurrection of the Body*, Boston, MA: Beacon Press, Inc.
685. Goldstein, B. (1992). *Reinscribing Moses. Heine, Kafka, Freud, and Schoenberg in a European Wilderness*, Cambridge, MA: Harvard University Press.
686. Goldstein, S. (2009). The parallel paths of psychoanalysis and spirituality: Convergences, divergences, transformations. *Psychoanalytic Perspectives, 6*: 45–66.
687. Gonçalves, N., Rita, H. & Chaves, W. C. (2011). "Paidescendo no paraíso": Uma investigação sobre o pai e a religião na teoria de Freud e Lacan. *Revista Mal-estar e Subjetividade, 11*: 335–367.
688. Gontijo, E. (1999). Limites e alcance da leitura freudiana da religião. In: M. Massimi & M. Madfoud (Eds.) *Diante do mistério* (pp. 143–162). São Paulo: Loyola.
689. González Guzzi, D. (2007). Lou Andreas-Salomé y la relación con lo divino. *Revista Carta Psicoanalítica, 11*. http://www.cartapsi.org/new/lou-andreas-salome-y-la-relacion-con-lo-divino/
690. Goodman, D. & Freeman, M. (2015). *Psychology and the Other*, New York, NY: Oxford University Press.
691. Goodman, D. & Severson, E. (2016). *The Ethical Turn: Otherness and Subjectivity in Contemporary Psychoanalysis*, London/New York, NY: Routledge.
692. Goodnick, B. (1995). Sigmund Freud and the countenance of Moses. *The Israel Journal of Psychiatry and Related Sciences, 32 (2)*: 669–682.

693. Gorog, J. J. (2010). La Religion du psychanalyste. *Champ lacanien, 8*: 100–107.
694. Görres, A. & Rahner, K. (1967). *Der Leib und das Heil*, Mainz: Matthias-Grünewald-Verlag.
695. Görres, A. & Rahner, K. (1982). *Das Böse. Wege zu seiner Bewältigung in Psychotherapie und Christentum*, Freiburg: Herder.
696. Görres, A. (1983). *Kennt die Religion den Menschen? Erfahrungen zwischen Psychologie und Glauben*, München: Serie Piper.
697. Görres, A. (1968). *An den Grenzen der Psychoanalyse*, München: Kössel.
698. Gorsuch, R. (1968). The conceptualization of God as seen in adjective ratings. *Journal for the Scientific Study of Religion*, 7: 56–64.
699. Gostečnik, C., Slavič, T. R., Lukek, S. P., Pate, T. & Cvetek, R. (2017). Emotional detachment of partners and the sanctity of the relationship with the analyst as the most powerful curative factor. *Journal of Religion and Health, 56 (4)*: 1123–1136.
700. Gostečnik, C. (2008). Redemptive experience in relational family therapy: A Christian perspective. *Journal of Religion and Health, 47 (3)*: 386–397.
701. Gottesfield, M. L. (1985). Mystical aspects of psychotherapeutic efficacy. *Psychoanalytic Review, 72*: 589–597.
702. Gottlieb, S. (2006). Some thoughts on Schreber (and Freud): depression, paranoia, and a delusional system. *British Journal of Psychotherapy, 22*: 427–428.
703. Grand, S. (2013). God at an Impasse: Devotion, social justice, and the psychoanalytic subject. *Psychoanalytic Dialogues, 23*: 449–463.
704. Granger, E. (1980). *Le croyant a l'épreuve de la psychanalyse*, Paris: Cerf.
705. Granqvist, P., Mikulincer, M. & Shaver, P. (2001). Religion as attachment: Normative processes and individual differences. *Personality and Social Psychology Review, 14*: 49–59.
706. Granqvist, P. (1998). Religiousness and perceived childhood attachment: On the question of compensation or correspondence. *Journal of Scientific Study of Religion, 37*: 350–367.
707. Granqvist, P. (2006). On the relation between secular and divine relationships: An emerging attachment perspective and a critique of "depth" approaches. *The International Journal for the Psychology of Religion, 16*: 1–18.
708. Granqvist, P. & Kirkpatrick, L. A. (1999). Attachment and religious representations and behavior. In: J. Cassidy & P. Shaver (Eds.) *Handbook of Attachment* (pp. 803–822). New York, NY: Guilford Press.
709. Grant Duff, I. F. (1976). Recherches psychanalytiques sur un cas de sainteté canonisé: Thérèse Martin (1873–1897). *Archives des Sciences Sociales des Religions, 41*: 109–136.
710. Grenz, S. J. (2001). *The Social God and the Relational Self: A Trinitarian Theology of the Imago Dei*, Louisville, KY: Westminster John Knox Press.
711. Gresser, M. (1994). *Dual Allegiance: Freud as a Modern Jew*, Albany, NY: State University of New York Press.
712. Griesl, G. (1980). Psychoanalyse in der Praktischen Theologie. *Archiv Für Religionspsychologie/Archive for the Psychology of Religion, 14 (1)*: 28–36.
713. Grinberg, L. (1960). La rivalidad en los sueños legendarios de José *Revista de Psicoanálisis*, 17: 27–45.
714. Grinberg, L. (1962). Psychoanalytic considerations on the Jewish Passover: Totemic sacrifice and meal. *American Imago, 19*: 321–424.
715. Grinberg, L. (1963). El duelo de Jacob. In: L. Grinberg (Ed.) *Culpa y depression* (pp. 263–273), Buenos Aires: Paidós 1978 (*Guilt and depression*, London: Karnac, 1992).
716. Grinberg, L. (1989). Freud y el judaísmo. *Raíces*, 7: 7–9.
717. Grollman, E. A. (1963). Some sights and insights of history, psychology and psychoanalysis concerning the Father-God and Mother-Goddess concepts of Judaism and Christianity. *American Imago, 20*: 187–209.
718. Grollman, E. A. (1966). *Judaism in Sigmund Freud's World*, New York, NY: Block Publishing.

719. Grossman, W. I. (1988). Some sources for a slip in a translation by Freud. *Journal of American Psychoanalytic Association, 36* (*3*): 729–739.
720. Grossman, W. I. (1998). Freud's presentation of 'The psychoanalytic mode of thought' in Totem and Taboo and his technical papers. *Journal of American Psychoanalytic Association, 79* (*3*): 469–486.
721. Grotstein, J. (1997). 'The sins of the fathers ...': human sacrifice and the inter- and trans-generational neurosis/psychosis. *International Journal of Psychotherapy, 2*: 11–26.
722. Grotstein, J. (2001). *Who Is the Dreamer Who Dreams the Dream? A Study of Psychic Presences*, Hillsdale, NJ: The Analytic Press.
723. Grotstein, J. (2006a). Bion, the pariah of 'O'. *British Journal of Psychotherapy, 14*: 79–90.
724. Grotstein, J. (2006b). Spirituality, religion, politics, history, apocalypse, and transcendence: An essay on a psychoanalytically and religiously forbidden subject. *International Journal of Applied Psychoanalytic Studies, 1*: 82–95.
725. Grotstein, J. (2007). *A Beam of Intense Darkness: Wilfred Bion's Legacy to Psychoanalysis*, London: Karnac.
726. Grotstein, J. (2008). The seventh servant: The implications of a truth drive in Bion's theory of 'O'. *The International Journal of Psychoanalysis, 85*: 1081–1101.
727. Grotstein, J. (2009). Waging holy war in the sacred body of the godhead. *International Journal of Applied Psychoanalytic Studies, 6*: 262–282.
728. Grotstein, J. (2017). Bion crosses the Rubicon: The fateful course -and curse- of "O" in psychoanalysis and the furies left in wake. In: A. Reiner (Ed.) *Of Things Invisible to Mortal Sight: Celebrating the Work of James S. Grotstein* (pp. 251–268). London: Karnac.
729. Groupe "Querinjean". (2003). Genre et religion. Une réflexion psychanalytique. In: C. Domínguez-Morano & R. Briones (Eds.) *Masculino-femenino y hecho religioso* (pp. 67–77). Granada: Universidad de Granada.
730. Grubrich-Simitis, I. (1991). *Freud's Moses-Studie als Tagtraum: Ein biographischer Essay*, Weinheim: Verlag Internationales Psychoanalyse.
731. Gruenbaum, G. (1970). *Psicoanalisi e teismo*, Napoli: ESE.
732. Grunberger, B. (1997). *Narcissisme, christianisme, antisémitisme*, Paris: Hébraïca Acte Sud.
733. Grupo Épsimo (1992). *Experiencia de Dios y psicoanálisis*, México: Promexa.
734. Grzymala-Moszczynska, H. & Bet-Hallahmi, B. (Ed.) *Religion, Psychopathology and Coping*. Amsterdam: Rodopi.
735. Guérin, N. (2004). *L'état de certitude: approche psychanalytique et modalités épistémiques des variétés De l'incroyance*, Aix en Provence: Université d'Aix-Marseille.
736. Guérin, N. (2005). Au-delà de la logique divine. *Psychanalyse, 2*: 5–17.
737. Guérin, N. (2006). La notion d'incroyance en psychanalyse: origine, réhabilitation et perspective. *L'évolution psychiatrique, 71*: 545–557.
738. Guérin, N. (2007). L'ombre blanche, ou le sens blanc de la croyance. *Essaim, 19*: 159–168.
739. Guimarães, A. E. (1999). *A paternidade no confronto entre psicanálise da religião e fé no "De l'intérpretation" de Paul Ricoeur*, Porto Alegre: EDIPUCRS.
740. Guimarães, M. A. & Bento, V. E. (2007). Seria a religião uma saída para a toxicomania? Uma abordagem psicanalítica. *Psychê. Revista de Psicanálise, 11*: 105–118.
741. Guimón, J. (2009). Religión y Psicoanálisis: De la sociogénesis al condicionamiento biológico. *Norte de Salud Mental, 34*: 65–74.
742. Guirdham, A. (1959). *Christ and Freud. A Study of Religious Experience and Observance*, London: George Allen & Unwin.
743. Guntrip, H. (1956a). *Psychotherapy and Religion*, New York, NY: Harper and Brothers.
744. Guntrip, H. (1956b). *Mental Pain and the Cure of Souls*, London: Independent Press.
745. Guntrip, H. (1969). Religion in relation to personal integration. *British Journal of Medical Psychology, 42*: 323–333.
746. Gurney, a. G. & Rogers, S. A. (2007). Objects-relations and spirituality: Revisiting a clinical dialogue. *Jour of Clinical Psycho-logy, 63*: 961–977.

747. Haas, E. T. (Ed.) (2012). *100 Jahre Totem und Tabu: Freud und die Fundamente der Kultur*, Giessen: Psychosozial-Verlag.
748. Hackett, C. D. (1986). Psychoanalysis and theology: Two dialectics. *Journal of Religion and Health, 25*: 29–45.
749. Hackett, C. D. (1982). Psychoanalysis and theology: Jacques Lacan and Paul. *Journal of Religion and Health, 21*: 184–192.
750. Haddad, G. (2021). *À l''origine de la violence. De Oedipe à Caïn, un erreur de Freud?* Paris: Salvator.
751. Hall, T. W. & Brokaw, B. F. (1995). The relationship of spiritual maturity to level of object relations development and God image. *Pastoral Psychology, 43*: 373–391.
752. Hall, T. W., Fujikawa, A., Halcrow, S., Hill, P. C. & Delaney, H. (2009). Attachment to God and implicit spirituality: Clarifying correspondence and compensation models. *Journal of Psychology and Theology, 37*: 227–242.
753. Hall, T. W. (2007). Psychoanalysis, attachment, and spirituality. *Journal of Psychology and Theology, 35*: 14–28, 29–42.
754. Hall, T. W., Brokaw, B. F., Edwards, K. J. & Pike, P. (1998). An empirical exploration of psychoanalysis and religion: Spiritual maturity and object relations development. *Journal for the Scientific Study of Religion, 37*: 303–313.
755. Hall, T. W. & Hill, C. P. (2002). Relational schemas in processing one's image of God and Self. *Journal of Psychology and Christianity, 21*: 365–373.
756. Halpern, J. R. (1999). Freud's intrapsychic use of the Jewish culture and religion. *Journal of the American Psychoanalytic Association, 47* (*4*): 1191–1212.
757. Hamon, M. C. (1980). El discurso de Santa Teresa. *Analítica, 3/4*: 21–31.
758. Handelman, S. (1981). Interpretation as Devotion: Freud's Relation to Rabbinic Hermeneutics. *Psychoanalytic Review, 68* (*2*): 201–208.
759. Handl, H. (Ed.) (2014). *Die Zukunft einer Illusion/Sigmund Freud. Die Illusion einer Zukunft/Oskar Pfister*, Drösing: Driesch.
760. Harding, C. (2014). Japanese psychoanalysis and Buddhism: the making of a relationship. *History of Psychiatry, 25* (*2*): 154–170.
761. Hark, H. (1985). Neurose und Religion: zur Korrelation zwischen Glaubensleben und seelischem Erleben. *Archiv Für Religionspsychologie/Archive for the Psychology of Religion, 17* (*1*): 21–73.
762. Harrison, I. B. (1979). On Freud's view of the infant-mother relationship and the oceanic feeling. Some subjective influences. *Journal of the American Psychoanalytic Association, 27*: 399–421.
763. Hart, C. W. (2011). Paul Tillich and psychoanalysis. *Journal of Religion and Health, 50*: 646–655.
764. Hartocollis, P. (1976). Aggression and mysticism. *Contemporary Psychoanalysis, 12*: 214–226.
765. Havens, J. (1965). Notes on Augustine's Confessions. *Journal for the Scientific Study of Religion, 5*: 141–143.
766. Hays, R. (2008). *Fashioning Our Own Freuds: Psychoanalysis and Religion*. PhD diss., Emory University.
767. Heimbrock, H. G. (1990). Ritual and transformation: A psychoanalytic perspective. In: H. G. Heimbrock & H. B. Boudewijnse (Eds.) *Current Studies on Ritual: Perspectives for the Psychology of Religion* (pp. 33–42). Amsterdam/Atlanta, GA: Rodopi.
768. Heimbrock, H. G. (1991). Psychoanalytic understanding of religion. *The International Journal for the Psychology of Religion, 1*: 71–89.
769. Held, R. (1962). Contribution à l'étude psychanalytique du phénomène religieux. *Revue Française de Psychanalyse, 26*: 211–266.
770. Helminiak, D. A. (2017). The problem of "God" in Psychology of Religion: Lonergan's "Common Sense" (Religion) versus "Theory" (Theology). *Zygon, 52*: 380–418.
771. Henrikson, J. O. (2013). *Relating God and the Self: Dynamic Interplay*, London/New York, NY: Routledge.

772. Herderson, J. (1975). Object relations and the doctrine of "original sin". *International Review of Psychoanalysis, 2*: 107–120.
773. Hermann, I. (1930). Two traditions from Pascal's childhood. *Imago XVI*, (*3*): 305–373.
774. Hernández Ramírez, V. (1999). Teología de la liberación y proyecto de sujeto. In: A. Avedaño, G. Montoya & I. H. Obregón (Eds.) (1999). *Psicología y religión. Tensiones y tentaciones* (pp. 151–158). Buenos Aires: Kairós.
775. Hernández Ramírez, V. (2020). Psicoanálisis y teología reformada. Diálogo y desafío. *Revista de información y análisis teológico. CMIRP, 11*: 45–52.
776. Hewitt, M. A. (2020). *Legacies of the Occult: Psychoanalysis, Religion, and Unconscious Communication*, Bristol, CT: Equinox.
777. Hewitt, M. A. (2014a). *Freud on Religion*, London/New York, NY: Routledge.
778. Hewitt, M. A. (2014b). Rivalry or difference? Contemporary psychospirituality and the psychoanalytic study of religion. *Religious Studies Review, 40*: 175–185.
779. Heyer, R. (2003c). Sur le prétendu déclin de la figure paternelle. *Revue des Sciences Religieuses, 77*: 75–84.
780. Heyer, R. (Ed.) (2003a). *Sujets à croire. Questions de théologie et de psychanalyse. Hommage a Roland Sublon*, Strasbourg: Presses Universitaires de Strasbourg.
781. Hill, P. C. & Hood, R. V. (2001). Affect, religion, and unconscious processes. *Journal of Personality, 67*: 1015–1046.
782. Hiltner, S. (1950). Religion and psychoanalysis. *Journal of Pastoral Care, 3*: 32–42.
783. Hirshbein, L. (2020). Religion and spirituality, meaning, and faith in American psychiatry from the 19th to the 21st century. *Journal of Nervous and Mental Disease, 208*: 582–586.
784. Hirt, J. M. (2008). La psychanalyse entre athéisme freudien et ouverture à l'écoute de l'évènement intérieur du sujet. *L'Évolution Psychiatrique, 73*: 93–103.
785. Hirt, J. M. (2006). Les trois despotes et l'infidèle. *Cliniques méditerranéennes: Psychanalyse et Psychopathologie Freudiennes, 73*: 9–23.
786. Hoch, S. & Lee, G. (1993). The significance of religious themes and fantasies during psychoanalysis. *Journal of the American Psychoanalytic Association, 41*: 755–764.
787. Hoffer, A. (2020). Psychoanalysis as a two-person meditation: free association, meditation and Bion. *American Journal of Psychoanalysis, 80* (*3*): 331–341.
788. Hoffer, A. (2015). *Freud and the Buddha. The Coach and the Cushion*, London: Karnac.
789. Hoffman, I. Z. (1998). *Ritual and Spontaneity in the Psychoanalytic Process*, Hillsdale, NJ: Analytic Press.
790. Hoffman, M. & Strawn, B. D. (Eds.) (2008). Transformation: Psychoanalysis and religion in dialogue. *Psychoanalytic Inquiry, 28*: 529–639.
791. Hoffman, M. (2004). From enemy combatant to strange bedfellow: The role of religious narratives in the work of W R D Fairbairn and D W. Winnicott. *Psychoanalytic Dialogues, 14*: 769–804.
792. Hoffman, M. (2007). From libido to love: Relational psychoanalysis and the redemption of sexuality. *Journal of Psychology and Theology, 35*: 74–82.
793. Hoffman, M. (2010). On Christianity, psychoanalysis, and the hope of eternal return. *Journal of Psychology and Christianity, 29*: 166–177.
794. Hoffman, M. (2011). *Toward Mutual Recognition: Relational Psychoanalysis and Christian Narrative*, London/New York, NY: Routledge.
795. Hoffman, M. (2019). Finding place for religion: A discussion of Lisa Cataldo's "Where God is Between Us: Religious Experience, Surrender, and the Third in Clinical Perspective". *Psychoanalytic Perspectives, 16*: 149–157.
796. Hoffman, M. T. (2020). Christianity and psychoanalysis: Orienting view and augmenting modality. *Psychoanalytic Inquiry, 40* (*6*): 395–407.
797. Holliman, P. J. (2002). Religious experience as selfobject experience. In: A.I. Goldberg (Ed.) *Progress in Self Psychology* (193–206), Vol. 18. London/New York, NY: Routledge.

798. Holliman, P. J. (2009). Why bother with God? *The Journal of American Academic for Psychoanalysis and Dynamic Psychiatry, 37 (1)*: 59–72.
799. Holm, N. (1997). Religionspsychologie gestern und heute: Einige Entwicklungslinien. *Rchiv Für Religionspsychologie/Archive for the Psychology of Religion, 22*: 15–27.
800. Holmes, J. (1997). Values in psychotherapy. *Australian and New Zealand Journal of Psychiatry, 31*: 331–339.
801. Homans, P. (1967). Toward a psychology of religion: by way of Freud and Tillich. *Zygon, 2*: 97–119.
802. Homans, P. (1970). *Theology after Freud: an interpretive inquiry*, New York, NY: Bobbs-Merrill Co.
803. Homans, P. (1987). Psychology and religion movement. In M. Eliade (Ed.) *Encyclopedia of Religion* (Vol. 12,pp. 66–75). New York, NY: Macmillan.
804. Homans, P. (1989). *The Ability to Mourn: Disillusionment and the Social Origins of Psychoanalysis*, Chicago, IL: University of Chicago Press.
805. Homans, P. (1998). We (not-so) happy few: Symbolic loss and mourning in Freud's psychoanalytic movement and the history of psychoanalysis. *Psychoanalysis and History, 1*: 69–86.
806. Homans, P. (Ed.) (1968). *The Dialogue Between Theology and Psychology*, Chicago, IL: University of Chicago Press.
807. Hood, R. W. Jr. (1992a). Mysticism, reality, illusion, and the Freudian critique of religion. *The International Journal for the Psychology of Religion, 2*: 141–159.
808. Hood, R. W. Jr. (2001). *Dimensions of Mystical Experiences: Empirical Studies and Psychological Links*, Amsterdam: Rodopi.
809. Hood, R. W. Jr. (2005). *The Psychology of Religious Fundamentalism*, New York, NY: Guilford Press.
810. Hood, R. W. Jr. (2008). *Them That Believe*, Oakland, CA: University of California Press.
811. Hood, R. W. Jr. (2012). Psychology of religion: A personal narrative. In: J. A. Belzen (Ed.) *Psychology of Religion: Autobiographical Accounts (Path in Psychology)* (pp. 107–131). New York, NY: Springer.
812. Hood, R. W. Jr. (1997). Psychoanalysis and fundamentalism: Lessons from a feminist critique of Freud. In: J. L. Jacobs & D. Capps (Eds.) *Religion, Society and Psychoanalysis* (pp. 42–67). Boulder, NV: Westview Press.
813. Hood, R. W., (Ed.) (1995). *Handbook of Religious Experience*, Birmingham, AL: Religious Education Press.
814. Hood, R. W. Jr. (1992b). *Sin and Guilt in Faith Traditions: Issues for Self-Esteem*, New York, NY: Oxford University Press.
815. Hopkins, B. (1989). Jesus and object-use: A Winnicottian account of the resurrection myth. *International Review of Psychoanalysis, 16*: 93–100.
816. Hopkins, B. (1997). Winnicott and the capacity to believe. *The International Journal of Psychoanalysis, 78*: 485–497.
817. Hopkins, P. (1940). Analytic observations of *scala perfectionis* of the mystics. *British Journal of Medical Psychology, 18*: 198–218.
818. Horney, K. (1950). The search for the Glory 2. *Pastoral Psychology, 1*: 31–38.
819. Horovitz, M. (2019). Stormy navigation with our 'secret sharer'. In: A. K. Alisobhani & G. Corstorphine (Eds.) *Explorations in Bion's 'O': Everything We Know Nothing About* (pp. 97–102). London/New York, NY: Routledge.
820. Horton, P. C. (1974). The mystical experience: Substance of an illusion. *Journal of the American Psychoanalytic Association, 22*: 364–380.
821. Hosteau, F. (2005). *Le désir filial dans l'expérience religieuse*, Paris: Harmattan.
822. Houck-Loomis, T. (2012). Good God?!? Lamentations as a model for mourning the loss of the good God. *Journal of Religion and Health, 51 (3)*: 701–708.
823. Houtsebaut, D. & Corveleyn (Eds.) (1994). *Belief and Unbelief: Psychological Perspectives*, Amsterdam: Rodopi.

824. Howard, P. (1974). *Freud and Religious Belief*, Santa Barbara, CA: Greenwood.
825. Huber, W. (1978). Katholiken und Psychoanalyse in Österreich bis zum Ständestaat. In: W. Huber, *Beiträge sur Gechichte der Psychanalyse in Österreich* (pp. 61–105).Wien/ Salzburg: Geyer.
826. Hulin, M. (1993). *La mystique sauvage*, Paris: PUF.
827. Hurtado, A. M. (2002). Reflexiones sobre el simbolismo de la cruz: A propósito de un caso clínico. *Trópicos: Revista de Psicoanálisis, 10*: 135–141.
828. Hutch, R. A. (1990). *Religious Leadership: Personality, History and Sacred Authority*, New York, NY: Peter Lang.
829. Infante, J. A. (1996). Dios y la religión en el psicoanálisis. *Teología y Vida, 37*: 47–56.
830. Irwin, J. (1968). *Ethical and Pastoral Aspects of Oskar Pfister's Correlation of Psychoanalysis and Religion*, STM-These, New York, NY: General Theological Seminary.
831. Irwin, J. (1973a). Pfister and Freud: the rediscovery of a dialogue. *Journal of Religion and Health, 12 (4)*: 315–327.
832. Irwin, J. (1973b). Oskar Pfister and the Taggart Report: The "First Pastoral Counselor" and today's role problems. *Journal of Pastoral Care, 27*: 189–195.
833. Isnard-Davezac, N. (2009). Le mal en ce jardin…20–27. *Le Coq-héron, 196*: 20–27.
834. Izcovich, L. (2010). Du Dieure au dire. *Champ lacanien, 8*: 85–91.
835. Jacobs, J. L. & Capps, D. (Eds.) (2018). *Religion, Society and Psychoanalysis: Readings in Contemporary Theory*, New York, NY/London: Routledge.
836. Jacques, J. R. (1998). Working with spiritual and religious themes in group therapy. *International Journal of Group Psychotherapy, 48 (1)*: 69.
837. Jager-Werth, H. U. (1974). Oskar Pfister and the beginning of religious socialism. *Journal of Religion and Health, 13 (1)*: 57–61.
838. Jeammet, N. (1993a). *Les destins de la culpabilité. Une lecture de l'histoire de Moïse aux frontières de la psychanalyse et de la théologie*, Paris: PUF.
839. Jeammet, N. (1993b). Le plaisir d'être insatisfait. Analyse psychologique de la morosité. *Christus, 157*: 39–50.
840. Jeammet, N. (1994). Ouvrir un espace au désir de vivre. *Christus, 164*: 401–411.
841. Jeammet, N. (1998). *Le plaisir et le péché. essai sur l'envie*, Paris: Desclée de Brouwer.
842. Jeammet, N. (2001). Sujet du désir, sujet de la foi. Après Freud, quelle religion? *Raisons Politiques, 4*: 71–82.
843. Jeammet, N. (2003). Après Freud, en quel dieu croire? Le paradoxe de la confiance. *Christus, 197*: 17–26.
844. Jiang, T. (2004). Storehouse consciousness and the unconscious: A comparative study of Xuang Zang and Freud on the subliminal mind. *Journal of American Academic of Religion, 72*: 119–139.
845. Jiang, T. (2006). *Contexts and Dialogue: Yogacara Buddhism and Modern Psychology on the Subliminal Mind (Monographs of the Society for Asian and Comparative Philosophy)*, Honolulu, HI: University of Hawaii Press.
846. Jochheim, M. (1998). *Seelsorge und Psychotherapie: historisch-systematische Studien zur Lehre von der Seelsorge bei Oskar Pfister, Eduard Thurneysen und Walter Uhsadel*, Bochum: Winkler.
847. Johnson, W. B. & Eastburg, M. C. (1992). God, parent, and self-concepts in abused and no abused children. *Journal of Psychology and Christianity, 11*: 235–243.
848. Jones, E. (1923). *Essays in Applied Psycho-Analysis*, London: International Psycho-Analytical Press.
849. Jones, E. (1953–1957). *Sigmund Freud: Life and Work* (Vols. 1–3), New York, NY: Basic Books.
850. Jones, E. (1958). The birth and death of Moses. *International Journal of Psychoanalysis, 39*: 1–4.
851. Jones, E. A. (2017). Freud's paternity crises. *The International Journal of Psychoanalysis, 98*: 961–1272.

852. Jones, J. W. (1982). The Delicate Dialectic: Religion and psychology in the modern world. *Cross Currents, 32*: 143–53.
853. Jones, J. W. (1991a). *Contemporary Psychoanalysis and Religion: Transference and Transcendence*, New Haven, CT: Yale University Press.
854. Jones, J. W. (1991b). The relational Self: Contemporary psychoanalysis reconsiders religion. *Journal of the American Academy of Religion, 59*: 119–135.
855. Jones, J. W. (1996a). *Religion and Psychology: Psychoanalysis, Feminism, and Theology*, New Haven, CT: Yale University Press.
856. Jones, J. W. (1996b). *Religion and Psychology in Transition*, New Haven, CT: Yale University Press.
857. Jones, J. W. (1997). Playing and believing: The uses of D. W. Winnicott in the psychology of religion. In: J. L. Jacobs & D. Capps (Eds.) *Religion, Society, and Psychoanalysis: Readings in Contemporary Theory* (pp. 106–126). Boulder, NV: Westview Press.
858. Jones, J. W. (2002). *Terror and Transformation: The Ambiguity of Religion in Psychoanalytic Perspective*, New York, NY: Brunner-Routledge.
859. Jones, J. W. (2006). Why does religion turn violent? A psychoanalytic exploration of religious terrorism. *Psychoanalytic Review, 93*: 167–90.
860. Jones, J. W. (2007). The return of the repressed: Narcissism, religion, and the ferment in psychoanalysis. *The Annual of Psychoanalysis, 35*: 47–60.
861. Jones, J. W. (2008). *Blood That Cries Out from the Earth: The Psychology of Religious Terrorism*, New York, NY: Oxford University Press.
862. Jones, J. W. (2010). Religie en het Relationele Zelf. Tillburg. Netherlands: KSGV.
863. Jones, J. W. (2012). The return of the repressed: Psychoanalysis as spirituality. *The Annual of Psychoanalysis, 34–35*: 47–60.
864. Jones, J. W. (2013). L'approche psychanalytique du développement religieux. In: P.Y. Brandt & J. M. Day (Ed.) *Psychologie du développement religieux: Questions classiques et perspectives contemporaines* (pp. 125–155). Genève: Labor et Fides.
865. Jones, S. L. (1994). A constructive relationship for religion with the science and profession of psychology: Perhaps the boldest model yet. In: J. A. Belzen (Ed.) *Hermeneutical Approach in Psychology of Religion* (pp. 51–54). Amsterdam/Atlanta, GA: Rodopi.
866. Jonte-Pace, D. & Parsons, W. B. (2001). *Religion and Psychology: Mapping the Terrain*, London/New York, NY: Routledge.
867. Jonte-Pace, D. (1992). Which Feminism, whose Freud? *Pastoral Psychology, 40*: 369–374.
868. Jonte-Pace, D. (1997). Julia Kristeva and the psychoanalytic study of religion: Rethinking Freud's cultural texts. In: J. L. Jacobs & D. Capps (Eds.) *Religion, Society and Psychoanalysis. Readings in Contemporary Theory* (pp. 240–268). Boulder, NV/Cumnor Hill: Westview Press.
869. Jonte-Pace, D. (1999a). "Legitimation of hatred or inversion into love": 'Religion in Kristeva' re-reading of Freud. *Journal of Research of the Social Scientific Study of Religion, 10*: 17–35.
870. Jonte-Pace, D. (1999b). In defense of an unfriendly Freud: Psychoanalysis, feminism, and theology. *Pastoral Psychology, 47*: 175–181.
871. Jonte-Pace, D. (2001a). *Speaking the Unspeakable: Religion, Misogyny, and the Uncanny Mother in Freud's Cultural Texts*, Berkeley, CA: University of California Press.
872. Jonte-Pace, D. (2001b). Turning away at the navel of the dream: Religion and the body of the mother at the beginning and end of interpretation. In: K. Bulkeley (Ed.) *Dreams: A Reader on Religious, Cultural, and Psychological Dimensions of Dreaming* (pp. 295–306). New York, NY: Palgrave Macmillan/Springer Nature.
873. Jonte-Pace, D. (2006). At home in the uncanny: Freudian representation of death, mothers, and the afterlife. *Journal of the American Academy of Religion, 64*: 61–88.
874. Jonte-Pace, D. (2010). When throne and altar are in danger: Freud, mourning, and religion in modernity. In: G. Kaplan & W. Parson (Eds.) *Disciplining Freud on Religion: Perspectives from the Humanities and Sciences* (pp. 59–83). Lanham, MD: Lexington.

875. Jonte-Pace, D. (Ed.) (2003). *Teaching Freud*, New York, NY: Oxford University Press.
876. Josephson, A. M., Nicholi, A., Tasman, A. (Ed.) (2010) Religion and Psychoanalysis: Past and present. In: P.J. Verhagen, H. M. Van Praag, J. J. López-Ibor, Jr. J. L. Cox, D. Moussaoui (Eds.) *Religion and Psychiatry: Beyond Boundaries* (283–303). Hoboken, NJ: Wiley-Blackwell.
877. Joyce, V. (2005). Faith links. In: M. B. Weiner, P. C. Cooper & C. Barbre (Eds.) *Psychotherapy and Religion: Many Paths, One Journey* (pp. 103–132). Lanham, MD: Jason Aronson.
878. Julien, P. (1973). Psychoanalysis and religion. *New Blackfriars, 54*: 196–201.
879. Julien, P. (1992). Pour une éthique de la perversion. *Lumière Et Vie, 215*: 35–41.
880. Julien, P. (2008). *La psychanalyse et le religieux: Freud, Jung, Lacan*, Paris: Cerf.
881. Júlio Costa, E. (2006). Ratio et fides no pensamento de Sigmund Freud. *Fides Reformata, 11*: 51–72.
882. Juni, S. & Fischer, R. E. (1985). Religiosity and preoedipal fixation. *The Journal of Genetic Psychology, 146*: 27–35.
883. Kaplan, A. (1963). Maturity in religion. *Bulletin of the Philadelphia Association for Psychoanalysis, 13*: 101–119.
884. Kakar, S. (1981). *The Inner World; A Psychoanalytic Study of Childhood and Society in India*, Oxford: Oxford University Press.
885. Kakar, S. (1982). *Shamans, Mystics and Doctors: A Psychological Inquiry Into India and Its Healing Traditions*, Chicago, IL: The University Chicago Press.
886. Kakar, S. (1995). *The Colors of Violence: Cultural Identities, Religion, and Conflict*, Chicago, IL: University of Chicago Press.
887. Kakar, S. (1997). *Culture and Psyche. Selected Essays*, New Delhi: Oxford University Press.
888. Kakar, S. (2003). Psychoanalysis and Eastern spiritual healing traditions. *The Journal of Analytical Psychology, 48 (5)*: 659–681.
889. Kakar, S. (2007). *The Analyst and the Mystic*, Gurugram: Penguin Books.
890. Kakar, S. (2009). *Mad and Divine: Spirit and Psyche in the Modern World*, Chicago, IL/London: University of Chicago Press.
891. Kakar, S. (2018). Re-reading Freud on religion in Hindu India. In: M. K. O'Neil & S. Akhtar (Eds.) *On Freud's "The Future of an Illusion"* (pp. 224–236). London/New York, NY: Routledge.
892. Kakar, S. & Kripal, J. J. (2012). *Seriously Strange: Thinking Anew About Psychical Experience*, New Delhi: Penguin Books.
893. Kaplan, K. J. (2002). Isaac versus Oedipus: an alternative view. *The Journal of American Academic for Psychoanalysis and Dynamic Psychiatry, 30*: 707–717.
894. Kaplan, K. J. (2007). Isaac and Ruth biblical: Resolutions of the Oedipus and Electra complexes. *The Annual of Psychoanalysis, 35*: 193–206.
895. Kaplan, R. (2009). Soaring on the wings of the wind: Freud, Jews, and Judaism. *Australasian Psychiatry: Bulletin of Royal Australian and New Zealand College of Psychiatrists, 17 (4)*: 318–325.
896. Kaplan, G. & Parsons, W. (Eds.) (2010). *Disciplining Freud on Religion: Perspectives from the Humanities and Sciences*, Lanham, MD: Lexington.
897. Kato, H. (2016). The relationship between the psychology of religion and Buddhist psychology. *Japanese Psychological Research, 58*: 70–84.
898. Katz, M. B. (2011). A rabbi, a priest, and a psychoanalyst: Religion in the early psychoanalytic case history. *Contemporary Jewry, 31 (1)*: 3–24.
899. Kaufman, M. R. (1939). Religions delusions on Schizophrenia. *International Journal of Psycho-Analysis, 20*: 363–376.
900. Kavaler-Adler, S. (2003). *Mourning, Spirituality and Psychic Change*, London/New York, NY: Routledge.
901. Kay O'Neil, M. & Akhtar, S. (Eds.) (2009). *On Freud's "The Future of an Illusion"*, London: Karnac.

902. Kay, P. (2020). *The Psychological Landscape of Spirituality and Religion: A Theoretical and Diagrammatic Exposition*, Washington, DC: George Washington University.
903. Keller, B. (2020). *Taking Psychoanalytic and Psychometric Perspectives Toward a Binocular Vision of Religion*, Leiden: Brill.
904. Keller, P. H. & Albarracin, D. (2012). An event in medical life, or the advent of a belief? *The International Journal of Psychoanalysis, 93*: 341–353.
905. Kelley, M. M. & Chan, K. T. (2012). Assessing the role of attachment to God, meaning, and religious coping as mediators in the grief experience. *Death Studies, 36*: 199–227.
906. Kennedy, R. (2014). *The Psychic Home: Psychoanalysis, Consciousness, and the Human Soul*, London/New York, NY: Routledge.
907. Kenny, D. (2015). *God, Freud, and Religion: The Origins of Faith, Fear, and Fundamentalism*, London/New York, NY: Routledge.
908. Kernberg, O. F. (2000). Psychoanalytic perspectives on the religious experience. *American Journal of Psychotherapy, 54*: 452–476.
909. Kessler, R. & Vandermeersch, P. (Eds.) (2001). *God, Biblical Stories and Psychoanalytic Understanding*, Frankfurt am Main: P. Lang.
910. Ketzer, E. (2019). Moisés e a máquina do tempo de Freud. *Tempo Psicanalítico, 51*: 185–210.
911. Kienast, H. W. (1973). Oskar Pfister's centennial. *The Proceedings of the Institute of Medicine of Chicago, 29 (10)*: 353.
912. Kienast, H. W. (1974). The significance of Oskar Pfister's in-depth pastoral care. *Journal of Religion and Health, 13 (2)*: 83–95.
913. Kilborne, B. & Langness, L. L. (Eds.) (1987). *Culture and Human Nature: Theoretical Papers of Melford E. Spiro*, Chicago, IL: University of Chicago Press.
914. Kirschmayr, A. (2020). Tiefenpsychologie und Religion. Anregungen und Annäherungsversuche. Zeitschrift für freie psychoanalytische. *Forschung und Individualpsychologie*, 7: 20–42.
915. Kirkpatrick, L. A., & Hood, R. W. (1990a). Intrinsic€xtrinsic religious orientation: The boon or bane of contemporary psychology of religion? *Journal for the Scientific Study of Religion, 29*(4), 442–462.
916. Kirkpatrick, L. A. & Shaver, P. R. (1990). Attachment theory and religion: Childhood attachments, religious beliefs, and conversion. *Journal for the Scientific Study of Religion, 29*: 3: 315–334.
917. Kirkpatrick, L. A. (2004). *Attachment, Evolution, and the Psychology of Religion*, New York, NY: Guilford Press.
918. Kirschner, S. R. (1996). *The Religious and Romantic Origins of Psychoanalysis: Individuation and Integration in Post-Freudian Theory*, New York, NY: Cambridge University Press.
919. Kirsner, D. (1990). Mystics and professionals in the culture of American psychoanalysis. *Free Association, 20*: 85–103.
920. Klass, D. (2014). Grief, consolation, and religions: A conceptual framework. *Omega, 69*: 1–18.
921. Klauber, J. (1974). Notes on the physical roots of religion, with particular reference to the development of Western Christianity. *International Journal of Psychoanalysis, 55*: 249–255.
922. Klein, D. (1985). *Jewish Origins of the Psychoanalytic Movement*, Chicago, IL: The University of Chicago Press.
923. Klein, M. (1961). *Narrative of a Child Analysis*, London: Hogarth.
924. Klepec, P. (2019). On Lacan's the triumph of religion and related matters. *Filozofski vestnik, 40*: 139–162.
925. Klessmann, M. (1994). *Pastoralpsychologie. Ein Lehrbuch*, Neukirchen-Vluyn: Neukichener Verlag.

926. Klimkov, O. (2017). E. Fromm religion psychology and its relevance for modern religious studies. *Traektoriâ Nauki, 3*: 1–19.
927. Klyman, C. M. (2014). A psychoanalytic perspective of women in the Bible. *Cross Currents, 64*: 135–152.
928. Koening, H. G., King, D. & Carson, V. B. (2012). *Handbook of Religion and Health*, New York, NY: Oxford University Press.
929. Koening, H. G. (1997). *Is Religion Good for Your Health? The Effects of Religion on Physical and Mental Health*, New York, NY/London: The Haworth Press.
930. Kohn, M. (1982). *Freud et le Yiddish: le Préanalytique*, Paris: Christian Bourgois.
931. Kohut, H. (1985). *Religion, ethics, values*. In: C. B. Strozier (Ed.) *Self-Psychology and the Humanities: Reflections on a New Psychoanalytic Approach* (pp. 261–262). New York, NY: W. W. Norton.
932. Koltai, C. (2010). *"Totem e tabu". Um mito freudiano*, Rio de Janeiro: Civilização Brasileira.
933. Koprowski, E. (2014). Freud, psychoanalysis, and the therapeutic effect of agapic love. *Issues in Mental Health Nursing, 35 (4)*: 314–315.
934. Kovel, J. (1990). Beyond the future of an illusion: further reflections on Freud and religion. *Psychoanalytic Review, 77 (1)*: 69–87.
935. Krapf, E. E. (1957) Psychoanalyse und Religion. In: Th. Adorno & W. Dirks (Ed.) *Freud in der Gegenwart* (pp. 231–245). Frankfurt: Europäische Verlagsanstalt.
936. Kristeva, J. (1987). *In the Beginning Was Love: Psychoanalysis and Faith*, New York, NY: Columbia University Press.
937. Kristeva, J. (1989). *Tales of Love*, New York, NY: Columbia University Press.
938. Kristeva, J. (1995). *New Maladies of the Soul*, New York, NY: Columbia University Press.
939. Kristeva, J. (2002). Le Cantique des cantiques. *Pardès, 32–33*: 65–78.
940. Kristeva, J. (2008). *Thérèse, mon amour*, Paris: Fayard.
941. Kristeva, J. (2009). *This Incredible Need to Believe*, New York, NY: Columbia University Press.
942. Kristeva, J. (2012). Daniel Widlöcher: L'imaginaire, les religions, la sublimation. *Annales Médico-Psychologiques, 170*: 440–443.
943. Kroeber, A. L. (1939). Totem and Taboo: An ethnologic psychanalysis. *American Anthropologist, 22*: 48–55.
944. Krull, M. (1986). *Freud and His Father*, New York, NY: Norton.
945. Kuchan, K. L. (2009). The metaphor of experience and the experience of metaphor: critical reflection on a contemplative process toward aliveness and compassion. *The Journal of Pastoral Care & Counseling, 63 (3–4)*: 1–13.
946. Kuchan, K. L. (2011). Prayer as therapeutic process toward transforming destructiveness within a spiritual direction relationship. *Journal of Religion and Health, 50 (1)*: 120–131.
947. Küchenhoff, J. (2021). Für Unverfügbares offen bleiben: Die gemeinsame Aufgabe von Religion und Psychoanalyse. *Zeitschrift für Psychoanalyse und ihre Anwendungen, 75*: 193–229.
948. Kugelmann, R. (2011). *Psychology and Catholicism: Contested Boundaries*, Cambridge: Cambridge University Press.
949. Kugelmann, R. (2005). Contradictions between Catholicism and psychology in the United States. *Passau Schriften zur Psychologiegeschischte, 13*: 13–33.
950. Kugelmann, R. (2014). Imprimi potest: Roman Catholic censoring of psychology and psychoanalysis in the early 20th century. *History of the Human Sciences, 27*: 74–90.
951. Küng, H. (1990). *Freud and the Problem of God*, New Haven, CT: Yale University Press.
952. Kurtz, S. N. (1992). *All the Mothers Are One: Hindu India and the Cultural Reshaping of Psychoanalysis*, New York, NY: Columbia University Press.

953. Kwilecki, S. (2004). Religion and coping: A contribution from religious studies. *Journal for the Scientific Study of Religion, 43*: 477–489.
954. Kyrillos Neto, F. & Drawin, C. R. (2019). Crença religiosa e final de análise: o sujeito frente à elaboração de saber. *Arquivos Brasileiros de Psicología, 2*: 99–113.
955. La Barre, W. (1958). The influence of Freud on anthropology. *American Imago, 15*: 275–328.
956. La Barre, W. (1959). Religion, Rorschach, and tranquillizers. *American Journal of Orthopsychiatry, 29*: 688–698.
957. La Barre, W. (1962). *They Shall Take Up Serpents: Psychology of the Southern Snake-Handling Cult*, Minneapolis, MN: University of Minnesota Press.
958. La Barre, W. (1970). *The Ghost Dance: The Origins of Religion*, New York, NY: Doubleday and Company.
959. La Barre, W. (1978). Freudian biology, magic, and religion. *Journal of American Psychoanalytic Association, 26* (*4*): 813–830.
960. La Barre, W. (1991). *Shadow of Childhood: Neoteny and the Biology of Religion*, Norman: University of Oklahoma Press.
961. Lacan, J. (1953–2005). *Le Séminaire (1953–2005)*, Paris: Seuil.
962. Lacan, J. (1982). God and the jouissance of the woman. In: J. Mitchell & J. Rose (Eds.) *Feminine Sexuality* (pp. 37–48). New York, NY: W. W. Norton.
963. Lacan, J. (2005). *Le triomphe de la religion. Précédé de: Discours aux catholiques*, Paris: Seuil.
964. Laing, R. D. (1970). Religious sensibility. *The Listener, 23*: 536–537.
965. Lamberetino, A. (1985). L'uomo Freud. Personalità morale e religiosa:. *Filosofía, 36*: 51–78.
966. Lambertino, A. (1987). *Psicoanalisi e morale in Freud*, Napoli: Guida.
967. Lamizet, B. (2011). Sémiotique du sacré. *Essachess, 4*: 47–57.
968. Lamontagne, D. (2003). Sainte Anne, épouse, mere et gran-mère ou le féminin qui résiste au Coeur du monothéisme? In: C. Domínguez-Morano & R. Briones (Eds.) *Masculino-femenino y hecho religioso* (pp. 247–361). Granada: Universidad de Granada.
969. Lamote, T. & Mary., A. (2010). Hypnose et fascination collective: Métapsychologie des processus d'adhésion à la scientologie—L'envers du discours psychanalytique. *Topique: Revue Freudienne, 112*: 143–160.
970. Lamote, T., Besson, D. G. & Sauret, M. J. (2021). From mystical quest to political movement: A Lacanian analysis of shia Islam. *Ágora. Estudos em Teoria Psicanalítica, 23* (*3*): 2–10.
971. Lamote, T., Besson, D. G. & Sauret, M.-J. (2020). From mystical quest to political movement: A Lacanian analysis of Shia Islam. *Ágora. Estudos em Teoria Psicanalítica, 23*: 2–10.
972. LaMothe, R. (1998b). Sacred objects as vital objects: Transitional objects reconsidered. *Journal of Psychology and Theology, 26*: 159–167.
973. LaMothe, R. (2003). Freud, religion, and the presence of projective identification. *Psychoanalytic Psychology, 20*: 287–302.
974. LaMothe, R. (2009). The clash of Gods: Changes in a patient's use of God representations. *Journal of American Academy of Psychoanalysis, 37*: 73–84.
975. LaMothe, R. (2014). Winnicott and helplessness: Developmental theory, religion, and personal life. *The Psychoanalytic Quarterly, 84* (*4*): 871–896.
976. LaMothe, R., Arnold, J. & Crane, J. (1998a). The penumbra of religious discourse. *Psychoanalytic Psychology, 15*: 63–73. *Psychoanalytic Review, 108*: 51–78.
977. Lang, B. (1910/11). Ein therapeutisches Christentum: Oskar Pfister und Eugen Drewermann. *Archiv für Religionspsychologie, 22*: 116–135.
978. Lang, R. (2007). *Beyond Yahweh and Jesus: Bringing Death's Wisdom to Faith, Spirituality, and Psychoanalysis*, New York, NY: Jason Aronson.
979. Langs, R. (2009). The role of religious imagery in adaptive psychotherapy. *The Journal of American Academic of Psychoanalysis and Dynamic Psychiatry, 37* (*1*): 85–98.

980. Laor, N. (1989). Psychoanalytic neutrality toward religious experience. *The Psychoanalytic Study of the Child, 44*: 211–230.
981. Läpple, V. & Scharfenberg, J. (1977). *Psychotherapie und Seelsorge*, Darmstadt: Wissenschaftliche Buchgesellschaft.
982. Larivée, S. (2017). Sexe, psychanalyse et religion. *Revue de Psychoéducation, 46*: 175–182.
983. Laval, G. (1997). Le travail de de-croyance. *Revue Française de Psychanalyse, 61*: 825–835.
984. Lavoie, G. (1978). Actes obsédants et exercices religieux. Un écrit freudien sur la religion. *Laval théologique philosophique, 34*: 247–260.
985. Le Bon, Y. (2010). De la sainte Trinité au nœud borroméen ou de la « croyance laïque ». *Champ lacanien, 8*: 117–122.
986. Le Brun, J. (2004). *Imago*, un laboratoire pour la science des religions. In: J. François (Ed.) *La Psychanalyse: chercher, inventer, réinventer* (pp. 39–49). Ramonville Saint-Agne: Erès.
987. Le Brun, J. (2010). Psychanalyse et mystique: quelques questions. *Champ lacanien, 8*: 127–147.
988. Le Rider, J. (1997). Jewish identity in "Moses and Monotheism". *The Psychohistory Review, 25*: 245–254.
989. Leavy, S. A. (1980). *The Psychoanalytic Dialogue*, New Haven, CT: Yale University Press.
990. Leavy, S. A. (1982). Questioning authority: The contribution of psychoanalysis to religion. *Cross Currents, 32*: 129–142.
991. Leavy, S. A. (1986). A Pascalian meditation on psychoanalysis and religious experience. *Cross Currents, 26*: 147–55.
992. Leavy, S. A. (1988). *In the Image of God. A Psychoanalytic View*, New Haven, CT: Yale University Press.
993. Leavy, S. A. (1990). Reality in religion and psychoanalysis. In: S. Smith & S. Handelman (Eds.) *Psychoanalysis and Religion* (pp. 43–59). Baltimore, MD: Johns Hopkins University Press.
994. Leavy, S. A. (2009). Psychoanalysis and religious mysticism. *Journal of American Psychoanalytic Association, 57 (2)*: 477–489.
995. Lebrun, J. P. & Wénin, A. (Eds.) (2008). *Des lois pour être humain*, Paris: Érès.
996. Lebzeltern, G. (1990). S. Freuds Bild vom Menschen: Das Moralische im Menschen. *Archiv Für Religionspsychologie/Archive for the Psychology of Religion, 19 (1)*: 126–145.
997. Lechat, F. (1950). Névrose et religiosité. *Revue Française de Psychanalyse, 14*: 90–105.
998. Lecuit, J. B. (2003). Désir de Dieu et sublimation. *Christus, 197*: 62–69.
999. Lecuit, J. B. (2007). *L'anthropologie théologique à la lumière de la psychanalyse. la contribution majeure d'Antoine Vergote*, Paris: Cerf.
1000. Lecuit, J. B. (2008). La mystique, entre régression et passion sublimatoire. *Adolescence, 26*: 143–157.
1001. Lecuit, J. B. (2010). Enjeux actuels de la "spiritualisation". Approche interdisciplinaire. In: L. Lemoine (Ed.) *Vérité, désir, expérience spirituelle et expérience psychanalytique* (pp. 55–83). Paris: Cerf.
1002. Lecuit, J. B. (2012). *Le défi de l'intériorité: Le carmel réformé en France 1611–2011*, Paris: Desclée de Brouwer.
1003. Ledoux, M. (1980). La relation d'absence. *Nouvelle Revue de Psychanalyse, 22*: 235–244.
1004. Ledure, Y. (1992). Potentialités de perversion dans le discours chrétien. *Lumière Et Vie, 215*: 43–50.
1005. Lee, R. S. (1949). *Freud and Christianity*, London: James Clark.
1006. Legendre, P. (1974). *L'amour du censeur. Essai sur l'ordre dogmatique*, Paris: Seuil.
1007. Lehmann, H. (1921). Zinzendorfs Frömmigkeit und ihre Bedeutung. *Zeitschrift Für Religionpsychologie, 5 (10)*: 284–300.

1008. Lehrman, N. S. (1963). Moses, Monotheism & Marital Fidelity. *Journal of Religion and Health, 3*: 70–89.
1009. Lemercier, G. (1966). *Dialogue avec le Christ. Moines en psychanalyse*, Paris: Grasset.
1010. Lemoine, L. (2002). Le dialogue foi chrétienne/Psychanalyse dans le discernement des vocations entre 1950 et 1975. *Le Supplément, 222*: 69–101.
1011. Lemoine, L. (2004). Louis Beirnaert, s.j. (1906–1985). La rencontre insolite et fructueuse entre éthique psychanalytique et éthique chrétienne. *Le Supplément, 229*: 89–114.
1012. Lemoine, L. (2005). Éthique chrétienne et psychanalyse aujourd'hui: "garder le débat vivant. *Revue d'Éthique et Théologie Morale, 233*: 85–112.
1013. Lemoine, L. (2008). Corps et Esprit: Quelles intrications sur le plan de la vie psychique? *La Vie Spirituelle, 88*: 523–538.
1014. Lemoine, L. (2010a). Le martyre: la dialectique du vivre et du mourir. *Topique: Revue Freudienne, 113*: 91–100.
1015. Lemoine, L. (Ed.) (2010b). *Vérité, désir expérience spirituelle et expérience psychanalytique*, Paris: Cerf.
1016. Leupin, A. (2004). *Lacan Today: Psychoanalysis, Science, Religion*, New York, NY: Other Press.
1017. Levin, J. (2010). Religion and mental health: theory and research. *International Journal of Applied Psychoanalytic Studies, 7*: 102–115.
1018. Levy, I. (2011). The Laius complex: From myth to psychoanalysis. *International Forum of Psychoanalysis, 20*: 222–228.
1019. Lewin, B. D. (1950). *The Psychoanalysis of Elation*, New York, NY: International University Press.
1020. Liebman, S. J. (2000). Reconstructing the sacred: Evolving conceptualizations of religious faith in psychoanalytic theory and practice. *Journal of Contemporary Psychotherapy, 30*: 7–25.
1021. Lietaer, H. & Corveleyn, J. (1995). Psychoanalytical interpretation of the demoniacal possession and the mystical development of Sister Jeanne des Anges from Loudun. *The International Journal for the Psychology of Religion, 5*: 259–276.
1022. Lijtmaer, R. M. (2009). The patient who believes and the analyst who does not. *The Journal of American Academic for Psychoanalysis and Dynamic Psychiatry, 37*: 99–110.
1023. Lima, J. G. (2017). *A grande tradição: Jacques Lacan, a filosofia antiga e o cristianismo*, Rio de Janeiro: Universidade Federal do Rio de Janeiro.
1024. Lippman, R. L. (2021). Freud's B'nai B'rith dream: Having lost his way, his "brethren … were unkind and scornful …". *The Psychoanalytic Review, 108 (3)*: 243–250.
1025. Litmanovich, J. A. (2015). *Un monasterio en psicoanálisis. Las operaciones psicoanalíticas al interior del monasterio Benedictino de Ahuacatitlán, Cuernavaca (1961–1967)*, México: Paradiso Ed.
1026. Loewenberg, P. (1971). Sigmund Freud as a Jew: A study in ambivalence and courage. *Journal of the Behavioral Sciences, 7*: 363–369.
1027. Loewenstein, R. M. (1951). *Christian and Jews: A Psychoanalytic Study*, New York, NY: International University Press.
1028. Lombillo, J. R. (1973). The soldier saint. A psychological analysis of the conversion of Ignatius of Loyola. *Psychiatric Quarterly, 47*: 386–418.
1029. Longhi, R. (2022). *Psicoanálisis y espiritualidad. Del diván a la meditación*, Barcelona: Herder.
1030. Lorand, S. (1962). Psychoanalytic therapy of religious devotees: A theoretical and technical contribution. *International Journal of Psychoanalysis, 43*: 50–55.
1031. Lowenfeld, H. (1969). The decline in belief on the devil. The consequences for group psychology. *The Psychoanalytic Quarterly, 38*: 455–462.
1032. Lust, J. (1989). Freud, Hosea and the murder of Moses; Hosea 12. *Ephemerides Theologicae Lovaniense, 65*: 81–93.

1033. Lustig, E. (1976). On the origin of Judaism: A psychoanalytic approach. *Psychoanalytic Study of Society, 7*: 359–367.
1034. Lutzky, H. (1991). The sacred and the maternal object: An application of Fairbairn's theory to religion. In: H. B. Siegelis, L. Barbanel, I. Hirsch, J. Lasky, H. Silverman & S. Warschau (Eds.) *Psychoanalytic Reflections on Current Issues* (pp. 25–44). New York, NY: New York University Press.
1035. Luyten, P. & Corveleyn, J. (2003). Mysticism, creativity, and psychoanalysis: Still crazy after all these years? *The International Journal for the Psychology of Religion, 13*: 97–109.
1036. Maciel, K. D. & Rocha, Z. (2008). Dois discursos de Freud sobre a religião. *Revista Mal-estar e Subjetividade, 8*: 729–754.
1037. Mack, M. (2006). The Savage Science: Sigmund Freud, psychoanalysis, and the history of religion. *Journal of Religious History, 30*: 331–353.
1038. Maclean, H. V. (1940). A few comments on *Moses and Monotheism*. *Psychoanalytic Quarterly, 9*: 207–213.
1039. Madonna, J. M. (2018). God in the hour: Religious faith in psychoanalytic treatment. *The Journal of Pastoral Care, 72*: 129–138.
1040. Magid, B. (2000). The couch and the cushion: integrating Zen and psychoanalysis. *The Journal of American Academy of Psychoanalysis and Dynamic Psychiatry, 28*: 513–526.
1041. Magid, B. (2004). Intrinsic opposition between the scientific nature of psychoanalytic inquiry and the nature of religious belief. *The Journal of American Academy of Psychoanalysis and Dynamic Psychiatry, 32* (2): 402–404.
1042. Maguire, U. (1969). La dernière cène. Étude de dynamique de groupe. *Le Supplément, 22*: 234–241.
1043. Mahlmann, T. (1994). Was genau verstand Sigmund Freud unter "Illusion" oder wie reicht di Religionkritik? *Wege zum Menschen, 46*: 79–101.
1044. Mahmood, K. (2015). Psychoanalysis, religion, and enculturation: Reflections through the life of Mother Teresa. *Journal of Religion and Health, 54* (2): 638–648.
1045. Mahon, E. (2006). The invention of purgatory: A note on the historical pedigree of the Superego. *The Psychoanalytic Study of the Child, 61*: 334–344.
1046. Maïdani Gerard, J. P. (2003). "Genre". "Sexe", "Sexuel" et le christianisme? In: C. Domínguez-Morano & R. Briones. *Masculino-femenino y hecho religioso* (pp. 101–114). Granada. Universidad de Granada.
1047. Main, R. (2006). Psychology of religion. In: R. A. Segal (Ed.) *The Blackwell Companion to the Study of Religion* (pp. 147–170). Malden, MA: Blackwell Publishing.
1048. Main, R. (2008). Psychology of religion: An overview of its history and current status. *Religion Compass, 2*: 708–733.
1049. Maître, J. (1981). Idéologie religieuse, conversion mystique et symbiose mère-enfant. Le cas de Thérèse Martin. *Archives des Sciences Sociales des Religions, 51*: 65–100.
1050. Maître, J. (1997). *Mystique et féminité: Essai de psychanalyse sociohistorique*, Paris: Editions du Cerf.
1051. Maître, J. (1999). Psychological history in France: 1968–1997. *Psychohistory Review, 27*: 23–48.
1052. Maître, J. (2000). *Anorexies religieuses, anorexie mentale. Essai de psychanalyse sociohistorique. de Marie de l'Incarnation à Simone Weil*, Paris: Cerf.
1053. Maître, J. & Saussure, T. (1972). Psychanalyse et sociologie religieuse. *Archives de Sociologie des Religions, 33*: 111–134.
1054. Maître, J., (1993). Une inconnue célèbre. *Madeleine Lebouc/Pauline Lair Lamotte (1853–1918)*. Paris: Antrhopos.
1055. Maître, J., (1995). L'Orpheline de la Bérésina. *Thérèse de Lisieux (1873–1897)*. Paris: Cerf.
1056. Malamoud, C. (2003). Psychanalyse et sciences des religions. In: P. Kaufmann (Ed.) *L'apport freudien: Eléments pour une encyclopédie de la psychanalyse* (pp. 584–593). Paris: Bordas.

1057. Malkwitz, L. (2003). 'Ich möchte an Sie glauben können!': Das Phänomen 'Religiosität' in der psychoanalytischen Praxis. *Forum der Psychoanalyse: Zeitschrift für klinische Theorie & Praxis, 19*: 343–361.
1058. Malone, K. & Friedlander, S. R. (2000). *Lacan's Social Psychoanalysis: Religion and Community in a Pluralistic Society*, New York, NY: State University of New York Press.
1059. Malony, H. & North, G. (1979). The Future of an Illusion-The Illusion of the Future: An historic dialogue on the value of religion between Oskar Pfister and Sigmund Freud. *Journal of the History of the Behavioral Sciences, 15* (*2*): 177–186.
1060. Malony, H. N. & Spilka, B. (Eds.) (1991). *Religion in Psychodynamic Perspective. The Contribution of Paul Pruyser*, New York, NY: Oxford University Press.
1061. Malony, H. N. & Shafranske, E. P. (Eds.) (2021). *Early Psychoanalytic Religious Writings*, Leiden: Brill Rodopi.
1062. Mangis, M. W. (2007). Kicking the patient: Immediacy in the consulting room. *Journal of Psychology and Theology, 35*: 43–51.
1063. Mann, J. (1962). Clinical and theoretical aspects of religious belief. *Journal of the American Psychoanalytic Association, 12*: 160–170.
1064. Mannoni, O. (1972). Freud y la religión. *Cuadernos Sigmund Freud, 2–3*: 57–72.
1065. Mannoni, O. (1976). L'athéisme de Freud. *Ornicar? 6*: 21–32.
1066. Manoussakis, J. P. (2016). On St. Augustine's body: The conversion of phenomenology, psychoanalysis, and theology. In: E. R. Severson, B. W. Becker & D. M. Goodman (Eds.) *In the Wake of Trauma: Psychology and Philosophy for the Suffering Other* (pp. 35–56). Pittsburgh, PA: Duquesne University Press.
1067. Marco, H. H. (2017). Religião, ciência e capitalismo: Sujeito massificado, objeto padrão e medida comum para o gozo. *Ágora. Estudos em Teoria Psicanalítica, 20*: 527–542.
1068. Marcos, C. M. (2006). O homem Moisés e a religião monoteísta. Da escrita do texto ao assasinato do pai. *Percurso, 36*: 101–108.
1069. Marcus, P. & Rosenberg, A. (1995). The value of religion in sustaining the Self in extreme situations. *Psychoanalytic Review, 82*: 81–105.
1070. Marcus, P. (2003). *Ancient Religious Wisdom, Spirituality, and Psychoanalysis*, Westport, CT: Praeger.
1071. Marcus, P. (2006). Religion without promises: the philosophy of Emmanuel Levinas and psychoanalysis. *Psychoanalytic Review, 93*: 923–951.
1072. Markez, I. (Ed.) (2015). *Religión y psicoanálisis en la obra de Ángel Garma*, Bilbao: Kimen-Core Academic.
1073. Marvaud, J. (2020). La peau et le toucher. *Annales médico-psychologiques, 178*: 137–144.
1074. Massad, J. (2009). Psychoanalysis, Islam, and the other of liberalism. *Psychoanalysis and History, 11*: 193–208.
1075. Massimi & Mahfoud (Eds.) (1999). *Diante de misterio: Psicologia e senso religioso*, São Paulo: Loyola.
1076. Masson, J. M. (1976). The psychology of the ascetic. *Journal of Asian Studies, 35*: 611–625.
1077. Masson, J. M. (1980). *The Oceanic Feeling. The Origins of Religious Sentiment in Ancient India*, Dordrecht: Springer.
1078. Matte Blanco, I. (1986). Psicoanalisi e teologia. In: N. Spaccapelo (Ed.) *Religione e psicoanalisi, una ricerca interdisciplinare* (pp. 23–58). Roma: Città Nuova.
1079. Matte Blanco, I. (1954). *Lo psíquico y la naturaleza humana*, Santiago de Chile: Universidad de Chile.
1080. Matte Blanco, I. (1975a). *The Unconscious as Infinite Sets*, London: Karnac.
1081. Matte Blanco, I. (1975b). Creatività e ortodossia. *Rivista di psicoanalisi, 21*: 225–289.
1082. Matte Blanco, I. (1988). *Thinking, Feeling and Being*, London/New York, NY: Routledge.

1083. Maurano, D. (2003). *A Tranfeêrencia. Uma viagem rumo ao continente Negro*, Rio de Janeiro: Zahar.
1084. Maurano, D. & Alburquerque, B. (2019). Lacan e a experiência mística à luz da psicanálise. *Revista Latinoamericana de Psicopatologia Fundamental, 22 (3)*: 439–456.
1085. Maurano, D. & Albuquerque, B. (2021). Feminino e mística: ressonâncias trágicas e barrocas do que ultrapassa o fio das palavras. *Revista Pistis&Praxis, 13*: 260–272.
1086. Mazzoti, M. (1993). Note sul problema dell'ateismo psicanalitico. *Agalma, 10*: 7–14.
1087. McBride, J. (1992). Missing bodies, missing persons: Detectives, analysts, and the quest for the Self. *Pastoral Psychology, 40*: 375–389.
1088. McDargh, J. (1992). Commentary on returning words to flesh and contemporary psychoanalysis and religion. *Pastoral Psychology, 40*: 391–399.
1089. McDargh, J. (1983). *Psychoanalytic Object Relations Theory and the Study of Religion: On Faith and the Imaging of God*, Lanham, MD: University Press of America.
1090. McDargh, J. (1986). God, mother, and me: An object relational perspective on religious material. *Pastoral Psychology, 34*: 251–263.
1091. McDargh, J. (1993). Concluding clinical postscript: On developing a psychotheological perspective. In: M. L. Randour (Ed.) *Exploring Sacred Landscape. Religious and Spiritual Experiences in Psychotherapy* (pp. 172–193). New York, NY: Columbia University Press.
1092. McDargh, J. (1997). Creating a new research paradigm for the psychoanalytic study of religion: The pioneering work of Ana-Maria Rizzuto. In: J. L. Jacobs & D. Capps (Eds.) *Religion, Society and Psychoanalysis. Reading in Contemporary Theory* (pp. 181–199). Boulder, NV/Cumnor Hill: Westview Press.
1093. McGrath, W. J. (1993). Retrospective medicine in Breuer and Freud's "Studies on Hysteria": The assault in medieval superstition. *The Annual of Psychoanalysis, 21*: 139–156.
1094. McGuire, W. (Ed.) (1974). *The Correspondence Between Sigmund Freud and C. G. Jung*, Princeton, NJ: Princeton University Press.
1095. Mead, M. (1963). *Totem y Taboo* reconsidered with respect. *Bulletin of the Menninger Clinic, 27*: 185–199.
1096. Medhi, Z. (2017). Phobia of religion: Religion as Islam a political argument and a psychoanalytic inquiry of Islamophobia in India. *International Journal of Applied Psychoanalytic Studies, 14*: 222–244.
1097. Meissner, W. W. (1961). *Annotated Bibliography in Religion and Psychology*, New York, NY: The Academy of Religion and Mental Health.
1098. Meissner, W. W. (1963–1964) Psychological notes on the *Spiritual Exercises. Woodstock Letters, 92*: 349–366, *93*: 31–58, 165–191.
1099. Meissner, W. W. (1964). Prolegomena of a psychology of Grace. *Journal of Religion and Health, 3*: 209–240.
1100. Meissner, W. W. (1965). *Group Dynamics in the Religious Life*, South Bend, IN: University of Notre Dame Press.
1101. Meissner, W. W. (1966). *Foundations for a Psychology of Grace*, New York, NY: Paulist Press.
1102. Meissner, W. W. (1973). Notes on the psychology of hope. *Journal of Religion and Health, 12*: 7–29, 120–139.
1103. Meissner, W. W. (1978). Psychoanalytic aspects of religious experience. *The Annual of Psychoanalysis, 6*: 103–142.
1104. Meissner, W. W. (1984). *Psychoanalysis and Religious Experience*, New Haven, CT: Yale University Press.
1105. Meissner, W. W. (1986). Aggression and theology. *Thought, 240*: 90–104.
1106. Meissner, W. W. (1987). *Life and Faith: Psychological Perspectives on Religious Experience*, Washington, DC: Georgetown University Press.

1107. Meissner, W. W. (1988a). The cult phenomenon and the paranoid process. In: L. B. Boyer & S. A. Grolnick (Eds.) *The Psychoanalytic Study of Society* (pp. 69–95). Hillsdale, NJ: Analytic Press, Inc.
1108. Meissner, W. W. (1990). The role of transitional conceptualization in religious thought. In: J. H. Smith & S. A. Handelman (Eds.) *Psychiatry and the Humanities, Vol. 11. Psychoanalysis and Religion* (pp. 95–116). Baltimore, MD: Johns Hopkins University Press.
1109. Meissner, W. W. (1992a). *Ignatius of Loyola: The Psychology of a Saint*, New Haven, CT: Yale University Press.
1110. Meissner, W. W. (1992b). Religious thinking as transitional conceptualization. *Psychoanalytic Review, 79* (*2*): 175–196.
1111. Meissner, W. W. (1992c). Medieval messianism and Sabbateanism. *Psychoanalytic Study of Society, 17*: 289–325.
1112. Meissner, W. W. (1995). *Thy kingdom Come: Psychoanalytic Perspectives on the Messiah and the Millennium*, Kansas City, MO: Sheed & Ward.
1113. Meissner, W. W. (1996). The pathology of beliefs and the beliefs of pathology. In: E. P. Shafranske (Ed.) *Religious and the Clinical Practice of Psychology* (pp. 241–268). Washington, DC: American Psychological Association Books.
1114. Meissner, W. W. (1999). *To the Greater Glory: a Psychological Study of Ignatian Spirituality*, Milwaukee, WI: Marquette University Press.
1115. Meissner, W. W. (2000a). *The Cultic Origins of Christianity: The Dynamics of Religious Development*, Collegeville, MN: Liturgical Press.
1116. Meissner, W. W. (2000b). *Freud and Psychoanalysis*, Notre Dame, IN: University of Notre Dame Press.
1117. Meissner, W. W. (2001). So, help me God! Do I help God or does God help me? In: S. Akhtar & H. Parens (Eds.) *Does God Help? Development and Clinical Aspects of Religious Belief* (pp. 77–126). Northvale, NJ/London: Jason Aronson.
1118. Meissner, W. W. (2005). On putting a cloud in a bottle: psychoanalytic perspectives on mysticism. *The Psychoanalytic Quarterly, 74*: 507–559.
1119. Meissner, W. W. (2007). Reflections on the love commandment. *The Annual of Psychoanalysis, 35*: 223–239.
1120. Meissner, W. W. (2008a). Psychoanalysis and Catholicism—Dialogues in transformation. *Psychoanalytic Inquiry, 28*: 80–89.
1121. Meissner, W. W. (2008b). A note on the use of the concept of the soul in psychoanalytic discourse. *Psychoanalytic Quarterly*, 77 (*1*): 327–340.
1122. Meissner, W. W. (2009a). Religion in the psychoanalytic relationship-some aspects of transference and countertransference. *The Journal of American Academic for Psychoanalysis and Dynamic Psychiatry, 37* (*1*): 123–136.
1123. Meissner, W. W. (2009b). The God question in psychoanalysis. *Psychoanalytic Psychology, 26*: 210–233.
1124. Meissner, W. W. (1988b). The origins of Christianity. In: L. B. Boyer & S. A. Grolnick (Eds.) *The Psychoanalytic Study of Society* (pp. 28–62). Hillsdale, NJ: Analytic Press, Inc.
1125. Meissner, W. W. (1991). Psychoanalytic hagiography: The case of Ignatius of Loyola. *Theological Studies, 52*: 3–33.
1126. Meissner, W. W. (2003). Methodological issues in the psychohistory- Psychobiography of religious figures. *The Annual of Psychoanalysis, 31*: 181–196.
1127. Mello Franco, O. (1998). Religious experience and psychoanalysis: from man-as-God to man-with God. *International Journal of Psychoanalysis, 79*: 113–131.
1128. Melman, C. (2009). O complexo de Moisés. In: M. Ch. (Ed.) *Para introduzir a psicanálise nos dias de hoje* (pp. 367–372). Porto Alegre: CMC.
1129. Meng, H. & Freud, E. (Eds.) (1963). *Psychoanalysis and Faith: the Letters of Sigmund Freud and Oskar Pfister*, New York, NY: Basic Books.

1130. Meng, W. (1997). *Narzissmus und christlische Religion: Selbstiliebe Nächstenliebe Gottesliebe*, Zurich: Theologicher Verlag.
1131. Merani, A. (1974). *Freud y el Talmud*, México: Grijalbo.
1132. Merkur, D. (1988a). The prophecies of Jeremiah. *American Imago, 42*: 1–37.
1133. Merkur, D. (1988b). Prophetic initiation in Israel and Judah. *Psychoanalytic Study of Society, 12*: 37–57.
1134. Merkur, D. (1989a). Unitive experience and the state of trance. In: M. Idel & Mc Ginn (Eds.) *Mystical Union and Monotheistic Faith* (pp. 125–153). New York, NY: Macmillan.
1135. Merkur, D. (1989b). The visionary practices of Jewish apocalyptists. *The Psychoanalytic Study of Society, 14*: 119–148.
1136. Merkur, D. (1999). *Mystical Moments and Unitive Thinking*, New York, NY: State University of New York Press.
1137. Merkur, D. (2005). Psychology of religion. In: J. R. Hillnes. *The Routledge Companion to the Study of Religion* (pp. 164–180), London/New York, NY: Routledge.
1138. Merkur, D. (2006). *Psychoanalytic Approaches to Myth*, London/New York, NY: Routledge.
1139. Merkur, D. (2010). *Explorations of the Psychoanalytic Mystic*, Amsterdam/New York, NY: Rodopi.
1140. Merkur, D. (2013). *Relating to God. Clinical Psychoanalysis, Spirituality, and Theism*, New York, NY: J. Aronson.
1141. Merot, P. (2008). Immateriality of the soul and unconscious material. *L'Évolution Psychiatrique, 73*: 79–91.
1142. Merot, P. (2011). Trace du maternel dans le religieux. *Revue Française de Psychanalyse, 75*: 1353–1433.
1143. Merzel, D. (1994). *Beyond Sanity and Madness: The Way of Zen Master Dogen*, Rutland, VT: Charles E. Tuttle.
1144. Mezan, R. (1987). *Psiconálise, judaísmo: Ressonâncias*, Campinas: Escuta.
1145. Michel, S. (1984). American conscience and the unconscious: Psychoanalysis and the rise of personal religion, 1906–1963. *Psychoanalysis and Contemporary Thought, 7*: 387–421.
1146. Mijolla-Mellor, S. (2006). Le progrès dans la spiritualité. *Cliniques Méditerranéennes, 73*: 61–72.
1147. Mijolla-Mellor, S. (2007). Le besoin de croire et ses sources océaniques. *Dialogue, 178*: 15–26.
1148. Mijolla-Mellor, S. (2004). *Le besoin de croire. Métapsychologie du fait religieux*, Paris: Dunod.
1149. Mijolla-Mellor, S. (2008). *Croire à l'épreuve du doute*, Paris: L'Atelier.
1150. Millar, D. (2008). A psychoanalytic view of biblical myth. *The International Journal of Psychoanalysis, 82*: 431–447.
1151. Miller, J. A. (2012). *Punto cenit. Política, religión y el psicoanálisis*, Buenos Aires: Diva.
1152. Miller, J. (1981). Interpretations of Freud's Jewishness, 1924–1974. *Journal of History of the Behavioral Sciences, 17*: 357–374.
1153. Miller, J. A. (2004). Religion, Psychanalyses. *Lacanian Ink, 23*: 8–39.
1154. Miller, J.-A. (2006a). Religião, psiconálise. *Opção lacaniana, 39*: 9–24.
1155. Miller, J. A. (2006b). Religión, psicoanálisis. In: D. Chorne & M. Goldenberg (Eds.) *La creencia y el psicoanálisis* (pp. 35–68). Buenos Aires: Fondo de Cultura Económica.
1156. Miller, M. E. (2005). Zen and Psychotherapy. From neutrality, through relationship, to the emptying place. In: P. Young-Eisendrath & S. Muramoto (Eds.) *Awakening and Insight Zen Buddhism and Psychotherapy* (pp. 89–99). Hove/New York, NY: Brunner-Routledge.
1157. Milner, M. (1969). *The Hands of the Living God*, London: Hogarth.
1158. Milner, M. (1987). *The Suppressed Madness of Sane Men: Forty-Four Years of Exploring Psychoanalysis*, London/New York, NY: Routledge.

1159. Molino, A. (Ed.) (1998). *The Couch and the Tree: Dialogues in Psychoanalysis and Buddhism*, New York, NY: North Point Press.
1160. Moller, H. (1965). Affective mysticism in Western Civilization. *Psychoanalytic Review, 52*: 259–338.
1161. Moloney, J. C. (1954). Mother, God, and Superego. *Journal of the American Psychoanalytic Association, 2*: 120–151.
1162. Mondello, M. L. (2001). Note sulla paternità in psicoanalisi. In: F. Ferrarotti (Ed.) *Le figure del padre* (pp. 133–168). Roma: Armando.
1163. Money-Kryle, R. (1929). *The Meaning of Sacrifice*, London: Hogarth.
1164. Money-Kryle, R. (1939). *Superstition and Society*, London: Hogarth.
1165. Moore, D. H. (1941). Freud and religion. *The Personalist, 22*: 169–173.
1166. Morandi, F. (1983). Confessione psicoanalitica e confessione sacramentale. *Revista Di Teologia Morale, 15*: 231–243.
1167. Moreau, C. H. (1976). *Freud et l'occultisme*, Paris: Privat.
1168. Moreira Silva, C. M. & Pinto, J. M. (2012). Para além da ilusão: Os limites da crítica freudiana à religião. *Ágora. Estudos em Teoria Psicanalítica, 15*: 389–404.
1169. Morel, F. (1923). Buddhistic training as artificial catatonia. *Psychoanalytic Review, 18*: 129–145.
1170. Morgan, N. (2021). Credo? Religion and psychoanalysis. *British Journal of Psychotherapy, 37*: 164–167.
1171. Moritz, M. C. (2012). Algunas ideas de Freud acerca de la religión. *Revista Pilquen. Sección Psicopedagogía, 14*: 1–9.
1172. Moscovici, M. (1980). Le monde réel. *Nouvelle Revue de Psychanalyse, 22*: 73–81.
1173. Moscovici, M. (1993). Les Préhistoires: pour aborder "Totem et Tabou". *Revue Française de Psychanalyse, 57*: 691–711.
1174. Moxon, C. (1926). *Freudian Essays on Religion and Science*, Boston, MA: The Gorham Press.
1175. Muensterberger, W. (1964). Remark on the function of mythology. *Psychoanalytic Quarterly, 3*: 94–97.
1176. Muensterberger, W. (Ed.) (1969). *Man, and His Culture: Psychoanalytic Anthropology after "Totem and Taboo"*, London: Rapp & Whiting.
1177. Muensterberger, W. (1972). The sources of Belief: A reappraisal of Geza Róheim's theory of religious origins. Introduction of G. Róheim. In *The Panic of Gods* (pp. ix–xxiii) New York, NY: Harper.
1178. Müller, J. (1927). Atheism in childhood and faulty character-development. *International Journal of Psychoanalysis, 8*: 521–522.
1179. Müller-Funk, W. (2013). *Monotheism and Morality:* The Sigmund Freud Museum Symposia 2009–2001, Leuven: Leuven University Press.
1180. N'Guyên, A. (2010). Se passer de croire à condition de s'en servir. *Champ lacanien, 8*: 59–66.
1181. Nachmani, G. (2009). Psychoanalysis and spirituality—Catastrophic change and becoming "O". *The Journal of American Academic of Psychoanalysis and Dynamic Psychiatry, 37 (1)*: 137–152.
1182. Najeeb, S. (2006). The religion of psychoanalysis, or Ode to a Nightingale. *Social Analysis, 50*: 224–238.
1183. Nase, E. (2000). Oskar Pfister's Challenge to Psychology of Religion in the Twenties. In: J. A. Belzen (Ed.) *The Psychology of Religion at the Crossroads* (pp. 45–89). Leiden-Boston-Köln: Brill.
1184. Nase, E. & Scharfenberg (Eds.) (1977). *Psychoanalyse und Religion*, Darmstadt: Wissenshaftliche Buchgesellschaft.
1185. Nase, E. (1993). *Oskar Pfister analytische Seelsorge*, Berlin: DeGruyteer.
1186. Nase, E. (2020). "Gesamtbibliographie Oskar Pfister". In: O. Pfisters (Ed.) *Analytische Seelsorge: Theorie und Praxis des ersten Pastoralpsychalogen* (pp. 494–506). Berlin/ Boston, MA: De Gruyter.

1187. Natanson, J. (2003). Lectures psychanalytiques de la Bible de Freud à nos jours. *Imaginarie & Inconscient, 3*: 7–16.
1188. Nay, J. Y. (2018). François Roustang (1923–2016) – jésuite, psychanalyste, hypnothérapeute. *Revue Medicale Suisse, 12 (543)*: 2190–2191.
1189. Nayar-Ahktar, M. C. (2022). The role of religious icons and mythological figures in traumatized individuals: A psychoanalytic perspective. In: P. L. Ellman, J. Basak & G. Schlesinger-Kipp (Eds.) *Psychoanalytic and Socio-Cultural Perspectives on Women in India: Violence, Safety and Survival* (pp. 49–59). London/New York, NY: Routledge.
1190. Neeser, M. (1920). *Les principes de la psychologie de la religion et la psychanalyse*, Neuchâtel: Attinger frères.
1191. Nelson, J. M. (2009). Psychodynamic and Relational Approaches. In: J. M. Nelson (Ed.) *Psychology, Religion and Spirituality* (pp. 143–174). New York, NY: Springer.
1192. Nelson, M. O. (1971). The concept of God and feelings toward parents. *Journal of Individual Psychology, 27*: 46–49.
1193. Neri, C. (2005). What is the function of faith and trust in psychoanalysis? *The International Journal of Psychoanalysis, 86 (1)*: 79–97.
1194. Nesci, D. A. (1991). *Collective Suicide at Jonestown: An Ethnopsychoanalytic Study of Leadership and Group Dynamics*, New York, NY: Plenum Press.
1195. Neumann, E. (1992). Freud und das Vaterbild. *Analytical Psychology, 23*: 100–108.
1196. Newman, J. W. (1996). *Disciplines of Attention. Buddhist Insight Meditation, the Ignacian Spiritual Exercises and Classical Psychoanalysis*, New York, NY: Peter Lang.
1197. Nichol, D. (2006). Buddhism and psychoanalysis: A personal reflection. *American Journal of Psychoanalysis, 66 (2)*: 157–172.
1198. Nicholi, A. (2002). *The Question of God: C.S. Lewis and Sigmund Freud Debate God, Love, Sex, and the Meaning of Life*, New York, NY: Free Press.
1199. Nields, J. A. (2003). From unity to atonement: Some religious correlates of Hans Loewald's developmental theory. *The International Journal of Psychoanalysis, 84*: 699–716.
1200. Noé, S. V. (2010). A vocação sublime: da relação entre religião e sublimação na definição da vocação religiosa. *Psicologia USP, 21*: 165–182.
1201. Noel, J. F. (2000). *Le point aveugle. L'intention imprévue de la psychanalyse*, Paris: Cerf.
1202. Nolan, E. (2009). *Film, Lacan, and the Subject of Religion: A Psychoanalytic Approach to Religious Film Analysis*, London: Continuum.
1203. Nolan, M. (1999). Situating *Totem and Taboo*. In: M. Nolan (Ed.) *Psychoanalyzing Colonialism, Colonizing Psychoanalysis: Re-reading Aboriginality* (pp. 16–75). Stirling: University of Stirling.
1204. Nominé, B. (2010). De la croyance en l'Autre au pari sur l'objet a. *Champ lacanien, 8*: 77–84.
1205. Noth, I. (2007a). Ein merkwürdiger Mann." Oskar Pfister und die Anfänge der analytischen Seelsorge. In: I. Noth & C. Morgenthaler (Eds.) *Seelsorge und Psychoanalyse* (pp. 15–33). Stuttgart: Kohlhammer.
1206. Noth, I. (2007b). "Deine Ehrfurcht und meine Liebe" – Oskar Pfister (1873–1956) und Albert Schweitzer. In: Noth & C. Morgenthaler (Ed.) *Seelsorge und Psychoanalyse.* (pp. 46–58). Stuttgart: Kohlhammer.
1207. Noth, I. (2008). Albert Schweitzer und die Psychoanalyse. *Luzifer-Amor. Zeitschrift zur Geschichte der Psychoanalyse, 43*: 133–143.
1208. Noth, I. (2010). Freud bleibenden Aktualität. Psychanalyse Rezeption in the Pastoral der Psychoanalyse in der Seelsorge. *Luzifer-Amor, 46*: 139–152.
1209. Noth, I. (2014). Un monde nouveau: L'importance de Oskar Pfister pour la psychanalyse en Suisse. *Le Coq-Héron, 218*: 81–85.
1210. Noth, I. & Morgenthaler, C. (Eds.) (2007). *Seelsorge und Psychoanalyse*, Stuttgart: Kohlhammer.
1211. Noth, I. & Morgenthaler, C. (Eds.) (2014a). *Sigmund Freud - Oskar Pfister. Briefwechsel 1909–1939*, Zürich: Theologischer Verlag.

1212. Noth, I. & Morgenthaler, C. (2014b). The friendship between Sigmund Freud and Oskar Pfister as seen in the correspondence between the Jewish atheist founder of psychoanalysis and the Swiss Pastor who pioneered Pastoral Psychology. *Pastoral Psychology, 63*: 81–90.
1213. Noth, I., Morgenthaler, C. & Greider, K. (Eds.) (2011). *Pastoral Psychology and Psychology of Religion in Dialogue: Implications for Pastoral Care*, Stuttgart: Kohlhammer.
1214. Novak, D. (2016). On Freud's theory of law and religion. *International Journal of Law and Psychiatry, 48*: 24–34.
1215. Novis-Deutsch, N. (2015). Identity conflicts and value pluralism—What can we learn from religious psychoanalytic therapists? *Journal for the Theory of Social Behaviour, 45*: 494–505.
1216. Nunberg, H. (1947). Circumcision and problems of bisexuality. *International Journal of Psychoanalysis, 28*: 145–179.
1217. Nurbakhsh, D. (1978). Sufism and psychoanalysis. Part one: what is Sufism? *The International Journal of Social Psychiatry, 24*: 204–212.
1218. Nurbakhsh, D. (1978). Sufism and psychoanalysis. Part two: A comparison between Sufism and psychoanalysis. *International Journal of Social Psychiatry, 24*: 213–219.
1219. Nuttin, J. (1950). *Psychanalyse et conception spiritualiste de l'homme*, Louvain: Publications Universitaires de Louvain.
1220. Nwoye, A. (2015). The multicultural relevance of Erikson's *Young Man Luther*: A study in psychoanalysis and history. *Psychotherapy and Politics International, 13*: 67–78.
1221. O'Connell, A. (2009). Man is born broken. He lives by mending. The grace of God is glue. How religion can enrich an analysis. *Journal of the American Academy of Psychoanalysis & Dynamic Psychiatry, 37*: 153–164.
1222. O'Neill, M. K. & Akhtar, S. (Eds.) (2018). *On Freud's "The Future of an Illusion"*, London/New York, NY: Routledge.
1223. Obeyesekere, G. (1981). *Medusa's Hair: An Essay on Personal Symbols and Religious Experience*, Chicago, IL: The University of Chicago Press.
1224. Obeyesekere, G. (1984). *The Cult of the Goddess Pattini*, Chicago, IL: The University of Chicago Press.
1225. Obeyesekere, G. (1991). *The Work of Culture: Symbolic Transformation in Psychoanalysis and Anthropology*, Chicago, IL: The University of Chicago Press.
1226. Oelschlegel, L. (1943). Regarding Freud's book on Moses. A religio-psychoanalytic study. *Psychoanalytic Review, 30*: 67–76.
1227. Oliveira de Aquino Pereira, M. (2006). *Que deus? Reflexão teológico-pastoral acerca da fé adulta no deus de Jesus em contraposição à fé no deus da onipotência infantil, conforme Domínguez Morano*, Rio de Janeiro: PUC.
1228. Oliveira, A. P. & Kupermann, D. (2022). Amizade e alteridade: Reflexões sobre psicanálise e religião a partir da relação entre Freud e Pfister. *Memorandum: Memória e História em Psicología, 39*: 1676–1669.
1229. Oliveira, S. N. (2012). Psicanálise da religiosidade: O marketing da intolerância ou de como a iurd oprime a umbanda. *Revista de Estudos da Religião (REVER), 12*: 111–122.
1230. Oliveira, T. A. (2021). Pulsão de morte: Um elemento propulsor da intolerância ideológico religiosa. *Revista Latinoamericana de Psicopatologia Fundamental, 24* (*1*): 92–114.
1231. Oppenheim, M. (2013). Langue, parole, et chanson: On language as song in psychoanalysis and Jewish Philosophy. *Pastoral Psychology, 62*: 403–421.
1232. Oraison, M. (1957). Le médecin psychanalyste et le confesseur. *Recherches et Débats du Centre Catholique des Intellectuels Français, 21*: 153–172.
1233. Ostow, M. & Scharfstein, B. A. (1954). *The Need to Believe: The Psychology of Religion*, New York, NY: International Universities Press.
1234. Ostow, M. (1955). The need to believe: Persistent religious behavior in non-believers. *International Record of Medicine and General Practice Clinics, 168*: 798–802.

1235. Ostow, M. (1958a). Biological basis of religious symbolism. *International Record of Medicine, 171*: 709–717.
1236. Ostow, M. (1958b). The nature of religious controls. *American Psychologist, 13*: 571–574.
1237. Ostow, M. (1986). Archetypes of Apocalypse in dreams and fantasies, and in religious scripture. *American Imago, 43*: 307–334.
1238. Ostow, M. (1988). Apocalyptic thinking in mental illness and social disorder. *Psychoanalysis and Contemporary Thought, 11*: 285–297.
1239. Ostow, M. (1989). Sigmund Freud and Jakob Freud and the Philipson Bible. *International Review of Psychoanalysis, 16*: 483–492.
1240. Ostow, M. (1995a). *Myth and Madness: The Psychodynamics of Anti-Semitism*, London/New York, NY: Routledge.
1241. Ostow, M. (1995b). *Ultimate Intimacy: The Psychodynamics of Jewish Mysticism*, London/New York, NY: Routledge.
1242. Ostow, M. (2006). Spirituality and religion: A psychoanalytic approach. *The Annual of Psychoanalysis, 35*: 69–81.
1243. Ostow, M. (2007). *Spirit, Mind, & Brain: A Psychoanalytic Examination of Spirituality and Religion*, New York, NY: Columbia University Press.
1244. Ostow, M. (Ed.) (1982). *Judaism and Psychoanalysis*, New York, NY: KTAV Publishing House.
1245. Padrón Estarriol, C. (1997). La croyance: *Revue Française de Psychanalyse, 56*: 787–810.
1246. Padvalskis, C. (2012). *Una lectura psicoanalítica de las "Meditaciones sobre los Cantares" de Teresa de Jesús*, Córdoba: Universidad Católica de Córdoba.
1247. Palmer, M. (1997). *Freud and Jung on Religion*, London/New York, NY: Routledge.
1248. Paloutzian, R. F. & Park, C. L. (Eds.) (2005). *Handbook of the Psychology of Religion and Spirituality*, New York, NY/London: Guilford Press.
1249. Paloutzian, R. F. (1996). *Invitation to the Psychology of Religion*, Boston, MA: Allyn and Bacon.
1250. Panajian, A. (2000). The challenge to stay open: Buber and Bion. In: D. Slattery, P. Dennis & L. Corbett (Eds.) *Depth Psychology: Meditations in the Field* (pp. 105–116). Einsiedeln: Daimon Verlag.
1251. Parat, C. (1988). *La dynamique du sacré*, Paris: Ed. Cesura.
1252. Parat, C. (2002). *L'Inconscient et le Sacré*, Paris: PUF.
1253. Parcells, F. H. & Segel, N. P. (1959). Oedipus and the prodigal son. *Psychoanalytic Quarterly, 28*: 213–227.
1254. Pargament, K. (2002). The bitter and the sweet: An evaluation of the costs and benefits of religiousness. *Psychological Inquiry, 13*: 168–181.
1255. Pargament, K. (2007). *Spiritually Integrated Psychotherapy: Understanding and Addressing the Sacred*, New York, NY: Guilford Press.
1256. Pargament, K. I. (2014). The role of religion and spirituality in mental health. *Current Opinion in Psychiatry, 27* (*5*): 358–363.
1257. Pargament, K. I. (1997). *The Psychology of Religious Coping: Theory, Research, Practice*, New York, NY: Guilford Press.
1258. Pargament, K. I. (1999). The psychology of religion and spirituality? Yes and No. *International Journal for the Psychology of Religion, 9*: 3–16.
1259. Pargament, K. I., Exline, J. J. & Jones, J. W. (Eds.) (2013). *APA Handbook of Psychology, Religion, and Spirituality (Vol 1): Context, Theory, and Research*, Washington, DC: American Psychological Association.
1260. Parker, I. & Siddiqui, S. (2018). *Islamic Psychoanalysis and Psychoanalytic Islam Cultural and Clinical Dialogues*, London/New York, NY: Routledge.
1261. Parker, S. (2009). Scriptural allusions in the writings of D. W. Winnicott. *Psychoanalytic Review, 96*: 597–612.

1262. Parker, S. (2012). *Winnicott and Religion*, Northvale, NJ: Jason Aronson.
1263. Parlow, s. B. (2008). Personal transformation in Karl Rahner's Christianity: Constructed by Love. *Psychoanalytic Inquiry, 28*: 570–579.
1264. Parsons, W. B. (1999). *The Enigma of the Oceanic Feeling. Revisioning the Psychoanalytic Theory of Mysticism*, New York, NY/Oxford: Oxford University Press.
1265. Parsons, W. B. (2006). Psychoanalytic spirituality. *The Annual of Psychoanalysis, 35*: 83–96.
1266. Parsons, W. B. (2007). Psychoanalytic spirituality. In: J. Winer & J. Anderson (Eds.) *Spirituality and Religion: Psychoanalytic Perspectives* (pp. 83–97). Catskill, NY: Mental Health Resources.
1267. Parson, W. B. (2010a). Of chariots, Navels, and Winged Steeds: The dialogue between psychoanalysis and Buddhism. In: G. Kaplan & W. B. Parson (Eds.) *Disciplining Freud on Religion: Perspectives from the Humanities and Sciences* (pp. 108–146). Lanham, MD: Lexington Books.
1268. Parsons, W. B. (2010b). *Disciplining Freud on Religion*, Lanham, MD: Lexington.
1269. Parsons, W. B. (2013). *Freud and Augustine in Dialogue: Psychoanalysis, Mysticism, and the Culture of Modern Spirituality*, Charlottesville, VA: University of Virginia Press.
1270. Parsons, W. B. (2021). *Freud and Religion: Advancing the Dialogue*, Cambridge: Cambridge University Press.
1271. Parsons, W. B. (Ed.) (2018). *Being Spiritual but Not Religious. Past, Present, Future (s)*, London/New York, NY: Routledge.
1272. Parsons, W. B., Jonte Pace, D. & Henking, S. (Eds.) (2008). *Mourning Religion*, Charlottesville, VA/London: University of Virginia Press.
1273. Pasqualini, M. (2016). Un enigma llamado Agostino Gemelli: catolicismo, fascismo y psicoanálisis en la Italia de entreguerras. *Historia, Ciencia, Saude-Manghinos, 23*: 1059–1075.
1274. Pasquarelli, B. (1960). Psychoanalysis and religion. A postulated autonomy in function. *Bulletin of the Philadelphia Association for Psychoanalysis, 10*: 10–17.
1275. Patuel, J. (2010). Psicoanàlisi i religió: ¿Debat actual? *Revista del COPC, 227*: 39–41.
1276. Paul, R. A. (1974). Did the primal crime take place? *Ethos, 4*: 311–352.
1277. Paul, R. A. (1976). The Sherpa temple as a model of the psyche. *American Ethnologist, 3*: 131–146.
1278. Paul, R. A. (1981). A mantra and its meaning. *The Psychoanalytic Study of Society, 9*: 85–94. New York, NY: Psychohistory Press.
1279. Paul, R. A. (1982). *The Tibetan Symbolic World: Psychoanalytic Explorations*, Chicago, IL: University of Chicago Press.
1280. Paul, R. A. (1996). *Moses and Civilization: The Meaning Behind Freud's Myth*, New Haven, CT: Yale University Press.
1281. Paul, R. A. (1994). Freud, Sellin and the death of Moses. *The International Journal of Psychoanalysis, 75 (4)*: 825–837.
1282. Pearson, W. & Maarlo, H. (Eds.) (2021). *The Spiritual Psyche in Psychotherapy. Mysticism, Intersubjectivity, and Psychoanalysis*, London/New York, NY: Routledge.
1283. Pelled, E. (2007). Learning from experience: Bion's concept of reverie and Buddhist meditation. A comparative study. *The International Journal of Psychoanalysis, 88*: 1507–1526.
1284. Perelberg, R. J. (2013). Paternal function and thirdness in psychoanalysis and legend: has the future been foretold? *The Psychoanalytic Quarterly, 82*: 557–585.
1285. Perestrello, M. (1996). Freud e a tradição judaica. In: M. Perestrello (Ed.) *A formação cultural de Freud* (pp. 43–72). Rio de Janeiro: Imago.
1286. Peri, T. (2012). Applied psychoanalysis in biblical interpretation. *International Journal of Applied Psychoanalytic Studies, 10*: 349–360.
1287. Perrière, N. (2009). Le temps dans la Bible et dans la cure psychanalytique. *Le Coq-Héron, 126*: 13–19.

1288. Pettet, J. R. (2009). Struggles with God: Transference and religious countertransference in the treatment of a trauma survivor. *Journal of American Academy of Psychoanalysis and Dynamic Psychiatry, 37*: 123–136.
1289. Pfister, O. (1903). Die Unterlassungssünden der Theologie gegenüber der modernen Psychologie. *Protestantische Monatshefte, 7*: 125–140.
1290. Pfister, O. Das Elend unserer wissenschaftlichen Glaubenslehre: *Schweizerische theologische Zeitschrift 22*: 209–212.
1291. Pfister, O. (1911). Hysterie and Mystik bei Margaretha von Ebner. *Zentral Psychoanalyse, 1*: 468–485.
1292. Pfister, O. (1910). *Die Frömmigkeit des Grafen Ludwig von Zinzendorf*, Leipzig/Viena: Deuticke.
1293. Pfister, O. (1912). *Die psychologische Enträtselung der religiöse Glossolalie und der automatischen Kryptographie*, Leipzig: Frank Deuticke.
1294. Pfister, O. (1913). *Die Psychoanalytische Methode*, Leipzig/Berlin: Julius Klinkhardt.
1295. Pfister, O. (1917). *Was bietet die Psychanalyse dem Erzieher?* Leipzig: Julius Klinkhardt.
1296. Pfister, O. (1920a). *Der psychologische und biologische Untergrund Expressionistischer Bilde*, Bern/Leipzig: Bircher Verlag.
1297. Pfister, O. (1920b). *Zum Kampf und die Psychoanalyse*, Wien: Internationaler Psychoanalytischer Verlag.
1298. Pfister, O. (1920c). Die Entwicklung des Apostels Paulus. Eine religionschitliche und psychologische Skizze. *Imago, 6*: 243–290.
1299. Pfister, O. (1921). Mission und psychoanalyse. *Zeitschrift für Missionkunde on Religionswissenschaft, 36*: 230–246, 265–280.
1300. Pfister, O. (1922). *Die Liebe des Kindes und ihre Fehlenwicklungen*, Bern: Bircher Verlag.
1301. Pfister, O. (1923a). *Die Aufgabe der Wissenschaft vom christlichen Glauben in der Gegenwart*, Zurich: Beer&Cie.
1302. Pfister, O. (1923b). *Some Applications of Psychoanalysis*, London: George Allen and Unwin.
1303. Pfister, O. (1924). *Die Liebe vor der Ehe und ihre Fehlentwicklungen*, Bern: Bircher Verlag.
1304. Pfister, O. (1926). *Die Legende Sundar Singhs: Eine auf Enthüllungen protestantischer Augenzeugen in Indien gegründete religionspsychologische Untersuchung*, Berna/Leipsig: P. Haupt.
1305. Pfister, O. (1927a). *Die Pädagogik der Gegenwart in Selbstdarstellungen*, Leipzig: Felix Meiner.
1306. Pfister, O. (1927b). *Analytische Seelsorge. Einführung in die praktische Psychoanalyse für Seelsorger und Laien*, Göttingen: Vandenhoeck und Ruprecht.
1307. Pfister, O. (1928a). Die Illusion einer Zukunft; Eine freundschaftliche Auseinandersetzung mit Prof. Sigmund Freud. *Imago, 14*: 149–184. Pfister, O. (1977) L'Illusion d'un avenir. *Revue Française de Psychanalyse, XLI* (*3*): 503–546.
1308. Pfister, O. (1928b). *Religiosität und Hysterie*, Leipzig/Zurich: Bircher Verlag.
1309. Pfister, O. (1928c). *Psychanalyse und Weltanschauung*, Leipzig/Zurich: Bircher Verlag.
1310. Pfister, O. (1934). *Zur Psychologie des philosophischen Denkens*, Bern/Leipzig: Bircher Verlag.
1311. Pfister, O. (1935). Die verschiedenen Arten des Unglaubens in psychoanalytischer Beleuchtung. *Zeitschrift für Religionspsychologie, 8*: 20–31.
1312. Pfister, O. (1943). *Religionshygiene: Die Psychohygienische Aufgabe des theologischen Seelsorgers*, Basel: Schwabe.
1313. Pfister, O. (1947). *Calvins Eingreifen in die Hexer und Hexenprozesse Von Peney 1545 nach seiner Bedeutung für Geschichte und Gegenwart*, Zurich: Artemis-Verlag, Zurich.
1314. Pfister, O. (1948). *Christianity and Fear. A Study in History and in the Psychology and Hygiene of Religion*, London: Allen & Unwin.

1315. Pfister, O. (1993) [1927]. The illusion of a future: A friendly disagreement with Prof. Sigmund Freud. *The International Journal of Psychoanalysis, 74*: 557–599.
1316. Pfrimmer, T. (1982). *Freud lecteur de la Bible*, Paris: PUF.
1317. Philip, H. C. (1956). *Freud and Religious Belief*, London: Rockliff.
1318. Philippo, M. (2001). Le biblique n'est pas accessible en solitaire. Comment Balmary relit la Bible: *Lumen Vitae, 56*: 401–412.
1319. Phillips, J. A. (1984). *Eve. The History of an Idea*, New York, NY: Harper&Row.
1320. Pires, R. E. (2007). Erotismo e religião: Um diálogo instigante. *Revista Brasileira de Psicanálise, 41*: 141–148.
1321. Plaut, F. (2002). Analyse und Religion als Übergangsphänomene. *Analytische Psychologie, 33*: 81–96.
1322. Plé, A. (1967). La religion, problème personnel de Freud. *Le Supplément, 83*: 575–593.
1323. Plé, A. (1968). *Freud et la Religion*, Paris: Cerf.
1324. Plé, A. (1969). *Freud et la Morale*, Paris: Cerf.
1325. Plé, A. (1973). La mise en question de la morale traditionnelle par la psychanalyse. In: Vergote, A., Ortigues, E., Trotignon, P. et al. *Problèmes de psychanalyse* (pp. 115–122). Paris: Desclée de Brouwer.
1326. Plé, A. (1974). Les variations de l'Église à l'égard de la psychanalyse. *Concilium, 99*: 119–124.
1327. Pohier, J. (1972). *Au nom du Père. Recherches théologiques et psychanalytiques*, Paris: Cerf.
1328. Pohier, J. (1973). L'interrogation de la psychanalyse. *Le Supplément de la Vie Spirituelle, 105*: 148–172.
1329. Pohier, J. (1974a). Les chrétiens devant les problèmes posés par la sexualité…aux chrétiens. *Le Supplément, 111*: 497–506.
1330. Pohier, J. (1974b). *Le chrétien, le plaisir et la sexualité*, Paris: Cerf.
1331. Pohier, J. (1974c). Le célibat consacré comme discours sur Dieu et la sexualité. *Le Supplément, 110*: 257–279.
1332. Pohier, J. (1977). *Quand je dis Dieu*, Paris: Seuil.
1333. Pohier, J. (1986). *God in Fragments*, London: SCM Press.
1334. Pollak, T. (2014). Psychoanalyse als Religion? Zur kirchlichen Verfasstheit psychoanalytischer Institutionen. *Psyche: Zeitschrift für Psychoanalyse und ihre Anwendungen, 68*: 1108–1131.
1335. Pontalis, J. B. (1971). L'illusion maintenue. *Nouvelle Revue de Psychanalyse, 4*: 3–11.
1336. Post, S. (Ed.) (1972). *Moral and Values and the Superego Concept in Psychoanalysis*, New York, NY: International University Press.
1337. Postle, B. (1947). Religion in the psychologies of Jung and Freud. *The Ohio State Medical Journal, 43*: 947–950.
1338. Pound, M. (2007a). *Theology, Psychoanalysis and Trauma*, London: SCM Press.
1339. Pound, M. (2007b). Towards a lacanian theology of religion. *New Blackfrears, 84*: 510–520.
1340. Prince, R. H. & Savage, C. (1972). Mystical states and the concept of regression. In: J. White (Ed.) *The Highest states of Consciousness* (pp. 114–134). New York, NY: Doubleday.
1341. Prokofyeva, D. (2020). Common ideals shared by eastern orthodoxy and Erich Fromm's humanism. *Journal for the Study of Religions & Ideologies, 19*: 158–172.
1342. Pruett, G. E. (1987). *The Meaning and End of Suffering for Freud and the Buddhist Tradition*, Lanham, MD: University Press of America.
1343. Pruyser, P. W. (1968). *A Dynamic Psychology of Religion*, New York, NY: Harper & Row.
1344. Pruyser, P. W. (1973). Sigmund Freud and his Legacy: Psychoanalytic psychology of religion. In: C. Glock & P. Hammond (Eds.) *Beyond the Classics? Essays in the Scientific Study of Religion* (pp. 243–290). New York, NY: Harper & Row.
1345. Pruyser, P. W. (1974). *Between Belief and Unbelief*, New York, NY: Harper & Row.

1346. Pruyser, P. W. (1977). The seamy side of current religious belief. In: H. N. Malony & B. Spilka (Eds.) (1991). *Religion in Psychodynamic Perspective. The Contributions of Paul W. Pruyser* (pp. 47–65). New York, NY: Oxford University Press.
1347. Pruyser, P. W. (1978). Narcissism in contemporary religion. *Journal of Pastoral Care, 32*: 219–231.
1348. Pruyser, P. W. (1979). Psychological roots and branches of belief. In: H. N. Malony & B. Spilka (Eds.) (1991). *Religion in Psychodynamic Perspective. The Contributions of Paul W. Pruyser* (pp. 155–169). New York, NY: Oxford University Press.
1349. Pruyser, P. W. (1983). *The Play of the Imagination: Toward a Psychoanalysis of Culture*, New York, NY: International Universities Press.
1350. Pruyser, P. W. (1991). A psychological view of religion in the 1970s. In: H. N. Malony & B. Spilka (Eds.) *Religion In Psychodynamic Perspective: The Contributions of Paul W. Pruyser* (pp. 23–44). New York, NY: Oxford University Press, 1991.
1351. Belzen, J. A. & Geels, A. (Ed.) (2008). *Psychic Functioning and Mental Health: The Role of Religion in Personal Life* (pp. 117–157). Amsterdam/New York, NY: Rodopi (International Series in the Psychology of Religion, Vol. 15).
1352. Quervain, P. F. (1977). *Psychoanalyse und dialektische Theologie: Zum Freud-Verständnis bei K. Barth, E. Thurneysen und P. Ricoeur* (Jahrbuch der Psychoanalyse, 3). Bern: Huber.
1353. Rabinovich, N. (2017). *El pecado original del psicoanálisis*, Buenos Aires: Letra viva.
1354. Racker, H. (1956). On Freud's position towards religion. *American Imago, 13*: 97–121.
1355. Racker, H. (1957). *Psicoanálisis del espíritu*, Buenos Aires: Nova. A.P.A.
1356. Raffani, L. E. (2008). El lugar del padre primordial en Moisés y la religión monoteísta. Algunas conclusiones. *Anuario de Investigaciones, 15*: 109–112.
1357. Raguse, H. (1992). Der Ödipus-Komplex und die depressive Position. Psychoanalytische Reflexionen zur Wirkungsgeschichte des 12. Kapitels der Apokalypse des Johannes. *Zeitschrift für Psychoanalytische Theorie und Praxis/Journal for Psychoanalytical Theory and Practice*, 7: 126–144.
1358. Raguse, H. (1993). *Psychoanalyse und biblische Interpretation: Eine Auseinandersetzung mit Eugen Drewermanns Auslegung der Johannes-Apokalypse*, Stuttgar: Kohlhammer.
1359. Raguse, H. (1997). Der zukünftige Sinn - Konstruktion und Rekonstruktion in der psychoanalytischen und in der theologischen Hermeneutik. *Zeitschrift für Psychoanalytische Theorie und Praxis/Journal for Psychoanalytical Theory and Practice, 12*: 213–226.
1360. Raguse, H. (2007). Freud-Pfister. Stationen einer unverbrüchlichen Freundschaft. In: C. Noth & Morgenthaler (Eds.) *Seelsorge und Psychoanalyse* (pp. 34–45). Stuttgart: Kohlhammer.
1361. Raguse, H. (2008). Religiöse Inhalte in der Psychoanalyse: Erwägungen zur psychoanalytischen Religionskritik und zur Technik der Psychoanalyse. *Psychotherapie Forum, 16*: 57–65.
1362. Rainey, R. (1975). *Freud as Student of Religion*, Atlanta, GA: Scholars Press, 1975.
1363. Ramey, S. W. (2015). *Writing Religion: The Case for the Critical Study of Religion*, Tuscaloosa, AL: University Alabama Press.
1364. Randall, S. L. (2004). *Minding Spirituality*, Hillsdale, NJ: Analytic Press.
1365. Randall, R. L. (1976). Religious ideation of a narcissistically disturbed individual. *Journal of Pastoral Care, 30*: 35–45.
1366. Randall, R. L. (1984). The legacy of Kohut for religion and psychology. *Journal of Religion and Health, 23*: 106–114.
1367. Randour, M. L. (1993). *Exploring Sacred Landscapes. Religious and Spiritual Experiences in Psychotherapy*, New York, NY: Columbia University Press.
1368. Rank, O. & Sachs, H. (1913). *Die Bedeutung der Psychoanalyse für die Geisteswissenschaften*, Wiesbaden: J.F. Bergmann.
1369. Rank, O. & Sachs, H. (1913). The significance of psychoanalysis for the humanities. *American Imago, 21 (1/2)*: 6–133.

1370. Rank, O. (1964) [1914]. *The Myth of the Birth of Heros and Other Writings*, New York, NY: Vintage Books/Random House.
1371. Rank, O. (1996). Psychology and the soul. *Journal of Religion and Health, 35 (3)*: 193–201.
1372. Raphael-Leff, J. (2007). Freud's prehistoric matrix-Owing 'nature' a death. *The International Journal of Psychoanalysis, 88*: 1345–1373.
1373. Rassial, J. J. (1975). *La psychanalyse: est-elle une histoire juive?* Paris: Seuil.
1374. Ray Chaudhuri, A. K. (1956). A psycho-analytic study of the Hindu Mother Goddess. *American Imago, 13*: 123–146.
1375. Recalcati, M. (2017). *Contro il sacrificio. Al di là del fantasma sacrificale*, Milano: Raffaello Cortina.
1376. Recalcati, M. (2020a). *Il gesto di Caino*, Milano: Einaudi.
1377. Recalcati, M. (2020b). *La notte del Getsemani*, Milano: Einaudi.
1378. Recalcati, M. (2022). *La Legge della parola. Radici bibliche della psicoanalisi*, Milano: Einaudi.
1379. Regan, C., Malony, H. N. & Beit-Hallahmi, B. (1980). Psychologists and religion: Professional factors and personal belief. *Review of Religious Research, 21*: 208–217.
1380. Reich, W. (2021) [1933]. The three foundational elements of religious feeling. In: H. N. Malony & E. P. Shafranske (Eds.) *Early Psychoanalytic Religious Writings* (pp. 152–158). Leiden: Brill Rodopi.
1381. Reichel, G. (1911). *Zinzendorfs Frömmigkeit im Licht der Psychoanalyse (Eine kritische Prüfung des Buchs von Dr. Oskar Pfister: "Die Frömmigkeit des Grafen Ludwig von Zinzendorf" und ein Beitrag zum Verständnis der extravaganten Lehrweise Zinzendorfs)*, Tübingen: Mohr.
1382. Reik, T. (1921). The science of religion. *International Journal of Psychoanalysis, 2*: 80–83.
1383. Reik, T. (1928). Bemerkungen zu Freuds "Zukunft einer Illusion". *Imago - Zeitschrift für Anwendung der Psychoanalyse auf die Natur- und Geisteswissenschaften, 2*: 185–198.
1384. Reik, T. (1929). The therapy of the neuroses and religion. *International Journal of Psychoanalysis, 10*: 292–302.
1385. Reik, T. (1931). *Ritual: Psychoanalytic Studies*, London: Hogarth Press.
1386. Reik, T. (1946). *The Psychological Problems of Religion*, New York, NY: Farrar, Straus & Co.
1387. Reik, T. (1951). *Dogma and Compulsion: Psychoanalytic Studies of Religion and Myth*, New York, NY: International University Press.
1388. Reik, T. (1953). *The Secret Self: Psychoanalytic Experiences in Life and Literature*, New York, NY: Farrar, Strauss and Young.
1389. Reik, T. (1955). From spell to prayer. *Psychoanalysis, 3*: 3–26.
1390. Reik, T. (1957). *Myth and Guilt: The Crime and Punishment of Mankind*, New York, NY: Braziller.
1391. Reik, T. (1959). *Mystery on the Mountain: The Drama of Sinai Revelation*, New York, NY: Harper and Brothers.
1392. Reik, T. (1960). *The Creation of Woman: A Psychoanalytic Inquiry into the Myth of Eve*, New York, NY: Braziller.
1393. Reik, T. (1961). *The Temptation*, New York, NY: Braziller.
1394. Reik, T. (1963). *Pagan Rites in Judaism*, New York, NY: Farrar.
1395. Reik, T. (1968). One's own and the foreign. *American Imago, 25*: 3–15.
1396. Reik, T. (1975). *Der einige und der fremde Gott. Zur Psychoanalyse der religiösen Entwicklung*, Frankfurt a. M: Shurkamp.
1397. Reiland, H. (2004). The object beyond objects and the sacred: Reflections on Freud's and Winnicott's contributions to the psychology of religion. *Scandinavian Psychoanalytic Review, 27*: 78–86.
1398. Reineke, M. J. & Goodman, D. M. (Eds.) (2017). *Ana-María Rizzuto and the Psychoanalysis of Religion. The Road to de Living God*, Lanham, MD: Lexington.

1399. Reineke, M. J. (2014). *Intimate Domain: Desire, Trauma, and Mimetic Theory*, East Lansing, MI: Michigan State University Press.
1400. Reiser, R. M. (1990). Postcritical religion and the latent Freud. *Zygon. Journal of Religion and Science, 25*: 369–525.
1401. Rempel, M. H. (1997). Understanding Freud's philosophy of religion. *Canadian Journal of Psychoanalysis, 5*: 215–242.
1402. Renik, O. (1991). The biblical book ofJob. Advise to clinicians. *Psychoanalytic Quarterly, 60*: 596–606.
1403. Restrepo Ramírez, A. (2018). La idea de Dios como sentido existencial y político: críticas desde la filosofía y el psicoanálisis. *Desde el jardín de Freud: Revista de psicoanálisis, ,18*: 275–290.
1404. Rey- Flaud, H. (2006). *Et Moïse créa les juifs… Le testament de Freud*, Paris: Aubier.
1405. Rhee, D. (1990). The Tao, psychoanalysis, and existential thought. *Psychotherapy and Psychosomatics, 53*: 21–27.
1406. Rice, E. (1999a). Religion and the adolescent: A psychodynamic perspective. *Psychoanalytic Psychology, 16*: 58–75.
1407. Rice, E. (1990). *Freud and Moses: The Long Journey Home*, Albany, NY: State University of New York Press.
1408. Rice, E. (1999b). Freud, religion, and science. *Journal of the American Academy of Psychoanalysis, 27*: 397–406.
1409. Richard, A. D. (2010). *The Jewish World of Sigmund Freud: Essays on Cultural Roots and the Problem of Religious Identity*, Jefferson, NC: McFarland & Co Inc.
1410. Richard, A. D. (2015). A genocide rooted in religion and culture. *Journal of American Psychoanalytic Association, 63*: 789–793.
1411. Richard, J. T. (1999). *Que reste-t-il de l'Amour après Freud? Questions aux sciences humaines et à la psychanalyse: des philosophes à Lacan, en passant par S. Freud*, Paris: L'Harmattan.
1412. Richards, A. D. (2009). The need not to believe: Freud's godlessness reconsidered. *Psychoanalytic Review, 96* (4): 561–578.
1413. Richardson, W. J. (1990). "Coufontaine, adsum!" Lacan and theological discourse. In: J. H. Smith & S. A. Handelman (Eds.) *Psychoanalysis and Religion* (pp. 60–73). Baltimore, MD: The Johns Hopkins University Press.
1414. Richardson, W. J. (1992). Love and the beginning: Psychoanalysis and religion. *Contemporary Psychoanalysis, 28*: 423–441.
1415. Ricoeur, P. (1966). The atheism of Freudian psychoanalysis. *Concilium, 16*: 59–72.
1416. Ricoeur, P. (1969). La paternité: du fantasme au symbolique. In: E. Castelli (Ed.) *L' analyse du langage théologique* (pp. 221–246). Paris: Aubier.
1417. Ricoeur, P. (1970). *Freud and Philosophy: An Essay on Interpretation*, New Haven, CT: Yale University Press.
1418. Ricoeur, P. (1974). *The Conflict of Interpretations: Essays in Hermeneutics*, Evanston, IL: Northwestern University Press.
1419. Rieff, P. (1961). *Freud: The Mind of the Moralist*, New York, NY: Anchor Books.
1420. Rieff, P. (1963). The meaning of history and religion in Freud's thought. In: B. Mazlish (Ed.) *Psychoanalysis and History*: Englewood Cliffs, NJ: Prentice Hall.
1421. Rieff, P. (1966). *The Triumph of the Therapeutic: Uses of Faith after Freud*, Chicago, IL: University of Chicago Press.
1422. Rieff, P. (2008). *The Jew of Culture: Freud, Moses, and Modernity*, Charlottesville, VA/London: University of Virginia Press.
1423. Rigby, P. (1985). Paul Ricoeur, Freudianism, and Augustine's Confession. *Journal of the American Academy of Religion, 53*: 93–114.
1424. Rivera, P. S. (2017). 'Freud's speculations in ethnology': A reflection on anthropology's encounter with psychoanalysis. *The International Journal of Psychoanalysis, 98*: 755–778.

1425. Rizq, E. (2017). On food, faith, and psychoanalysis: Isak Dinesen's Babette's Feast. *British Journal of Psychotherapy, 33*: 537–554.
1426. Rizq, E. (2019). The wager of faith in fiction and psychoanalysis: Reading Colm Tóibín's the Testament of Mary. *British Journal of Psychotherapy, 35*: 610–627.
1427. Rizzuto, A. M. (1974). Object relations and the formation of the image of God. *The British Journal of Medical Psychology, 47 (1)*: 83–99.
1428. Rizzuto, A. M. (1976). Freud, God, the devil, and the theory of object representation. *International Review of Psychoanalysis, 3*: 165–180.
1429. Rizzuto, A. M. (1979). *The Birth of the Living God: A Psychoanalytic Study*, Chicago, IL: University of Chicago Press.
1430. Rizzuto, A. M. (1980). The psychological foundation of belief in God. In: J. Fowler & A. Vergote (Eds.) *Toward Moral and religious Maturity* (pp. 115–135). Morristown, NJ: Silver Burdett.
1431. Rizzuto, A. M. (1982). The father and the child representation of God: A developmental approach. In: S. H. Cath, A. R. Gurwitt & J. M. Ross (Eds.) *Father and Child: Developmental and Clinical Perspectives* (pp. 357–381). Boston, MA: Little: Brown and Co.
1432. Rizzuto, A. M. (1991). Religious development: A psychoanalytic point of view. *New Directions for Child and Adolescent Development, 52*: 47–60.
1433. Rizzuto, A. M. (1992). Afterword. In: M. Finn & J. Gartner (Eds.) *Object Relations Theory and Religion. Clinical Applications* (pp. 155–175). Westport, CT/ London: Praeger.
1434. Rizzuto, a. M. (1996)[1997]. Belief as a psychic function. *Newsletter. Psychology of Religion. American Psychological Association Division, 36*: 1–7.
1435. Rizzuto, A. M. (1996a). Psychoanalytic psychotherapy and religious person. In: E. Shafranske (Ed.) *Religion and the Clinical Practice of Psychology* (pp. 409–431). Washington, DC: American Psychological Association.
1436. Rizzuto, A. M. (1996b). Christian worshipping and psychoanalysis in spiritual truth. In: J. T. Chirban (Ed.) *Personhood: Orthodox Christianity and the Connection between Mind, Body, and Soul* (pp. 51–59). New Haven, CT: Yale University Press.
1437. Rizzuto, A. M. (1996c). Reflexiones psicoanalíticas acerca de la experiencia mística. *Teología y Vida, 37*: 27–38.
1438. Rizzuto, A. M. (1998b). Psychoanalytic psychotherapy and pastoral guidance. *Journal of Pastoral Care, 52 (1)*: 69–78.
1439. Rizzuto, A. M. (1998c). *Conocimiento científico, creencia religiosa y convicción psicológica. Psicodinámica del conocer*, Pelotas: Simpósio Transdisciplinar de Cone Sul.
1440. Rizzuto, A. M. (2001a). Does God help? What God? Helping Whom? The Convolutions of Divine Help. In: S. Akhart & H. Parens (Eds.) *Does God Help? Development and Clinical Aspects of Religious Belief* (pp. 19–51). Northvale, NJ/London: Jason Aronson.
1441. Rizzuto, A. M. (2001b). Religious development beyond the modern paradigm discussion. The psychoanalytic point of view. *The International Journal for the Psychology of Religion, 11*: 201–214.
1442. Rizzuto, A. M. (2001c). Vicissitudes of Self, object, and God representations during psychoanalysis. In: M. Aletti & G. Rossi (Eds.) *Illusione religiosa: rive e deriva* (pp. 22–55). Torino: Centro Scientifico Editore.
1443. Rizzuto, A. M. (2002a). Technical approach to religious issues in psychoanalysis. In: M. Aletti & F. De Nardi (Eds.) *Psicoanalisi e religione. Nuove prospettive clinico-ermeneutiche* (pp. 1184–216). Torino: Centro Scientifico Editore.
1444. Rizzuto, A. M. (2002b). Believing and personal and religious beliefs: Psychoanalytic considerations. *Psychoanalysis and Contemporary Thought, 25*: 433–63.
1445. Rizzuto, A. M. (2003a). Un Dios y dos géneros. In: C. Domínguez-Morano & R. Briones (Eds.) *Masculino-femenino y hecho religioso* (pp. 147–155). Granada: Universidad de Granada.

1446. Rizzuto, A. M. (2004). Roman Catholic background and psychoanalysis. *Psychoanalytic Psychology, 21*: 436–441.
1447. Rizzuto, A. M. (2007b). Réflexions psychanalytiques sur les expériences religieuses: description et interprétation dynamiques. In: C. A. Brandt- & Fournier (Eds.) *Fonctions psychologiques du religieux* (pp. 67–86). Genève: Labor et Fides.
1448. Rizzuto, A. M. (2009a). Sacred space, analytic space, the Self, and God. *Journal of the American Academy of Psychoanalysis, 37 (1)*: 175–188.
1449. Rizzuto, A. M. (2009b). One hundred years after Freud declared that religion was a universal obsessional neurosis. In: J. A. Belzen (Ed.) *Changing the Scientific Study of Religion: Beyond Freud? Theoretical, Empirical and Clinical Studies from Psychoanalytic Perspectives* (pp. 35–55). New York, NY: Springer.
1450. Rizzuto, A. M. (2012). An accidental psychologist of religion. In: J. Belzen (Ed.) *Psychology of Religion: Autobiographical Accounts* (pp. 185–200). New York, NY: Springer.
1451. Rizzuto, A.-M. (1993). Exploring sacred landscapes. In: M. L. Randour (Ed.) *Exploring Sacred Landscapes: Religious and Spiritual Experiences in Psychotherapy* (pp. 16–33). New York, NY: Columbia University Press.
1452. Rizzuto, A. M. (1998a). *Why Did Freud Reject God? A Psychodynamic Interpretation*, New Haven, CT: Yale University Press.
1453. Rizzuto, A. M. (2003b). Believing, personal beliefs, and transformational processes: psychoanalytic considerations. In: W. W. Meissner & C. R. Schlauch (Eds.) *Psyche and Spirit: Dialectics of Transformation* (pp. 1–25). Lanham, MD: University Press of America.
1454. Rizzuto, A. M. (2005). Psychoanalytic considerations about spiritually oriented psychotherapy. In: L. Sperry & E. P. Shafranske (Eds.) *Spiritually Oriented Psycho-Therapy* (pp. 31–50). Washington, DC: American Psychological Association.
1455. Rizzuto, A. M. (2007a). God in the mind: The psychodynamic of an unusual relationship. *The Annual of Psychoanalysis, 35*: 25–46.
1456. Rizzuto, A. M. & Shafranske, E. P. (2013). Addressing religion and spirituality in treatment from a psychodynamic perspective. In K. Pargament, A. Mahoney & E. P. Shafranske (Ed.) *APA Handbook of Psychology, Religion and Spirituality* (Vol. 2, pp. 125–146). Washington, DC: American Psychological Association.
1457. Roback, A. A. (1918). Freudian psychology and Jewish commentators of the Bible. *Jewish Forum, 1*: 528–533.
1458. Roback, A. A. (1926). *Freud, Chassid, or Humanist*: *B'nai B'rith Magazine, 40*: 129–130.
1459. Robert, M. (1977). *From Oedipus to Moses*, Garden City, NY: Doubleday.
1460. Roberts, D. (1950). *Psychotherapy and a Christian View of Man*, New York, NY: Charles Scribner's Sons.
1461. Robertson, R. (1991). My true enemy: Freud and the Church 1927–1939. In: K. Segar & J. W. Riverside (Eds.) *Austria in the Thirties. Culture and Politics Studies in Austrian Literature, Culture and Thought* (pp. 328–344). Riverside, CA: Ariadne Press.
1462. Robertson, R. (1993). Freud und Pater Wilhelm Schmidt. In: J. P. Nautz & R. Vahrenkamp (Eds.) *Die Wiener Jahrhundertwende* (pp. 360–376). Wien, Köln, Graz: Böhlau.
1463. Robinson, L. H. (1985). The illusion of no future: Psychoanalysis and religion. *The Journal of American Academy of Psychoanalysis, 13*: 211–228.
1464. Robinson, L. H. (Ed.) (1986). *Psychiatry and Religion: Overlapping Concerns*, Washington, WA: American Psychiatric Press.
1465. Rocha, Z. (1992). O Deus de Freud. *Estudos de Psicanálise, 14*: 69–94.
1466. Rodríguez Amenábar, S. M. (1979). *Metapsicología y hecho religioso*, Buenos Aires: Eudeba.
1467. Rodríguez Amenábar, S. M. (1995). *Psicoanálisis, cristianismo y religiosidad*, Buenos Aires: Paulinas.

1468. Rof Carballo, J. (1969). Psicoanálisis y religión. Estudio Introductorio. In: A. Plé (Ed.) *Freud y la religión* (pp. 3–93). Madrid: BAC.
1469. Rogers, W. R. (1974). Dependence and counterdependency in psychoanalysis and religious faith. *Zygon, 9*: 190–210.
1470. Rohrbacher, P. (2020). Pater Wilhelm Schmidt und Sigmund Freud: Gesellschaftliche Kontexte einer religionsethnologischen Kontroverse in der Zwischenkriegszeit. *Cultura & psyché, 1*: 53–68.
1471. Róheim, G. (1925). *Australian Totemism: a Psychoanalytic Study in Anthropology*, London, UK: Allen and Unwin.
1472. Róheim, G. (1930). *Animism, Magic, and the Divine King*, London: Kegan Paul and Co.
1473. Róheim, G. (1932). Animism and religion. *Psychoanalytic Quarterly, 6*: 59–112.
1474. Róheim, G. (1934a). *The Riddle of the Sphinx*, London: Hogarth Press.
1475. Róheim, G. (1934b). Primitive high gods. *Psychoanalytic Quarterly, 3*: 1–133.
1476. Róheim, G. (1939). The covenant of Abraham. *International Journal of Psychoanalysis, 20*: 452–459.
1477. Róheim, G. (1940). The Garden of Eden. *Psychoanalytic Review, 27*: 1–26.
1478. Róheim, G. (1945). *The Eternal One of the Dream: A Psychoanalytic Interpretation of Australian Myth and Ritual*, New York, NY: International University Press.
1479. Róheim, G. (1955a). *Magic and Schizophrenia*, New York, NY: New York University Press.
1480. Róheim, G. (1955b). Some aspects of Semitic monotheism. *Psychoanalysis and the Social Sciences, 4*: 169–192.
1481. Róheim, G. (1971). *The Origin and Function of Culture*, Garden City: NY: Doubleday.
1482. Róheim, G. (1972). *The Panic of the Gods*, New York, NY: Harper.
1483. Roland, A. (1972). Imagery and symbolic expression in dreams and art. *International Journal of Psychoanalysis, 53*: 531–539.
1484. Roland, A. (1988). *In Search of Self in India and Japan: Toward a Cross-Cultural Psychology*, Princeton, NJ: Princeton University Press.
1485. Roland, A. (1996). *Cultural Pluralism and Psychoanalysis: The Asian and North American Experience*, London/New York, NY: Routledge.
1486. Roland, A. (1999). The spiritual Self and psychopathology: Theoretical reflections and clinical observations. *Psychoanalysis and Psychotherapy, 16*: 211–234.
1487. Roland, A. (2005). Psychoanalysts and the spiritual quest: Framing a new paradigm. In A. Roland, B. Ulanov & C. Barbre (Ed.) *Creative Dissent: Psychoanalysis in Evolution*. New York, NY: Praeger.
1488. Roland, A. (2011). *Journeys to Foreign Selves: Asians and Asian Americans in a Global Era*, New York, NY: Oxford University Press.
1489. Roland, A. (2017). Erich Fromm's involvement with Zen Buddhism: Psychoanalysts and the spiritual quest in subsequent decades. *Psychoanalytic Review, 104 (4)*: 503–522.
1490. Rolnik, E. (2010). Therapy and ideology: Psychoanalysis and its vicissitudes in pre-state Israel (including some hitherto unpublished letters by Sigmund Freud and Albert Einstein). *Science in Context, 23*: 473–506.
1491. Rolnik, E. (2012). *Freud in Zion*, London: Karnac.
1492. Roos, J. A. (2010). *"Sacred Psychoanalysis" – An Interpretation of the Emergence and Engagement of Religion and Spirituality in Contemporary Psychoanalysis*, Birmingham: University of Birmingham.
1493. Roquefort, D. (1986). Rom. 7/7 selon Jacques Lacan. *Etudes théologiques et religieuses, 3*: 343–352.
1494. Roquefort, D. (2002). *L'envers d'une illusion. Freud et la religion revisités*, Paris: Érès.
1495. Rosa Sousa, P. L. & Martínez de Oliveira, P. (1998–1999). Dios: ¿Representable o irrepresentable? Ensayo interdisciplinario sobre las representaciones de Dios en el psicoanálisis y en la teología. *Revista de Psicoanálisis, 6*: 273–299.

1496. Rosenberg, A. E. (1980). *Freudian Theory and American Religious Journals 1900–1965. (Studies in American History and Culture)*, Michigan, MI: UMI Research Press.
1497. Rosmarin, T. W. (1939). *The Hebrew Moses: An Answer to Sigmund Freud*, New York, NY: Jewish Club Book.
1498. Rosolato, G. (1969). *Essais sur le symbolique*, Gallimard: Paris.
1499. Rosolato, G. (1987). *Le sacrifice*, Paris: P.U.F.
1500. Rosolato, G. (1980). Présente mystique. *Nouvelle Revue de Psychanalyse, 22*: 5–36.
1501. Ross, M. E. & Ross, C. L. (1983). Mothers, infants, and the psychoanalytic study of ritual. *Journal of Women in Culture and Society, 9*: 26–39.
1502. Ross, M. E. (2001). The humanity of the Gods: The past and future of Freud's psychoanalytic interpretation of religion. *The Annual of Psychoanalysis, 29*: 263–277.
1503. Ross, N. (1958). Psychoanalysis and religion. *Journal of the American Psychoanalytic Association, 6*: 519–539.
1504. Ross, N. (1968). Beyond 'The Future of an Illusion'. *Journal of the Hillside Hospital, 17*: 259–276.
1505. Ross, N. (1975). Affect as cognition: With observations on the meanings of mystical states. *International Review of Psychoanalysis, 2*: 79–93.
1506. Rossi, G. & Aletti, M. (Eds.) (2009). *Psicologia della religione e teoria dell'attaccamento*, Torino: Aracne, Torino.
1507. Rossi, G. (1992). Lettura psicoanalitica della Bibbia. *La Civiltà Cattolica, 4*: 476–487.
1508. Roth, M. (1993). Freud's Jewish identity: A case study in the impact of ethnicity. *Journal of the American Academy of Psychoanalysis, 21*: 161–162.
1509. Roth, M. (2000). Oskar Pfister - der Beginn einer problematischen Freud-Rezeption innerhalb der Theologie. Eine Problemanzeige. *Praktische Theologie, 35*: 40–57.
1510. Roudinesco, E. & Borossa, J. (2009). Humanity and its gods: Atheism. *Psychoanalysis and History, 11* (2): 251–261.
1511. Rowatt, W. C. & Kirkpatrick, L. A. (2002). Two dimensions of attachment to God and their relation to affect, religiosity, and personality constructs. *Journal for the Scientific Study of Religion, 41* (4): 637–651.
1512. Rubenstein, R. L. (1963a). The significance of castration anxiety in rabbinic mythology. *Psychoanalytic Review, 50*: 289–312.
1513. Rubenstein, R. L. (1963b). A note on research lag in psychoanalytic studies in religion. *Jewish Social Studies, 25*: 133–144.
1514. Rubenstein, R. L. (1967a). *The Religious Imagination*, New York, NY: Bobbs-Merrill.
1515. Rubenstein, R. L. (1967b). Freud and Judaism: A review article. *The Journal of Religion, 47*: 39–44.
1516. Rubin, J. B. (1992). *Psychoanalytic Treatment with a Buddhist Meditator*, Westport, CT: Praeger Publishers/Greenwood Publishing Group, Inc.
1517. Rubin, J. B. (1996). *Psychotherapy and Buddhism: Toward an Integration*, New York, NY: Plenum Press.
1518. Rubin, J. B. (2009). Deepening psychoanalytic listening: The marriage of Buddha and Freud. *American Journal of Psychoanalysis, 69* (2): 93–105.
1519. Rudin, J. (1968). *Psychotherapy and Religion*, Notre Dame, IN: University of Notre Dame.
1520. Rudin, J. (1969). *Fanaticism: A Psychological Analysis*, Notre Dame, IN: University of Notre Dame.
1521. Rudnytsky, P. L. (2008). Inventing Freud. *American Journal of Psychoanalysis, 88* (2): 117–127.
1522. Ruff, W. (2015). "An infidel Jew"? Zur Religiosität von Sigmund Freud. *Forum Der Psychoanalyse, 31*: 415–431.
1523. Ruff, W. (2017). *Perspektivenwechsel in Psychoanalyse und Religion. Reflexionen über ethische Fragen und Weltanschauungen*, Berlin: Psychosozial Verlag.
1524. Rümke, H. C. (1952). *The Psychology of Unbelief: Character and Temperament in Relation to Unbelief*, London: Rockliff.

1525. Runestam, A. (1958). *Psychoanalysis and Christianity*, Rock Island, IL: Augustana.
1526. Rupolo, H. (1991). *Un estudio sobre el Moisés de Freud*, Buenos Aires: Ed. Nacal.
1527. Saarinen, J. A. (2012). The oceanic state: A conceptual elucidation in terms of modal contact. *The International Journal of Psychoanalysis, 93*: 939–9361.
1528. Sabbadini, A.-D. & Ceglie, G. (2013). A camera inside a monastery: Reflections on of Gods and Men [Des Hommes et des Dieux]. *The International Journal of Psychoanalysis, 92*: 745–754.
1529. Sachs, H. (1941). "The Man Moses" and the man Freud. *Psychoanalytic Review, 28*: 156–162.
1530. Sachs, H. (1947). At the Gates of Heaven. *American Imago, 4*: 15–32.
1531. Sack, H. L. (1979). The effects of spiritual exercises on the integration of the Self-system. *Journal for the Scientific Study of Religion, 18*: 46–50.
1532. Saffady, W. (1976). New developments in the psychoanalytic study of religion: A bibliographic survey of the literature since 1960. *Psychoanalytic Review, 63*: 291–299.
1533. Safran, J. D. (Ed.) (2003). *Psychoanalysis and Buddhism: An Unfolding Dialogue*, Boston, MA: Wisdom Publications.
1534. Sagne, J. C. (1971a). *Péché, culpabilité, pénitence*, Paris: Cerf, Paris.
1535. Sagne, J. C. (1971b). La psychanalyse, la foi et la théologie. *Le Supplément, 97*: 176–191.
1536. Sagne, J. C. (1996). Oui, je viens bientôt: le désir et l'espérance. *Lumière et Vie, 227*: 43–54.
1537. Salazar, C. (2014). *Antropologías de las creencias. Religión, simbolismo e irracionalidad*, Barcelona: Fragmenta.
1538. Sales, M. (1979). Possibilités et limites d'une lecture psychanalytique de la Bible. *Nouvelle Revue Théologique, 101*: 699–723.
1539. Salman, D. H. (1967). La régression au service du moi dans l'expérience religieuse: *Archiv für Religionspsychologie, 9*. Gottingen: Vandenhoeck & Ruprecht.
1540. Sanders, B. G. (1949). *Christianity after Freud. An Interpretation of the Christian Experience in the Light of Psycho-Analytic Theory*, London: Geoffrey Bles.
1541. Saroglou, V. (1997). *Structuration psychique de l'expérience religieuse. La fonction paternelle*, Paris-Montreal: L'Harmattan.
1542. Saroglou, V. (2003). Spiritualité moderne. Un regard de psychologie de la religion. *Revue Théologique de Louvain, 34*: 473–504.
1543. Satish, R. (2014). Spiritual conversion in The Bhagavad Gita: A psychoanalytic study. In: J. Gale, M. Robson & G. Rapsomaioti (Eds.) *Insanity and Divinity: Studies in Psychosis and Spirituality* (pp. 131–152). London/New York, NY: Routledge.
1544. Saur, M. & Saur, W. (1993). Transitional phenomena as evidenced in prayer. *Journal of Religion and Health, 32*: 55–65.
1545. Sauret, M.-J. (2008). Topologie, religion, psychanalyse. *Psychanalyse, 11*: 5–23.
1546. Sauret, M. J. (1982). *Croire? Approche psychanalytique de la croyance*, Toulouse: Privat.
1547. Saussure, T. (1984). Sentiments de culpabilité et signification du péché. *Revue de théologie et de philosophie, 116*: 201–215.
1548. Saussure, T. (1987). Psychanalyse et christianisme: où en sommes-nous? *Le Supplément, 163*: 61–73.
1549. Saussure, T. (1989). *Psychanalyse et christianisme aujourd'hui*, Barcelona: Fundació Vidal i Barraquer.
1550. Saussure, T. (1992). Institution ecclésiale et perversion. *Lumière et Vie, 215*: 23–34.
1551. Saussure, T. (1997). Psychanalyse et religion: deux oreilles pour un désir et une parole. *Études théologiques et religieuses, 72*: 259–266.
1552. Saussure, T. (2003). Un mythe originaire de la honte: Adam et Ève. *Revue Française de Psychanalyse, 67*: 1849–1854.
1553. Saussure, T. (2009). *L'inconscient, nos croyances et la foi chrétienne. Études psychanalytiques et bibliques*, Paris: Cerf.

1554. Saussure, T. (2012). Fruit défendu et fruit partagé: De la Chute à l'Eucharistie.... In: M. Vaucher, D. Bourdin, M. Durrerm & O. Revaz (Eds.) *Foi de canniabale! La dévoration, entre religion et psychanalyse* (pp. 227–241). Genève: Labor et fides.
1555. Saussure, T. et al. (Ed.) (1993). *Les miroirs du fanatisme. Integrisme, narcissisme et alteriré*,Genève: Labor et Fides.
1556. Sauty, R. (2016). *Psychanalyse et religion*, Paris: Perret-Gentil.
1557. Sayers, J. (2002). Marion Milner, mysticism, and psychoanalysis. *The International Journal of Psychoanalysis, 82*: 105–120.
1558. Sayers, J. (2007). Beyond abjection: Art, religion, psychoanalysis. *The Annual of Psychoanalysis, 35*: 165–177.
1559. Schaap-Jonker, H., Eurelings-Bontekoe, E., Verhagen, P. J. & Zock, H. (2002). Image of God and personality pathology: An exploratory study among psychiatric patients. *Mental Health, Religion and Culture, 5*: 55–71.
1560. Schade, S. (2018). Feminism, Islam, and psychoanalysis—A psychoanalytic case study. *Psychotherapy and Politics International, 16*: 1 1459.
1561. Schär, H. (1950). *Erlösungsvorstellungen und ihre psychologischen Aspekte*, Zurich: Rascher.
1562. Scharfenberg, J. (1970). Zum Religionbregriff Sigmund Freud. *Evangelische Theologie, XXX*: 367–378.
1563. Scharfenberg, J. (1972a). *Religion zwischen Wahn und Wirklichkeit: gesammelte Beiträge zur Korrelation von Theologie und Psychoanalyse*, Hamburg: Furche.
1564. Scharfenberg, J. (1972b). Die Begegnung von Psychoanalyse und Theologie: eine Zwischenbilanz. In: H. Zahrnt (Ed.) *Jesus und Freud* (pp. 93–107). München: Piper.
1565. Scharfenberg, J. (1980). *Mit Symbolen leben: soziologische, psychologische und religiöse Konfliktbearbeitung*, Olten: Walter.
1566. Scharfenberg, J. (1985). *Einführung in die Pastoralpsychologie*, Göttingen: Vandenhoeck & Ruprecht.
1567. Scharfenberg, J. (1987). *Pastoral Care as Dialogue*, Philadelphia, PA: Fortress Press.
1568. Scharfenberg, J. (1988). *Sigmund Freud and His Critique of Religion*, Philadelphia, PA: Fortress Press.
1569. Scharfenberg, J. (2012). Anthropology as a voyage of discovery: Or everything that finds expression in humans merits reflection. In: J. A. Belzen (Ed.) *Psychology of Religion: Autobiographical Accounts* (pp. 201–213). New York, NY: Springer Science.
1570. Schjelderup, H. & Schjelderup, K. (1932). *Über drei Haupttypen der religiösen Erlebnisformen und ihre psychologische Untersuchung*, Berlin: Walter de Gruyter.
1571. Schjelderup, K. (1928). *Die Askese; Eine Religionspsychologie Untersuchung*, Berlin: Walter de Gruyter.
1572. Schlauch, C. R. (1993). The intersecting overlapping Self: Contemporary psychoanalysis reconsiders religion again. *Pastoral Psychology, 42*: 21 43.
1573. Schlauch, C. R. (1999). Rethinking Selfobject and Self: Implications for understanding and studying religious matters. *Pastoral Psychology, 48*: 57–78.
1574. Schlauch, C. R. (2007). Being-there-with-and-for: Contemporary psychoanalysis characterizes notions of being religious. *Pastoral Psychology, 56*: 199–221.
1575. Schlauch, C. R. (2016). Readings of Winnicott II. *Pastoral Psychology, 65*: 395–426.
1576. Schmidl, F. (1972). Problems of method in applied psychoanalysis. *The Psychoanalytic Quarterly, 41*: 402–419.
1577. Schmidt, W. (1928–1929) Eine wissenschaftliche Abrechnung mit der Psychoanalyse. *Das Neue Reich*: 266–277.
1578. Schmidt, W. (1929a). Prof. Dr. Freud's psychoanalytische Theorie zum Ursprung der. Familie und der Religion. *Schönere Zukunft, 4*: 263–265. *14*: 287–289, *1515*.
1579. Schmidt, W. (1929b). *der Ödipus-Komplex der Freud'schen Psychoanalyse und die Ehegestaltung des Bolschewismus*, Berlin: Nationalwirtschaft.
1580. Schimmel, I. (1982). Le déluge, la Tour de Babel et autres histoires. *Revue Française de psychanalyse, 41*: 464–467, 472–482.

1581. Schimmel, I. (1998). *Créations, psychanalyse*, Paris: PUF.
1582. Schneider, S. & Berke, J. H. (2008). The oceanic feeling, mysticism, and Kabbalah: Freud's historical roots. *Psychoanalytic Review, 95* (*1*): 131–156.
1583. Schnittker, J. (2001). When is faith enough? The effects of religious involvement on depression. *Journal for the Scientific Study of Religion, 40*: 393–411.
1584. Schoenfeld, C. G. (1962). God the father-and mother: Study and extension of Freud's conception of God as an exalted father. *American Imago, 19*: 214–233.
1585. Schoenfeld, C. G. (1966). Psychoanalysis and antisemitism. *Psychoanalytic Review, 53*: 24–37.
1586. Schossman, H. H. (1966). Circumcision as defense. A study in psychoanalysis and religion. *Psychoanalytic Quarterly, 35*: 340–356.
1587. Schossmann, H. H. (1972). God the father and his son. *American Imago, 29*: 35–52.
1588. Schreiber, J. (1967). Freud als Theologue. *Theologia Practica, 192*: 3.
1589. Schroeder, T. (1914). The Wildisbuch crucified saint: A study in the erotogenesis of religion. *The Psychoanalytic Review, 1*: 129–148.
1590. Schroeder, T. (1922). Prenatal psychism and mystical Pantheism. *International Journal of Psychoanalysis, 3*: 445–466.
1591. Schroeder, T. (1929a). Guilt and inferiority. Feeling as creator of religious experience. *The Psychoanalytic Review, 16*: 46–54.
1592. Schroeder, T. (1929b). The psychoanalytic approach to religious experience. *The Psychoanalytic Review, 16*: 361–376.
1593. Schroeder, T. (1932). A "Living God" incarnate. *Psychoanalytic Review, 19* (*1932*): 36–46.
1594. Schroeder, T. (1936). One religio-sexual maniac. *Psychoanalytic Review, 23*: 26–45.
1595. Schulman, M. A. & Kaplan, R. S. (2015). Homosexuality as an issue in the psychoanalytic treatment of Lubavitch Chassidim. *International Forum of Psychoanalysis, 24*: 153–161.
1596. Schulman, M. A. (2013). Transference and "the Rebbe" idiographic and nomothetic factors in the psychoanalysis of Lubavitch Chassidim. *Journal of Religion and Health, 52*: 1267–1280.
1597. Schulman, R. (2006). Psychotherapy and religion – A paradox? *International Journal of Applied Psychoanalytic Studies, 1*: 73–81.
1598. Schumaker, J. F. (1990). *Wings of Illusion. The Origin, Nature, and Future of Paranormal Belief*, Buffalo, NY: Prometheus Book.
1599. Schumaker, J. F., (Ed.) (1992). *Religion and Mental Health*, Oxford: Oxford University Press.
1600. Schwab., E. (2011). *Croire avec Freud? Quête de l'origine et identité*, Genève: Labor et Fides.
1601. Schwartz, P. J. (2016). The psychogenetic legacy of Freud's totem proto-God. *The International Journal of Psychoanalysis, 97*: 187–188.
1602. Seafeld, H. (1928). *Das Christentum in der Beleuchtung der Psychanalyse*, Gütersloh: Beterlsmann.
1603. Sedat, J., Vermorel, H. & Cazenave, M. (2002). Freud et le "sentiment océanique". In: M. Cazenave (Ed.) *Bible et religion: Les vivants et les Dieux* (pp. 117–138). Paris: Desclée de Brouwer.
1604. Segal, R. A. (2011). Mysticism and psychoanalysis. *Religious Studies Review, 37*: 1–18.
1605. Selz, M. (2009). Sur l'interdit du regard. *Le Coq-Héron, 126*: 49–58.
1606. Selz, M. (2011). "Le sauveur". *Revue Française de Psychanalyse, 75*: 1719–1723.
1607. Shaffi, M. (1988). *Freedom from the Self: Sufism, Meditation, and Psychotherapy*, New York, NY: Human Sciences Press, Inc.
1608. Shafranske, E. P. & Cummings, J. P. (2013b). Religious and spiritual beliefs, affiliations, and practices of psychologists. In: K. I. Pargament, A. Mahoney & E. P. Shafranske (Eds.) *APA Handbook of Psychology, Religion, and Spirituality (Vol 2): An Applied Psychology of Religion and Spirituality* (pp. 23–41). Washington, DC: American Psychological Association.

1609. Shafranske, E. P. (1992). God-representation as a transformational object. In: M. Finn & J. Gartner (Eds.) *Objects Relations Theory and Religion, Clinical Applications* (pp. 52–72). Westport, CT/London: Praeger.
1610. Shafranske, E. P. (1995). Freudian theory and religious experience. In: R. W. Hood (Ed.) *Handbook of Religious* Experience (pp. 200–230). Birmingham, AL: Religious Education Press.
1611. Shafranske, E. P. (Ed.) (1996). *Religion and the Clinical Practice of Psychology*, Washington, DC: American Psychological Association Books.
1612. Shafranske, E. P. (2000). Religious involvement and professional practices of psychiatrists and other mental health professionals. *Psychiatric Annals*, *30*: 1–8.
1613. Shafranske, E. P. (2002). The meaning of religious experience in psychoanalytic treatment. In: M. Aletti & F. De Nardi (Eds.) *Psicoanalisi e religione. Nuove prospettive clinico-ermeneutiche* (pp. 147–160). Torino: Centro Scientifico Editore.
1614. Shafranske, E. P. (2005). Psychoanalytic approach. In: L. Sperry & E. P. Shafranske (Eds.) *Spiritually Oriented Psychotherapy* (pp. 105–130). Washington, DC: American Psychological Association.
1615. Shafranske, E. P. (2009). Spiritually oriented psychodynamic psychotherapy. *Journal of Clinical Psychology*, *65*: 147–157.
1616. Shafranske, E. P. (2013a). Addressing religiousness and spirituality in psychotherapy: Advancing evidence-based professional practice. In: R. Paloutzian & C. Park (Eds.) *The Handbook of the Psychology of Religion and Spirituality* (pp. 595–616). New York, NY: Guilford Press.
1617. Shafranske, E. P. (2014a). Addressing religiousness and spirituality as clinically relevant cultural features in supervision. In C. A. Falender, E. P. Shafranske & C. Falicov (Eds.) *Diversity and Multiculturalism in Clinical Supervision: A Competency-Based Approach* (pp. 181–207). Washington, DC: American Psychological Association.
1618. Shafranske, E. P. (2014b). Psychotherapy with Roman Catholics. In: P. S. Richards (Ed.) *Handbook of Psychotherapy and Religious Diversity* (2nd ed.) (pp. 59–88). Washington, DC: American Psychological Association.
1619. Shafranske, E. P. & Malony, H. N. (1990). California psychologists' religiosity and psychotherapy. *Journal of Religion and Health*, *29* (*3*): 219–231.
1620. Sharvit, G. (2015). *Freud, Religion, and Messianism.* Working Paper, 146, Wien: Wien Kultur.
1621. Sharvit, G. & Feldman, K. S. (Eds.) (2018). *Freud and Monotheism. Moses and the Violent Origins of Religion*, New York, NY: Fordham University Press.
1622. Shaw, J. (2005). Psychoanalysis, meet religion: And this time, get it right. *Contemporary Psychoanalysis*, *41* (*2*): 352–359.
1623. Sherman, M. H. (1957). Values, religion, and the psychoanalyst. *Journal of Social Psychology*, *45*: 261–269.
1624. Sholham, S. G. (1976). The Isaac syndrome. *American Imago*, *33*: 329–349.
1625. Shuter, W. (2006). Sharing our humanity: The psychological power of the Catholic Mass. *American Imago*, *63* (*1*): 7–23.
1626. Sibony, D. (2001). *Psychanalyse et judaïsme*, Paris: Flammarion.
1627. Sibony, D. (2002). *Nom de Dieu: Par-delà les trois monothéismes*, Paris: Points-Essais. *Lectures bibliques*. Paris: Odile Jacob.
1628. Sibony, D. (2013). *Islam, phobie, culpabilité*, Paris: Odile Jacob.
1629. Sibony, D. (2016). *Coran et Bible en questions et réponses*, Paris: Odile Jacob.
1630. Siddiqui, S. (2016). *Religion and Psychoanalysis in India*, London/New York, NY: Routledge.
1631. Siddiqui, S. (2018). Devi possession: At the intersections of religion, culture, and psychoanalysis. In: M. Kumar, A. Dhar & A. Mishra (Eds.) *Psychoanalysis from the Indian Terroir: Emerging Themes in Culture, Family, and Childhood* (pp. 19–36). New York, NY/London: Lexington.

1632. Siebert, R. (1982). Psychoanalysis and religion: European situation. *Concilium, 18*: 27–37.
1633. Siegmann, A. W. (1961). An empirical investigation of the psychoanalytic theory of religious behavior. *Journal for the Scientific Study of Religion, 1*: 74–78.
1634. Sillman, L. R. (1949). Monotheism and the sense of reality. *International Journal of Psychoanalysis, 30*: 124–132.
1635. Silva, A. & Blanco, A. (2009). O Moisés de Freud: saber e transmissão na psicanálise. *Estilos Da Clínica, 14*: 216–235.
1636. Silva, G. (1966). *O ateísmo de Freud*, Rio de Janeiro: Zahar.
1637. Simitis, I. G. (2006). *El estudio de Freud sobre Moisés; un sueño diurno. un ensayo bibliográfico*, Buenos Aires: Imago Mundi.
1638. Simmonds, J. G. (2006b). The oceanic feeling and a sea change: Historical challenges to reductionist attitudes to religion and spirit from within psychoanalysis. *Psychoanalytic Psychology, 23*: 128–142.
1639. Simmonds, J. G. (2004). Heart and spirit: Research with psychoanalysts and psychoanalytic psychotherapists about spirituality. *The International Journal of Psychoanalysis, 85*: 951–971.
1640. Simmonds, J. G. (2005). Other than "the set pattern:" developing one's own thoughts about spirituality and religion. *Mental Health, Religion, and Culture, 8*: 239–251.
1641. Simmonds, J. G. (2006a). Freud and the American physician's religious experience. *Mental Health, Religion, and Culture, 9*: 401–405.
1642. Simmonds, J. G. (2006c). Being and potential: Psychoanalytic clinicians' concepts of God. *International Journal of Applied Psychoanalytic Studies, 3*: 221–241.
1643. Simmonds, J. G. (2006d). The Oceanic Feeling and a sea change: Historical challenges to reductionist attitudes to religion and spirit from within psychoanalysis. *Psychoanalytic Psychology, 23*: 128–142.
1644. Simmonds, J. G. (2008). Heart and spirit. *International Journal of Psychoanalysis, 85*: 951–971.
1645. Simmonds, J. G. (2015). Forerunner of the science of psychoanalysis? An essay on the Spanish and Portuguese inquisition. *The Journal of Psychohistory, 42*: 295–309.
1646. Simon, E. (1957). *Sigmund Freud, the Jew*, London: Leo Baeck Institute.
1647. Skinner, J. (1961). Ritual matricide: A study of the origin of sacrifice. *American Imago, 18*: 71–102.
1648. Slattery, M. (2002). How Françoise Dolto links Lacanian psychoanalysis with the Christian Gospels. *The Journal of Pastoral Care & Counseling, 56*: 363–375.
1649. Slavet, E. (2009). *Racial Fever. Freud and the Jewish Question*, New York, NY: Fordham University Press.
1650. Smith, J. H. & Handelman, S. A. (Eds.) (1990). *Psychoanalysis and Religion*, Baltimore, MD: The Johns Hopkins University Press.
1651. Snoeck, A. (1964). *Confession and psychoanalysis*, Westminster: Newman Press.
1652. Sochaczewski, J. (2017). Psychoanalysis and religion in the 21st century: Examining the possibility of integration. *Contemporary Psychoanalysis, 53*: 247–268.
1653. Soler, C. (2010). L'exit de Dieu, ou pire. *Champ Lacanien, 8*: 23–32.
1654. Sorenson, A. L. (1990). Psychoanalytic perspectives on religion: The illusion has a future. *Journal of Psychology and Theology, 18*: 209–217.
1655. Sorenson, R. L. (1994a). Ongoing change in psychoanalytic theory: Implications for analysis of religious experiences. *Psychoanalytic Dialogues, 4*: 631–660.
1656. Sorenson, R. L. (1994b). Therapists' (and their therapists') God representation in clinical practice. *Journal of Psychology and Theology, 22*: 325–344.
1657. Sorenson, R. L. (1997). Transcendence and intersubjectivity: The patient's experience of the analyst's spirituality. In: C. Spezzano & G. L. Gargiulo (Eds.) *Soul on the Couch: Spirituality, Religion, and Morality in Contemporary Psychoanalysis* (pp. 163–199). Hillsdale, NJ: Analytic Press, Inc.

1658. Sorenson, R. L. (2004). Kenosis and alterity in Christian spirituality. *Psychoanalytic Psychology, 21*: 458–462.
1659. Sorenson, R. L. (2014). *Minding Spirituality*, London/New York, NY: Routledge.
1660. Sorter, D. (1995). Principles of Self psychological treatment. Prague symposium: Contemporary perspectives in psychotherapy and psychoanalysis. *International Forum of Psychoanalysis, 4*: 247–254.
1661. Spaccapelo, N. (Ed.) (1986). *Religione e psicoanalisi*, Roma: Città Nova.
1662. Spero, M. H. (1985). The reality of the image of God in psychotherapy. *American Journal of Psychology, 39*: 75–85.
1663. Spero, M. H. & Cohen, M. (2009). Discussion of a symposium: The God representation in the psychoanalytic relationship: When is three a crowd? *The Journal of American Academic for Psychoanalysis and Dynamic Psychiatry, 37 (1)*: 219–239.
1664. Spero, M. H. (1977). Religious anxiety and the experience of God. *Judaism, 26*: 206–216.
1665. Spero, M. H. (1980). *Judaism and Psychology: Halakhic Perspectives*, New York, NY: Yeshiva University Press.
1666. Spero, M. H. (1981). Countertransference in religious therapists of religious patients. *American Journal of Psychoanalysis, 35*: 565–576.
1667. Spero, M. H. (1992). *Religious Objects as Psychological Structures: A Critical Integration of Object Relations Theory, Psychotherapy, and Judaism*, Chicago, IL: The University of Chicago Press.
1668. Spero, M. H. (1993). The concept of iconic mental representation as anticipated by the Talmudic term *De'mut De'yukon*. *Psychoanalysis and Contemporary Thought, 16*: 233–296.
1669. Spero, M. H. (1995). Countertransference-derived elaboration of religious conflicts and representational states. *American Journal of Psychotherapy, 49*: 68–94.
1670. Spero, M. H. (1996). Original sin, the symbolization of desire and the development of mind. *Psychoanalysis and Contemporary Thought, 19*: 499–562.
1671. Spero, M. H. (1998). Brilliantly lit streets': Oedipal and preoedipal influences on the transformation of God representations in a schizoid male. *Psychoanalysis & Contemporary Thought, 21*: 521–591.
1672. Spero, M. H. (1999). Metapsychological dimensions of religious suffering: Common ground between Halakhic Judaism and psychoanalysis. In: S. Carmy (Ed.) *Jewish Perspectives on the Experience of Suffering* (pp. 213–176). New York, NY: Aronson.
1673. Spero, M. H. (2002). What con-verges and what di-verges when religious object representations transform? An annotated critique of Cohen (2002). *The Journal of American Academic for Psychoanalysis and Dynamic Psychiatry, 32 (4)*: 669–708.
1674. Spero, M. H. (2004). Hearing the faith in time: countertransference and religious metaphor in an oncology patient's psychotherapy. *Psychoanalytic Quarterly, 73 (4)*: 971–1021.
1675. Spero, M. H. (2008). The experience of religious transformation during psychoanalysis as an event horizon. *Psychoanalytic Inquiry, 28*: 622–637.
1676. Spero, M. H. (2009). When the light shed by God is dimmer than the light shed upon God: countertransference illumination of latent religious object representations of a Jewish patient in psychoanalysis. *The Journal of American Academic for Psychoanalysis and Dynamic Psychiatry, 37 (1)*: 189–218.
1677. Spero, M. H. (2010). Moses lactans: Evidence in support of the latent mythic value of Freud's 1914 'Moses of Michelangelo'. *American Imago, 67*: 183–242.
1678. Spero, M. H. (2012). Touched by grace during the psychoanalytic hour: the transformation of a religious resistance. *The Psychoanalytic Quarterly*, 77: 283–325.
1679. Sperry, L. & Shafranske, E. P. (Eds.) (2005). *Spiritually Oriented Psychotherapy*, Washington, DC: American Psychological Association.
1680. Spezzano, C. & Gargiulo, G. J. (Eds.) (2003). *Soul on the Couch: Spirituality, Religion, and Morality in Contemporary Psychoanalysis*. Hillsdale, NJ: Analytic Press, Inc.

1681. Spiegel, Y. (1972). *Psychoanalytische Interpretationen biblischer Texte*, München: Kaiser.
1682. Spiegel, Y. (1978). *Doppeldeutlich, Tiefendimensionen biblischer Texte*, München: Kaiser.
1683. Spilka, B. & McIntosh, D. N. (Eds.) (1996). *The Psychology of Religion: Theoretical Approaches*, Boulder, NV: Westview Press.
1684. Spilka, B., Addison, J. & Rosensohn, M. (1975). Parents, Self, and God: A test of competing theories of individual-religion relationships. *Review of Religious Research*: 154–165.
1685. Spilka, B., Armatas, P. & Nussbaum, J. (1964). The concept of God: A factor analytic approach. *Review of Religious Research, 6*: 28–36.
1686. Spilka, B., Hood, R. W. Jr., Hunsberger, B. & Gorsuch, R. (2003). *The Psychology of Religion: An Empirical Approach* (3rd ed.). New York, NY: Guilford Press.
1687. Spira, N. (2007). Psychoanalysis and the disavowed religious impulse. *The Annual of Psychoanalysis, 35*: 137–147.
1688. Spiro, M. (1965). Religious systems as culturally constituted defense mechanisms. In: M. Spiro (Ed.) *Context and Meaning in Cultural Anthropology* (pp. 100–113). Glencoe, IL: The Free Press.
1689. Spitz, R. A. (1972). The genesis of magical and transcendent cults. *American Imago, 29*: 2–10.
1690. Springett, J. (2003). Religious fundamentalism and primitive projective processes. *Psychoanalytic Psychotherapy, 17*: 325–341.
1691. Squverer, A. (2015). Epistemological controversies in the analytic field elucidated by the theological realm. *International Journal of Psychoanalysis, 96*: 1025–1039.
1692. St. Clair, M. (1994). *Human Relationships and the Experience of God: Object Relations and Religion*, Mahwah, NJ: Paulist Press.
1693. St. Clair, M. (2006). Fundamentalism, psychoanalysis, and psychoanalytic theories. *Psychoanalytic Review, 93*: 329–352.
1694. Stålsett, G., Austad, A. & Engedal, L. G. (2017). The persecuting God and the Crucified Self. In: M. J. Reineke & D. M. Goodman (Eds.) *Ana-María Rizzuto and the Psychoanalysis of Religion. The Road to the Living God* (pp. 65–91). Lanham, MD: Lexington.
1695. Stein, D. (1985). *Lectures psychanalytiques de la Bible*, Paris: Cerf.
1696. Stein, R. (2002). Evil as love and liberation. *Psychoanalytic Dialogues, 12*: 393–420.
1697. Stein, R. (2006). Father regression: Clinical narratives and theoretical reflections. *International Journal of Psychoanalysis*: 1005–1027.
1698. Stein, S. (Ed.) (1999). *Beyond Belief. Psychotherapy and Religion*, London: Karnac.
1699. Steiner, R. (1990). *Psychoanalysis and Spiritual Psychology. Five Lectures Held in Dornarch and Munich Between February 25, 1912, and July 2, 1921*, New York, NY: Anthropology Press.
1700. Stern, K. (1954). *The Third Revolution: A Study of Psychiatry and Religion*, New York, NY: Harcourt, Brace.
1701. Stettner, J. (1973). Pfister as Pastoral Theologian. *Journal of Religion and Health, 12 (3)*: 211–222.
1702. Stickler, G. (1998). Dall'esperienza oggetuale all'esperienza simbolica e sviluppo della fede religiosa. In: D. Fagnani & M. T. Rossi (Eds.) *Ricerca di sé e trascendenza. Aprocci psicologici all'identità religiosa in una società pluralista* (pp. 1676–210). Torino: Centro Scientifico Editore.
1703. Stickler, G. (1999). Ferite narcisistiche e dinamiche dell'evoluzione religiosa. In: M. Aletti & G. Rossi (Eds.) *Ricerca di sé e trascendenza. Aprocci psicologici all'identità religiosa in una società pluralista* (pp. 45–64). Torino: Centro Scientifico Editore.
1704. Stokes, A. (1985). *Ministry After Freud*, New York, NY: Pilgrim Press.
1705. Stoloff, J. C. (2009). *Pourquoi l'antisémitisme? Et si Freud s'était trompé … Freud, la question paternelle et l'antisémitisme*, Paris: Pascal.
1706. Stoloff, J.-C. (2011). Croyance religieuse et narcissisme. *Revue Française de Psychanalyse, 75*: 1545–1552.

1707. Storfer, A. J. (1928). Einige Stimmen zu Sigmund Freud "Zukunft einer Illusion". *Imago, 14*: 377–382.
1708. Strachey, J. (1939). Preliminary notes upon the problem of Akhenaten. *International Journal of Psychoanalysis, 20*: 33–42.
1709. Sträuli, D. (2008). 'Ein stilles, sanftes sausen': Psychotherapie, psychoanalyse und religion. *Psychotherapie Forum, 16* (*2*): 74–80.
1710. Strauss, M. (2010). Les deux faces de Dieu. *Champ lacanien, 8*: 67–75.
1711. Strawn, B. D. (2007). Slouching toward integration: Psychoanalysis and religion in dialogue. *Journal of Psychology and Theology, 35*: 3–13.
1712. Strozier, C. (1994). *Apocalypse: On the Psychology of Fundamentalism in America*, Boston, MA: Beacon Press.
1713. Strozier, C. (2003). Kohut and God. In: A. Roland, B. Ulanov & C. Barbre (Eds.) *Creative dissent: Psychoanalysis in Evolution* (pp. 245–255). Westport, CT: Praeger Publishers.
1714. Strunk, 0 (1959). Perceived relationships between parental and deity concepts. *Psychological Newsletter, 10*: 222–226.
1715. Sublon, R. (1975). *Le temps de la mort: savoir, parole, désir*, Strasbourg: Cerdic Pub.
1716. Sublon, R. (1982). *Fonder l'éthique en psychanalyse*, Paris: Fac. Ed.
1717. Sublon, R. (1993). *La Lettre ou l'Esprit - Une lecture psychanalytique de la théologie*, Paris: Cerf.
1718. Sublon, R. (2007). Freud i la religió. *Aloma. Revista de Psicologia i Ciencies de l'Educació, 20*: 109–127.
1719. Sublon, R. (2008). Freud et la religion ou le choix du commencement. *Revue des sciences religieuses, 82*: 65–79.
1720. Sublon, R. (2009). L'impossible concordisme enre théologie et psychanalyse. *Revue de droit canonique, 57* (*2*): 389–408.
1721. Sugar, M. (2002). Commonalities between the Isaac and Oedipus myths: A speculation. *The Journal of American Academic for Psychoanalysis and Dynamic Psychiatry, 30*: 691–706.
1722. Suler, J. (1965). In search of the Self: Zen Buddhism and psychoanalysis. *Psychoanalytic Review, 82* (*3*): 407–426.
1723. Šumiga, D. (2020). Fromm's understanding of the Buddhist philosophical theory and psychoanalysis: From the phenomenal ego to the authentic being. *International Forum of Psychoanalysis, 29* (*1*): 50–61.
1724. Sundén, H. (1959). Über den Beitrag der Psychoanalyse zur Religionpsychologie. In: H. Sundén, *Die Religion und die Rollen: Eine Spychologische Untersuchung* (Kapitel 3). Berlin: Töpelman.
1725. Suzuki, D., Fromm, E. & De Martino, R. (1963). *Zen Buddhism and Psychoanalysis*, New York, NY: Harper Collins.
1726. Swisher, W. S. (1920). *Religion and the New Psychology; a Psycho-analytic Study of Religion*, Boston, MA: Marshall Jones.
1727. Symington, N. (1999). Religion and science in psychoanalysis. In: S. M. Stein (Ed.) *Beyond Belief: Psychotherapy and Religion* (pp. 162–178). London: Karnac.
1728. Symington, N. (2004b) [2004c]. The spirituality of natural religion. *International Journal of Applied Psychoanalytic Studies, 1*: 61–72.
1729. Symington, N. (1985). The survival function of primitive omnipotence. *International Journal of Psychoanalysis, 66*: 481–487.
1730. Symington, N. (1993). Is psychoanalysis a religion? In: D. M. Black, N. Coltart, J. Kristeva et al. (Eds.) *Is Psychoanalysis Another Religion? Contemporary Essays on Spirit, Faith, and Morality in Psychoanalysis*. London: Freud Museum.
1731. Symington, N. (1994a). *Emotion and Spirit: Questioning the Claims of Psychoanalysis and Religion*, London: Cassels.
1732. Symington, N. (1994b). *Psychoanalysis and Religion*, New York, NY: Cassell.

1733. Symington, N. (2004a). *The Blind Man Sees: Freud's Awakening and Other Essays*, London/New York, NY: Routledge.
1734. Symington, N. (2008). Generosity of heart: Source of sanity. *British Journal of Psychotherapy, 24*: 488–500.
1735. Tamayo, A. & Desjardins, L. (1976). Belief systems and conceptual images of parents and God. *Journal of Psychology, 92*: 131–140.
1736. Tamayo, A. & Dugas, A. (1977). Conceptual representation of mother, father, and God according to sex and field of study. *Journal of Psychology, 97*: 9–84.
1737. Tamayo, L. (2009). El psicoanálisis: sin "religio", pero con espíritu. *Litoral, 42*: 73–90.
1738. Tan., P. B. (2016). Evaluating the "Unconscious in Dream" between Sigmund Freud and the Buddhist Tipiṭaka. *Journal of the International Association of Buddhist Universities, 9*: 36–46.
1739. Tapia, N. (1995). La crítica de Freud a la religión. *Revista de Ciencias Sociales de Costa Rica, 67*: 15–26.
1740. Tarachow, S. (1960). Judas, the beloved executioner. *Psychoanalytic Quarterly, 29*: 528–554.
1741. Taubes, J. (1956). Religion and the future of psychoanalysis. *Psychoanalysis, 4–5* (*57*): 136–142.
1742. Taubes, J. (2022). Religion and the future of psychoanalysis. In: S. Gourgouris (Ed.) *Freud and Fundamentalism* (pp. 138–144). New York, NY: Fordham University Press.
1743. Taylor, G. (1978). Demoniacal possession and psychoanalytic theory. *British Journal of Medical Psychology, 51*: 53–60.
1744. Taylor, G. J. (1984). Judith and the infant Hercules: Its iconography. *American Imago, 41*: 101–115.
1745. Teixeira, L. C., Cavalcante, M. M., Barreira, K. S., Aguiar, A. C., Shirley., D. & Aquino, E. C. (2010). Figurações do corpo nos ex-votos: a devoção entre psicanálise e antropologia. *Revista Mal-estar e Subjetividade, 10*: 283–301.
1746. Thayer, N. S. (1979). Perspectives on contemporary mysticism. *Journal of Religion and Health, 18* (*3*): 230–240.
1747. Theissen, G. (1987). *Psychological Aspects of Pauline Theology*, Philadelphia, PA: Fortress Press.
1748. Thevenot, X. (1980). Emmaüs, une nouvelle Genèse? Une lecture psychanalytique de Genèse 2–3 et Luc 24, 13–35. *Mélanges de Science Religieuse, 37*: 3–18.
1749. Tillich, P. (1984). *The Meaning of Health: Essays in Existentialism, Psychoanalysis, and Religion*, Chicago, IL: Exploration Press.
1750. Tisdale, T. C. (2007). From the shadow of the object to the shadow of the almighty: A story of transformation. *Journal of Psychology and Theology, 37*: 52–64.
1751. Tisdale, T. C., Key, T. L., Edwards, K. J. & Brokaw, B. F. et al. (1997). Impact of treatment on God image and personal adjustment and object relations development. *Journal of Psychology and Theology, 25*: 227–239.
1752. Tisdale, T. C. (2022). The name of God is mercy': Reflections on suffering, healing, and growth from a Roman Catholic, contemplative, mystic psychoanalyst. In: J. S. Sandage & B. D. Strawn (Eds.) *Spiritual Diversity in Psychotherapy: Engaging the Sacred in Clinical Practice* (pp. 185–219). Washington, DC: American Psychological Association.
1753. Todd, W. H. (1995). The relationship of spiritual maturity to level of object relations development and God image. *Pastoral Psychology, 43*: 373–391.
1754. Tofighi, F. (2013). Psychoanalytic theories of religion in Protestant contexts. *Religious Inquiries, 2* (*4*): 57–75.
1755. Torno, A. (1976). La fe vista desde el psicoanálisis. *Proyección, 101*: 151–154.
1756. Tornos, A. (1968). *Psicoanálisis y Dios*, Bilbao: Mensajero.
1757. Tornos, A. (1986). *Psicoanálisis y confesión*, Madrid: Fundación Santa María.

1758. Tornos, A. (1987). Freud y la identidad cristiana. *Madrid: Instituto Fe y Secularidad. Memoria académica*, 1986–87: 74–82.
1759. Torri de Araújo, R. (2000). Os Exercícios Espirituais e a psicanálise; a ordenação afetiva como reconversão libidinal. *Itaici*, *42*: 5–15.
1760. Torri de Araújo, R. (2006). Experiência Cristã de Deus e Complexo de Édipo. *Itaici*, *16*: 5–24.
1761. Torri de Araújo, R. (2008). Acompanhamento espiritual e transferência. *Itaici*, *73*: 21–34.
1762. Torri de Araújo, R. (2014). *Deus analisado. Os católicos e Freud*, São Paulo: Loyola.
1763. Torri de Araujo, R. (2015). *Experiência mística e psicanalise*, São Paulo: Ed. Loyola.
1764. Tort, M. (2017). Aux filles et aux fils des dieux du carnage. Filiations religieuses dans la psychanalyse. *Cliniques méditerranéennes: Psychanalyse et Psychopathologie Freudiennes*, *95*: 89–108.
1765. Tractenberg, M. (1990). *Psicanálise da circuncisão. Povos africanos, judaísmo, cristianismo, islamismo*, Porto Alegre: Sagra.
1766. Trovato Gomez, M. T. (2000). O pastor psicanalista Oskar Pfister: Um legado de desconforto. *Psicologia: ciência e profissão*, *20* (*3*): 34–41.
1767. Tummala-Narra, P. (2009). The relevance of a psychoanalytic perspective in exploring religious and spiritual identity in psychotherapy. *Psychoanalytic Psychology*, *26*: 83–95.
1768. Tummala-Narra, P. (2022). Hindu spirituality and psychoanalytic psychotherapy. In: J. S. Sandage & B. D. Strawn (Eds.) *Spiritual Diversity in Psychotherapy: Engaging the Sacred in Clinical Practice* (pp. 19–46). Washington, DC: American Psychological Association.
1769. Turner, J. J. (2002). A brief history of illusion: Milner, Winnicott and Rycroft. *The International Journal of Psychoanalysis*, *83*: 1063–1082.
1770. Tyler, P. (2016). *The Pursuit of the Soul: Psychoanalysis, Soul-Making and the Christian Tradition*, London: Bloomsbury.
1771. Ulanov, A. B. (2005). *Finding Space. Winnicott, God and Psychic Reality*, Louisville, KY: Westminster John Knox Press.
1772. Ullman, C. (1989). *The Transformed Self: The Psychology of Religious Conversion*, New York, NY: Plenum Press.
1773. Ullman, V. Z. & Keini, N. L. (2021). Intrapsychic conflicts arising while meeting ultraorthodox patients. *Journal of Religion and Health*, *60*: 2620–2631.
1774. Underwood, R. L. (1986). The presence and absence of God in object relational and theological perspectives. *Journal of Psychology and Theology*, *14*: 298–305.
1775. Uribe, J. G. (2014). Psicoanálisis y budismo. *Affectio Societatis*, *11*: 96–107.
1776. Urtubey, L. (1983). *Freud et le Diable*, Paris: P.U.F.
1777. Utsch, M., Bonelli, R. M. & Pfeifer, S. (2014). *Psychotherapie und Spiritualität. Mit existenziellen Konflikten und Transzendenzfragen professionell umgehen*, Berlin: Springer.
1778. Utsch, M. (1998). *Religionpsychologie: Voraussetzungen, Grundlagen, Forschungsüberblick*, Stuttgar: Kohlhamer.
1779. Utsch, M. (2013). Religião e Psicologia. *Estudos teológicos*, *2* (*53*): 364–381.
1780. Valas, P. (2010). Dieu, le retour? *Champ lacanien*, *8*: 93–100.
1781. Valle, E. (1998). *Psicologia e experiência religiosa*, São Paulo: Loyola.
1782. Valle, E. (2002). Ilusão e desejo: chaves para a compreensão do dilema ateísmo-devoção. In: G. J. Paiva & W. Zangari (Eds.) *A representação na religião* (pp. 277–298). São Paulo: Loyola.
1783. Van del Kleij, G. (1993). Group analysis and religion: Is there a common ground? Ideas arising from paper by Gregory Van der Kleij. *Group Analysis*, *26* (*1*): 39–53.
1784. Van del Kleij, G. (1993). Religion and Freud and groups. *Group Analysis*, *26* (*1*): 27–37.
1785. Van Herik, J. (1982). *Freud on Femininity and Faith*, Berkeley, CA: University of California Press.

1786. Vande Kemp, H. (1984). *Psychology and Theology in Western Thought 1672–1965*, New York. NY: Kraus Int. Publ.
1787. Vandermeersch, P. & Westerink, H. (2007). *Godsdienstpsychologie in cultuurhistorisch perspectief*, Amsterdam: Boom.
1788. Vandermeersch, P. (1991a). The victory of psychiatry over demonology. The origin of the nineteenth century myth. *History of Psychiatry, 2*: 351–363.
1789. Vandermeersch, P. (1991b). *Unresolved Questions in the Freud/Jung Debate. On Psychosis, Sexual Identity and Religion*, Leuven: Leuven University Press.
1790. Vandermeersch, P. (1992). *Het voetstuk van het weten: over psychologie, psychoanalyse en theologie*, Nijmegen: SUN.
1791. Vandermeersch, P. (1995). Du bon usage de la flagellation et des problèmes posés par son interprétation: Corp et sacré. *Religionlogiques, 12*: 215–242.
1792. Vandermeersch, P. (1996). Passions and Virtues. In: K.-W. Merks & F. Vosman (Eds.) *Aiming al Happiness. The Moral Teaching in the Catechism of the Catholic Church* (pp. 93–112). Kampen: Pharos.
1793. Vandermeersch, P. (1998). Et si, finalement, ça pissait seulement dru? Réflexions d'un psychanalyste au sujet du Déluge: *Gradiva. Revue Européenne d'Anthropologie Littéraire, 3*: 21–53.
1794. Vandermeersch, P. (2002). *La chair de la Passion. Une histoire de foi: la flagellation, (Passages)*, Paris: Cerf.
1795. Vargas Castro, D. A. (2018). Del trazo de la No-Fe de la verdad, o por qué el psicoanálisis no es una religión. *Desde el Jardín de Freud, 18*: 49–62.
1796. Vasse, D. (1969). *Les temps du désir*, Paris: Seuil.
1797. Vasse, D. (1978). *Un parmi d'autres*, Paris: Seuil.
1798. Vasse, D. (1983). *Le poids du réel. La suffrance*, Paris: Seuil.
1799. Vasse, D. (1989). Une demande d'amour: "Que ta volonté soit faite". *Christus, 144*: 402–413.
1800. Vasse, D. (1991). *L'autre du désir et le Dieu de la foi: Lire aujourd'hui Thérèse d'Avila*, Paris: Seuil.
1801. Vasse, D. (2001). *La vie et le vivants. Conversations avec Françoise Muckensturn*, Paris: Seuil.
1802. Vasse, D. (2003). La parole, la chair et le nom. Reconaître sa filiation. *Christus, 197*: 70–78.
1803. Vasse, D. (2007a). La souffrance: alteration, alterité. *Christus, 214*: 68–82.
1804. Vasse, D. (2007b). La foi en la promesse. *Christus, 214*: 219–230.
1805. Vasse, D. (2008). *La Souffrance sans jouissance ou le Martyre de l'amour. Thérèse de l'Enfant-Jésus et de la Sainte-Face*, Paris: Seuil.
1806. Vaucher, M., Bourdin, D., Durrer, M. & Revaz, O. (Eds.) (2012). *Foi de canniabale! La dévoration, entre religion et psychanalyse*, Genève: Labor et fides.
1807. Vázquez, A. (1982). *Notas para una lectura de las "Moradas" de Santa Teresa desde la psicología profunda*, Salamanca: Universidad Pontificia.
1808. Vázquez, A. (2014). Teresa de Lisieux (1873–1897). In: Diego Tolsada Peris (Ed.), *Maestros y testigos* (pp. 83–110). Valencia: Tirant lo Blanch.
1809. Végsö, R. (2006). Freud and the prophetic. *Psychoanalysis, Culture & Society, 11*: 265–281.
1810. Veliq, F. (2016). Religião e projeção em Freud: elementos para o debate entre psicanálise e religião. *Synesis, 8 (2)*: 49–65.
1811. Veliq, F. (2017a). O totem e o desamparo: duas chaves de leitura para a religião no pensamento freudiano. *Analytica – Revista de Psicanálise, 6 (10)*: 28–45.
1812. Veliq, F. (2017b). Oskar Pfister e a crítica à concepção freudiana de Religião. *Revista de Filosofia, 46*: 93–104.
1813. Veliq, F. (2018a). Feuerbach, Marx, Nietzsche e Freud: a crítica da religião no século XXI. *Sapere aude, 9 (18)*: 285–306.

1814. Veliq, F. (2018b). O homem sem inconsciente de Massimo Recalcati. Elementos para o debate entre Psicanálise e Religião. *Numen: Revista de estudos e pesquisa da religião, 21*: 66–80.

1815. Veliq, F., Drawin, C. R., Moreira, J. O. & Paiva, M. A. (2015). *Os destinos da religião na Contemporaneidade. Um diálogo com a psicanálise, a filosofia e as ciências da religião*, Curitiba: CRV.

1816. Ventimiglia, G. (2008). Martin Buber, God, and psychoanalysis. *Psychoanalytic Inquiry, 28*: 612–621.

1817. Vergote, A. (1999). Psicologia dell'identità religiosa: struttura, processi, problema. In: M. Aletti & G. Rossi (Eds.) *Ricerca di sé e trascendenza. Aprocchi psicologici all'identità religiosa in Una società pluralista* (pp. 3–15). Torino: Centro Scientifico Editore.

1818. Vergote, A. (2003). Psicanálise e religião: nas encruzilhadas da palavra pessoal. *Revista Portuguesa de filosofia, 1 (2)*: 573–585.

1819. Vergote, A. (1960). Le nom du Père et l'écart de la topographie symbolique. In: A. Gaillard (Ed.) *L'analyse du langage théologique* (pp. 257–269). Paris: Aubier.

1820. Vergote, A. (1969). *The Religious Man. A Psychological Study of Religious Attitudes*, Dayton, OH: Pflaum Publishing.

1821. Vergote, A. (1971). Apports des données psychanalytiques à l'exégèse. Vie, loi et clivage du Moi dans l'épître aux Romains. In: R. Barthes (Ed.) *Exégèse et herméneutique* (pp. 109–147). Paris: Seuil.

1822. Vergote, A. (1972a). Approche psychologique de la prière. *La Maison-Dieu, 109*: 72–86.

1823. Vergote, A. (1972b). *Religion, foi et incroyance*, Bruxelles: P. Mardaga.

1824. Vergote, A. (1985). Le temps du désir de Saint Augustin à J. Lacan. In: E. Jeddi (Ed.) *Psychose, famille et culture. Recherches en psychiatrie sociale* (pp. 115–133). Paris: L'Harmattan.

1825. Vergote, A. (1988). *Guilt and Desire: Religious Attitudes and their Pathological Derivatives*, New Haven, CT: Yale University Press.

1826. Vergote, A. (1990). *Explorations de l'espace théologique*, Leuven: University Press.

1827. Vergote, A. (1991). Visions et apparitions. Approche psychologique. *Revue Théologique de Louvain, 22*: 202–225.

1828. Vergote, A. (1993a). What the psychology of religion is and what is not. *The International Journal of Psychology of Religion, 3 (2)*: 73–86.

1829. Vergote, A. (1993b). Psychanalyse et religion. In: J. Florence, A. Vergote, et al. (Eds.) *Psychanalyse. L'homme et ses destins* (pp. 311–333). Louvain/Paris: Ed. Peeters.

1830. Vergote, A. (1995a). Debate concerning the psychology of religion. *The International Journal of Psychology of Religion, 5 (2)*: 119–123.

1831. Vergote, A. (1995b). Religion, pathologie, guérison. *Revue Théologique De Louvain, 26*: 3–30.

1832. Vergote, A. (1996). *Religion, Belief and Unbelief: A Psychological Study*, Leuven/Atlanta, GA: Leuven University Press/Rodopi Press.

1833. Vergote, A. (1997a). *La psychanalyse à l'épreuve de la sublimation*, Paris: Cerf.

1834. Vergote, A. (1997b). Neither masterly nor ancillary. In: A. Belzen & O. Wikström (Eds.) *Taking a Step Back. Assessments of the Psychology of Religion* (pp. 159–169). Upsala: Acta Universitatis.

1835. Vergote, A. (1997c). Religion et psychanalyse. In: *Encyclopaedia Universalis. Dictionnaire de la psychanalyse* (pp. 731–737). Paris: Albin Michel.

1836. Vergote, A. (1997d). Psychologie et religion. Dieu, Mère, Père et Amant. In: J. P. Rosa (Ed.) *Encyclopédie des Religions* (Vol. II, pp. 2275–2288). Paris, Bayard.

1837. Vergote, A. (1998a). Religion after the critique of psychoanalysis. The scope of psychoanalysis In: J. Corveleyn & D. Hutsebaut (Eds.) *Psychoanalysis, Phenomenological Anthropology and Religion*. Amsterdam/Atlanta, GA: Leuven University Press.

1838. Vergote, A. (1999b). Condition monothéiste du péché. In: E. Blattchen et al. (Eds.) *Où va Dieu?* (pp. 63–72). Bruxelles: Éditions Complexe.

1839. Vergote, A. (1999c). L'esprit de la psychanalyse. In: J. F. Rey (Ed.) *Spiritualités du temps présent. Fragments d'une analyse, jalons pour une recherche* (pp. 111–125). Paris/Montréal: L'Harmattan.
1840. Vergote, A. (2000). *Le président Schreber revisité*, Leuven: Leuven University Press.
1841. Vergote, A. (2001a). A key conflict questioning religion and its psychology. In: M. Aletti & G. Rossi (Eds.) *L'Illusione religiosa: rive e derive* (pp. 281–288). Torino: Centro Scientifico Editore.
1842. Vergote, A. (2001b). Non necéssaire, mais pouvant être bénéfique ou ambivalente pour la santé mentale. In: M. Aletti & G. Rossi (Eds.) *L'Illusione religiosa: rive e derive* (pp. 1–12). Torino: Centro Scientifico Editore.
1843. Vergote, A. (2001c). Necessidade et desejo da religião na ótica da psicología. In: G. J. Pavia (Ed.) *Necessidade e desejo. Diálogos da psicologia com a religião* (pp. 9–24). São Paulo: Loyola.
1844. Vergote, A. (2001d). Processos psicológicos. Vergonha, sentimento de culpa e sentido bíblico do pecado em particular em Romanos 7. In: G. J. Pavia (Ed.) *Necessidade e desejo. Diálogos da psicologia a religião* (pp. 127–157). São Paulo: Loyola.
1845. Vergote, A. (2002). At the crossroads of the personal word. In: M. Aletti & F. De Nardi (Eds.) *Psicoanalisi e Religione. Nuove Prospettive Clinico-Ermeneutiche* (pp. 5–34). Torino: Centro Cientifico Editore.
1846. Vergote, A. (2012). How and why I became interested in the psychology of religion. In: J. A. Belzen (Ed.) *Psychology of Religion: Autobiographical Account* (pp. 243–248). New York, NY: Springer Science.
1847. Vergote, A., Bonami, M., Custers, A. & Pattyn, M. R. (1967). Le symbole paternel et sa signification religieuse. *Archiv für Religionspsychologie, 9*: 118–140.
1848. Vergote, A. & Aubert, C. (1972). Parental images and representations of God. *Social Compass, 19*: 431–444.
1849. Vergote, A. & Tamayo, A. (1980). *The Parental Figures and the Representation of God: A Psychological and Cross-cultural Study*, The Hague: Mouton.
1850. Vergote, A., Tamayo, A., Pasquali, L., Bonami, M., Pattyn, M. & Custers, A. (1969). Concept of God and parental images. *Journal for the Scientific Study of Religion, 8*: 79–87.
1851. Vergote, A. & Van der Lans, J. M. (1986b). Two opposed viewpoints concerning the object of the psychology of religion. Introductory statement and plenary debate. In: J. Belzen & J. M. Van der Lans (Eds.) *Currents Issues in the Psychology of Religion. Proceedings of the Third Symposium on the Psychology of Religion in Europe* (pp. 67–81). Amsterdam: Rodopi.
1852. Vermorel, H. & Vermorel, M. (1993a). *Sigmund Freud et Romain Rolland, correspondance 1923–1936: de la sensation océanique au "Trouble du souvenir sur l'Acropole*, Paris: PUF.
1853. Vermorel, H. & Vermorel, M. (1993b). De l'avenir d'une illusion au Malaise dans la culture. *Revue Française de Psychanalyse, 57* (4): 1095–1111.
1854. Vinnai, G. (1999). *Jesus und Ödipus: zur Psychoanalyse der Religion*, Frankfurt am Main: Fischer.
1855. Vitz, P. C. & Gartner, J. (1984a). Christianity and psychoanalysis: I. Jesus as Anti-Oedipus. *Journal of Psychology and Theology, 12* (1): 4–14.
1856. Vitz, P. C. & Gartner, J. (1984b). Christianity and psychoanalysis: II. Jesus the transformer of the super-ego. *Journal of Psychology and Theology, 12* (2): 82–90.
1857. Vitz, P. C. (1977). *Psychology as Religion*, Grand Rapids, MI: Eerdmans.
1858. Vitz, P. C. (1983). Sigmund Freud's attraction to Christianity. Biographical evidence. *Psychoanalysis and Contemporary Thought, 6*: 73–183.
1859. Vitz, P. C. (1988). *Sigmund Freud's Christian Unconscious*, New York, NY: Guilford Press.
1860. Vitz, P. C. & Felch, S. M. (2006). *The Self: Beyond the Postmodern Crisis*, Wilmington, DE: ISI Books.

1861. Vitz, P. C. (1999). *Faith of the Fatherless: The Psychology of Atheism*, Dallas, TX: Spence.
1862. Vitz, P. C. (2013). *Faith of the Fatherless: The Psychology of Atheism*, San Francisco, CA: Ignatius Press.
1863. Vogt, P. (2015). The Masculinity of Christ according to Zinzendorf: Evidence and Interpretation. *Journal of Moravian History, 15 (2)*: 97–135.
1864. Volney, G. (1992). *Freud on Sublimation*, Albany, NY: State University of New York.
1865. Vosman, F. (2003). Zin in werkelijkheid: Psychoanalyse en Katholieke moraaltheologie over seks en over liefde. *Psyche en Geloof, 14*: 26–42.
1866. Waelhens, A. (1960). La paternité et le complexe d'Œdipe en psychanalyse. In: E. Castelli (Ed.) *L'analyse du langage théologique* (pp. 247–256). Paris: Aubier.
1867. Wahl, W. H. (2008). Pathologies of desire and duty: Freud, Ricoeur, and Castoriadis on transforming religious culture. *Journal of Religion and Health, 47 (3)*: 398–414.
1868. Waitz, C. (2019). Immersion in the Mother: Lacanian Perspectives on Borderline States. *Psychoanal. Rev.106 (1)*: 29–47
1869. Waitz, C. & Tisdale, T. C. (2021). *Lacanian Psychoanalysis and Eastern Orthodox Christian Anthropology in Dialogue*, London/New York, NY: Routledge.
1870. Waldenmaier, J. (2017). J. Ana-María Rizzuto and the new atheism. Science and religion in the light of psychoanalysis. In: M. J. Reineke & D. M. Goodman (Eds.) *Ana-María Rizzuto and the Psychoanalysis of Religion. The Road to the Living God* (pp.139–182). Lanham, MD: Lexington.
1871. Wallace, E. R. (1979). Freud and Religion. *The American Journal of Psychiatry, 136 (2)*: 237–238.
1872. Wallace, E. R. (1983). Reflections on the relationship between psychoanalysis and Christianity. *Pastoral Psychology, 33*: 215–243.
1873. Wallace, E. R. (1984). *Freud and Religion: A History and Reappraisal*, New York, NY: International Universities Press.
1874. Wallace, E. R. (1985). Further reflections on the relationship between psychoanalysis and religion. *Listening: Journal of Religion and Culture, 20*: 175–194.
1875. Wallace, E. R. (1991). Psychoanalytic perspectives on religion. *International Review of Psychoanalysis, 18*: 265–278.
1876. Wallace, W. H. (1977). The psychodynamic determinants of Moses and Monotheism. *Psychiatry, 40 (1)*: 79–87.
1877. Wallace, W. H. (1978). Freud's mysticism and its psychodynamic determinants. *Bulletin of Menniger Clinic, 42*: 203–222.
1878. Wallwork, E. & Wallwork, A. S. (1990). Psychoanalysis and religion: Current state of a historical antagonism. In: J. H. Smith & S. A. Handelman (Eds.) *Psychoanalysis and Religion* (pp. 160–171). Baltimore, MD: Johns Hopkins University Press.
1879. Wang, J., Goodman, D. & Freeman, M. (2015). The melancholy of psychoanalysis: Marion, Kristeva, and the difference of theology. In: D. Goodman & M. Freeman (Eds.) *Psychology and the Other* (pp. 94–111). Straw. New York, NY: Oxford University Press.
1880. Ward, I. (Ed.) ((1993). *Is Psychoanalysis Another Religion?* London: Freud Museum Publications.
1881. Watson, R. A. (2007). Ready or not, here I come: Surrender, recognition, and mutuality y psychotherapy. *Journal of Psychology and Theology, 35*: 65–73.
1882. Webb, R. E. & Sells, M. A. (1995). Lacan and Bion: psychoanalysis and the mystical language of 'unsaying'. *Theory and Psychology, 5*: 195–215.
1883. Webster, R. (1995). *Why Freud Was Wrong. Sin, Science and Psychoanalysis*, New York, NY: Basic Books.
1884. Weinmann, A., Medeiros, R. & Mano, G. C. (2010). Deus está morto. Viva o autômato! *Estudos e Pesquisas em Psicologia, 17*: 225–237.
1885. Weinstein, J. J. (1958). Religion looks at psychiatry. *Pastoral Psychology, 9*: 25–32.

1886. Weinstein, J. J. (1991). Psychoanalytic perspectives on religion. *International Review of Psychoanalysis, 18*: 265–278.
1887. Weintraub, W. & Aronson, H. (1974). Patients in psychoanalysis: Some findings related to sex and religion. *American Journal of Orthopsychiatry, 44*: 102–108.
1888. Weiss, S. A. (1959). The biblical story of Ruth: Analytic implications of the Hebrew Masoretic Text. *American Imago, 16*: 195–209.
1889. Weiss-Rosmarin, T. (1939). *The Hebrew Moses: An Answer to Sigmund Freud*, New York, NY: The Jewish Book Club.
1890. Wellisch, E. (1954). *Isaac and Oedipus. A Study in Biblical Psychology of the Sacrifice of Isaac. The Akedah*, London: Routledge & Kegan Paul.
1891. Werbner, P. (2008). Arguing sainthood: Modernity, psychoanalysis, and Islam. *American Ethnologist, 26*: 1035–1036.
1892. Werman, D. S. (1977). Sigmund Freud and Romain Roland. *International Review of Psychoanalysis, 4*: 225–242.
1893. Werman, D. S. (1979). On the nature of oceanic experience. *Journal of American Psychoanalytic Association, 27*: 123–139.
1894. Westendorp, F. (1974). The value of Freud's illusion. *Journal of Psychology and Theology, 3*: 82–89.
1895. Westerink, H. (2011). Eternal hate and conscience: on the filiation between Freudian psychoanalysis and sixteenth and early seventeenth century Protestant thought. *Psychoanalysis and History, 13 (1)*: 5–24.
1896. Westerink, H. (2007a). The great man from Tarsus: Freud on the apostle Paul. *The Psychoanalytic Quarterly*, 76:1, 217–235.
1897. Westerink, H. (2009a). *Controversy and Challenge. The Reception of Sigmund Freud's Psychoanalysis in German and Dutch-Speaking Theology and Religious Studies*, Vienna: LIT Verlag.
1898. Westerink, H. (2009b). *A Dark Trace. Sigmund Freud on the Sense of Guilt*, Leuven: Leuven University Press.
1899. Westerink, H. (2010). Unter Verdacht. Bemerkungen zu Paul Ricoeurs Symbolbegriff und Freud Interpretation. *Wiener Jahrbuch für Theologie, 8*: 123–134.
1900. Westerink, H. (2012a). *The Heart of Man's Destiny. Lacanian Psychoanalysis and Early Reformation Thought*, London/New York, NY: Routledge.
1901. Westerink, H. (2012b). Eine Wende des Denkens. Jacques Lacan und die kulturelle Vaterschaft zwischen Psychoanalyse und Reformation. *Psyche: Zeitschrift für Psychoanalyse und ihre Anwendungen, 66*: 506–521.
1902. Westerink, H. (2013a). *Pathology and Moral Courage in Freud's Early Case Histories*, Leuven: Leuven University Press.
1903. Westerink, H. (2013b). *Constructs of Meaning and Religious Transformation: Current Issues in the Psychology of Religion*, Vienna: Vienna University Press.
1904. Westerink, H. (2014). Demonic possession and the historical construction of melancholy and hysteria. *History of Psychiatry, 25 (3)*: 335–349.
1905. Westerink, H. (2015). Theology after Lacan. The passion for the real. *Mental Health, Religion & Culture, 18*: 316–317.
1906. Westerink, H. (2017). *Lust en onbehagen. Over psychoanalyse, Mystiek, subjectiviteit en psychopathologie*, Amsterdam: Sjibbolet.
1907. Westerink, H. (2020). Pathoanalysis of existence and the study of religion - An unfinished freudian project. *Psychoanalytic Quarterly, 89*: 583–611.
1908. Westerink, H. & Vandermeersch, P. (2007b). *Godsdienstpsychologie in cultuurhistorisch perspectief*, Amsterdam: Boom.
1909. Westerink, H., Scholz-Strasser, I. & Müller-Funk, W. (2013). *Psychoanalysis, Monotheism and Morality: The Sigmund Freud Museum Symposia 2009–2011*, Leuven: Leuven University Press.
1910. Whachul, O. (2021). Understanding of Self: Buddhism and psychoanalysis. *Journal of Religion and Health, 8*: 1–12.

1911. White, S. (1984). Imago Dei and object relations theory: Implications for a model of human development. *Journal of Psychology and Theology, 12*: 286–293.
1912. Whitebook, J. (2006). Wissenschaft und religion: Zur problematic von objektivität und kritik der psychoanlyse. *Psyche: Zeitschrift für Psychoanalyse und ihre Anwendungen, 60 (9–10)*: 1018–1039.
1913. Whitebook, J. (2008). Hans Loewald, psychoanalysis, and the project of autonomy. *Journal of American Psychoanalytic Association, 56 (4)*: 1161–1187.
1914. Whitebook, J. (2014). "Imagine": Zur Verteidigung des Säkularismus der Psychoanalyse. *Psyche: Zeitschrift für Psychoanalyse und ihre Anwendungen, 68*: 1167–1195.
1915. Whitebook, J. (2017a). Leaving heaven to the angels and the sparrows: Freud's critique of religion. In: J. Whitebook (Ed.) *Freud. An Intellectual Biography* (pp. 377–406). Cambrige: Cambridge University Press.
1916. Whitebook, J. (2017b). *"Geistigkeit: A Problematic Concept," Violent Origins: On Freud and Moses*, New York, NY: Fordham University Press.
1917. Whitebook, J. (2017c). *Freud: An Intellectual Biography*, New York, NY: Cambridge University Press.
1918. Whitney, L. (2017). Jung in dialogue with Freud and Patañjali: Instinct, affective neuroscience, and the reconciliation of science and religious experience. *Cosmos and History: The Journal of Natural and Social Philosophy, 13*: 298–312.
1919. Wiessenhütter, E. (1977). *Religion und Tiefenpsychologie. Echnaton, Mose, Christus, Freud*, Gütersloh: Gütersloher Verlagshaus Mohn.
1920. Wilkinson, H. (2003). Psychoanalysis as finite, psychoanalysis as infinite? Psychoanalysis' religious potential. *The International Journal of Psychotherapy, 8*: 147–168.
1921. Will, H. (2012a). Freuds Atheismus im Kontext betrachtet. *Psyche, 68*: 1–30.
1922. Will, H. (2012b). Gewalt, Schuldgefühl und Religionsbildung - 100 Jahre nach Totem und Tabu. In: T. Haas Eberhard (Ed.) *100 Jahre Totem und Tabu. Freud und die Fundamente der Kultur* (pp. 151–176). Gießen: Psychosozial.
1923. Will, H. (2014). *Freuds Atheismus im Widerspruch. Freud, Weber und Wittgenstein im Konflikt zwischen säkularem Denken und Religion*, Stuttgart: Kohlhammer.
1924. Williams, M. H. (1999). Psychoanalysis: an art or a science? A review of the implications of the theory of Bion and Meltzer. *British Journal of Psychotherapy, 16*: 127–135.
1925. Williams, M. H. (2006). The three vertices: Science, art and religion. *British Journal of Psychotherapy, 21*: 429–441.
1926. Williams, M. H. (2015). The infant and the infinite: On psychoanalytic faith – Bion, Meltzer and Kierkegaard. *Psychodynamic Practice, 21*: 112–125.
1927. Winborn, M. (Ed.) (2014). *Shared Realities: Participation Mystique and Beyond*, Carmel, CA: Fisher King Press.
1928. Winer, J. & Anderson, J. (Ed.) *Spirituality and Religion: Psychoanalytic Perspectives.* Catskill, NY: Mental Health Resources.
1929. Winnicott, D. W. (1953). Transitional objects and transitional phenomena. *International Journal of Psychoanalysis, 34*: 89–97.
1930. Winnicott, D. W. (1965). *The Maturational Process and the Facilitating Environment*, New York, NY: International Universities Press.
1931. Winton, S. (2013). Religion in the consulting room. *British Journal of Psychotherapy, 29*: 346–357.
1932. Wittgenstein, L. (2007). *Lectures and Conversations on Aesthetics, Psychology and Religious Belief*, Berkeley, CA: University of California Press.
1933. Wolf, M. A. (2005). *Un psychiatre lit la Bible*, Paris: Cerf, Paris.
1934. Wolman, B. (Ed.) (1976). *Psychoanalysis and Catholicism*, New York, NY: Gardner.
1935. Wondracek, K. H. K. (1999). Psicanálise e religião. Abismo escancarado ou útil variação? Reflexões sobre a correspondência entre Freud e o pastor Pfister. *Estudos Teológicos, 39 (2)*: 186–191.

1936. Wondracek, K. H. K. (2003a). *O futuro e a ilusão. Um embate com Freud sobre Psicanálise e Religião*, Petrópolis, RJ: Vozes.
1937. Wondracek, K. H. K. (2003b). Freud, Pfister e suas ilusões – Que ciência? Que religião? In: O. Pfister (Ed.) *O futuro e a ilusão: um embate com Freud sobre psicanálise e religião* (pp. 167–200). Petrópolis: Vozes.
1938. Wondracek, K. H. K. (2005a). *O amor e seus destinos: a contribuição de Oskar Pfister para o diálogo entre teologia e psicanálise*, São Leopoldo: Sinodal.
1939. Wondracek, K. H. K. (2005b). Entre o desamparo humano e o amparo divino: Um caso clínico numa ótica interdisciplinar. *Estudos de psicanálise. Rio De Janeiro, 28*: 75–82.
1940. Wondracek, K. H. K. (2011). Freud e sua genealogia: implicações para clínica do religioso. *Pistis & Praxis, 3 (2)*: 383–403.
1941. Wondracek, K. H. K., Albuquerque, B., Jávera, J. P. & Caon, J. L. (2018). As raízes religiosas de Freud, Pfister, Winnicott e Lacan. In: A. Antúnez & G. Safra (Eds.) *Psicologia clínica da graduação à pós-graduação* (pp. 341–348). Rio de Janeiro: Atheneu.
1942. Wright, J. (1994). *Freud's War with God: Psychoanalysis Versus Religion*, Lafayette, CO: Huntington House.
1943. Wright, J. E. (1982). *Erikson, Identity and Religion*, New York, NY: Seabury Press.
1944. Wright, R. W. & Strawn, B. D. (2010). Grief, hope, and prophetic imagination: Psychoanalysis and Christian tradition in dialogue. *Journal of Christianity and Psychology, 29*: 149–157.
1945. Wulff, D. M. (1997). *Psychology of Religion. Classic and Contemporary Views*, New York, NY: John Wiley & Sons.
1946. Wulff, D. M. (1999). Psychologists define religion. Patterns and prospects of a century quest. In: G. Platvoet & A. L. Molendijk (Eds.) *The Pragmatics of Defining Religion. Contexts, Concepts and Contents* (pp. 207–224). Leiden/Boston/Köln: Brill.
1947. Leon, W. (2007). Thoughts of a psychoanalyst about Jewish mysticism. *The Annual of Psychoanalysis, 35*: 207–221.
1948. Yarom, N. (1992). *Body, Blood and Sexuality*, New York, NY: Peter Lang.
1949. Yerushalmi, Y. H. (1989). Freud on the Historical Novel: From the manuscript draft (1934) of Moses and Monotheism. *International Journal of Psychoanalysis, 70*: 375–395.
1950. Yerushalmi, Y. H. (1991). *Freud's Moses: Judaism Terminable and Interminable*, New Haven, CT: Yale University Press.
1951. Yerushalmi, Y. H. (1992). The Moses of Freud and the Moses of Schoenberg. On words, idolatry, and psychoanalysis. *The Psychoanalytic Study of the Child, 47*: 1–20.
1952. Young, B. (2011). The psychological life, religion, and immortality: Musings of a venerable psychoanalyst. *International Journal of Applied Psychoanalytic Studies, 8*: 288–300.
1953. Zanocco, G. C. (1988). *Sulle tracce del padre*, Roma: Borla.
1954. Zaretsky, E. (2006). The place of psychoanalysis in the history of the Jews. *Psychoanalysis and History, 8*: 235–253.
1955. Zelig, D. F. (1974). *Psychoanalysis and the Bible: A Study in Depth of Seven Leaders*, New York, NY: Bloch.
1956. Zharnt, H. (Ed.) (1974). *Jesús de Nazaret y Sigmund Freud*, Estella: Verbo Divino.
1957. Zilboorg, G. (1955a). Some denials and affirmations of religious faith. In: F. Braceland (Ed.) *Faith, Reason and Modern Psychiatry* (pp. 99–121). New York, NY: P.J. Kennedy & Sons.
1958. Zilboorg, G. (1938). The sense of immortality. *Psychoanalytic Quarterly, 12*: 465–475.
1959. Zilboorg, G. (1953). L'amour et Dieu chez Freud. *Le Supplément, 24*: 5–30.
1960. Zilboorg, G. (1955b). *Faith, Reason, and Modern Psychiatry: Sources for a Synthesis*, New York, NY: Kennedy.
1961. Zilboorg, G. (1962). *Psychoanalysis and Religion*, New York, NY: Farrar, Straus, & Cudahy.

1962. Zilboorg, G. (1964). *Freud and Religion: A Social and Cultural History of Psychoanalysis*, New York, NY: The Newman Press.
1963. Zilles, U. (1996). Freud: Provocação do ateísmo psicanalítico. In: U. Zilles (Ed.) *Filosofia da religião* (pp. 137–162). São Paulo: Paulus.
1964. Zimmerman, F. (1951). Origin and significance on the Jewish rite on circumcision. *Psychoanalytic Review, 38*: 103–112.
1965. Ziparri, S. (2000). *Nel nome del Padre e di Edipo. Appunti di psicoanalisi e religione per il Nuevo millennio*, Roma: Armando.
1966. Zizek, S. (2001). *On Belief*, London/New York, NY: Routledge.
1967. Zizek, S. (2003a). O real da ilusão cristã. Notas sobre Lacan e religião. In: V. Safatle (Ed.) *Um limite tenso. Lacan entre a filosofia e a psicanálise* (pp. 169–187). São Paulo: Unesp.
1968. Zizek, S. (2003b). The *Puppet and the Dwarf: The Perverse Core of Christianity*, Cambridge, MA/London: MIT Press.
1969. Zizek, S. (2004). Jews, Christians, and other monsters. *Lacanian Ink, 23*: 83–99.
1970. Zizek, S. (2006). *Il cuore perverso del cristianismo*, Roma: Meltemi.
1971. Zizek, S. (2007). Anxiety: Kierkegaard with Lacan. *The Annual of Psychoanalysis, 35*: 179–189.
1972. Zock, H. (1990). *A Psychology of Ultimate Concern: Erik H. Erikson's Contribution to the Psychology of Religion*, Atlanta, GA: Rodopi Press.
1973. Zock, H. (1997). Religie als Transitionael Fenomeen: Her Belang van D. W. Winnicott voor de Godsienstpsychologie. *Nederlands Theologisch Tijdsvrift, 51 (1)*: 31–48.
1974. Zock, H. (1999). Religions as the realization of faith. The conceptualization of religion in relational psychoanalysis. In: G. Platvoet & A. L. Molendijk (Eds.) *The Pragmatics of Defining Religion. Contexts, Concepts and Contents* (pp. 433–459). Leiden/Boston/Köln: Brill.
1975. Zock, H. & Erikson, E. H. (2022). Young Man Luther: A Study in Psychoanalysis and History (1958): A psychosocial interpretation of Luther and its relevance for understanding religious identity formation today. *Journal for Theology and the Study of Religion, 76 (1)*: 61–75.
1976. Zulliger, H. (1966). Oskar Pfister, Psychoanalysis and Faith. In: F. Alexandre, S. Eisenstein & M. Gotjahn (Eds.) *Psychoanalytic Pioneers* (pp. 169–179). New York, NY: Basic Books.
1977. Zwart, H. (Ed) (2019a) *Psychoanalysis of Technoscience. Symbolization and Imagination* (Vol. 1), Wien: Lit Verlag.
1978. Zwart, H. (Ed.) (2019b) *Philosophy and Psychology in Dialogue. Symbolization and Imagination* (Vol. 1), Wien: Lit Verlag.
1979. Zwiebel, R. & Weischede, G. (2015). *Buddha und Freud. Präsenz und Einsicht: Über buddhistisches und psychoanalytisches Denken*, Göttingen: Vandenhoek & Ruprecht.
1980. Zwiebel, R. & Weischede, G. (2017). *Die Suche nach dem Stillen Ort. Filmpsychoanalytische Betrachtungen zum Buddhismus*, Göttingen: Vandenhoeck & Ruprecht.

BIBLIOGRAPHIC SUBJECT INDEX

The endless character of the psychoanalysis-faith dialogue initiated by Sigmund Freud and Oskar Pfister manifests itself in the immense bibliography accumulated and still appearing today. The present one responds to the same purpose as those classical ones by W. W. Meissner in 1961 (*Annotated Bibliography in Religion and Psychology*) and B. Beit-Hallahmi in 1996 (*Psychoanalytic Studies of Religion: A Critical Assessment and Annotated Bibliography*). We offer an update to our present times, including essential contributions in Spanish, French, Italian, German, Portuguese, etc., mostly missing in the ones mentioned above.

Additionally, a 20-section subject index can help the readers choose their specific interests among the numerous titles. The thematic limits are not always clear and definite, and some titles will appear in more than one thematic field. The numbers refer to the BIBLIOGRAPHY given after the book's CONCLUSION.

Sigmund Freud's writings on religion

Oskar Pfister's writings on religion

On Sigmund Freud's texts

On the psychoanalytic interpretation of religion

On the texts by Oskar Pfister

Writings of the first generation of psychoanalysts

From the object relations approach

Religion from the Lacanian approach

Bion's psychoanalysis and religion

Mysticism and psychoanalysis

Spirituality and psychoanalysis

Psychoanalytic therapy and religious experience

Health and illness in religion

INDEX

Note: Page references with "n" denote endnotes.

For Product Safety Concerns and Information please contact our EU representative GPSR@taylorandfrancis.com
Taylor & Francis Verlag GmbH, Kaufingerstraße 24, 80331 München, Germany

www.ingramcontent.com/pod-product-compliance
Ingram Content Group UK Ltd.
Pitfield, Milton Keynes, MK11 3LW, UK
UKHW020009200926
475702UK00015B/2562
* 9 7 8 1 0 3 2 4 8 2 6 2 0 *